Study Guide for

Wong's Nursing Care of Infants and Children

Tenth Edition

Marilyn J. Hockenberry, PhD, RN, PNP-BC, FAAN
David Wilson, MS, RNC (NIC)

By

David Wilson, MS, RNC (NIC)
Staff
Children's Hospital at Saint Francis
Tulsa, Oklahoma

Linda Sawyer McCampbell, MSN, APRN, BC
Family Nurse Practitioner
Laguna Vista, Texas

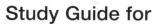

ELSEVIER
MOSBY

3251 Riverport Lane
St. Louis, Missouri 63043

STUDY GUIDE FOR

WONG'S NURSING CARE OF INFANTS AND CHILDREN, TENTH EDITION   ISBN: 978-0-323-22242-6

Notices

Knowledge and best practice in this field are constantly changing. As new research and experience broaden our understanding, changes in research methods, professional practices, or medical treatment may become necessary.

Practitioners and researchers must always rely on their own experience and knowledge in evaluating and using any information, methods, compounds, or experiments described herein. In using such information or methods they should be mindful of their own safety and the safety of others, including parties for whom they have a professional responsibility.

With respect to any drug or pharmaceutical products identified, readers are advised to check the most current information provided (i) on procedures featured or (ii) by the manufacturer of each product to be administered, to verify the recommended dose or formula, the method and duration of administration, and contraindications. It is the responsibility of practitioners, relying on their own experience and knowledge of their patients, to make diagnoses, to determine dosages and the best treatment for each individual patient, and to take all appropriate safety precautions.

To the fullest extent of the law, neither the Publisher nor the authors, contributors, or editors, assume any liability for any injury and/or damage to persons or property as a matter of products liability, negligence or otherwise, or from any use or operation of any methods, products, instructions, or ideas contained in the material herein.

Content Development Manager: Michele D. Hayden
Content Development Specialist: Emily Vaughters
Content Coordinator: Hannah Corrier
Publishing Services Manager: Hemamalini Rajendrababu
Project Manager: Jayashree Balasubramaniam
Design Direction: Amy Buxton

Printed in the United States of America

Last digit is the print number: 9 8 7 6 5 4 3 2 1

Working together
to grow libraries in
developing countries

www.elsevier.com • www.bookaid.org

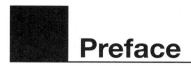

Preface

This Study Guide accompanies the tenth edition of Wong's Nursing Care of Infants and Children. Students may use the Study Guide not only to review content but also to enhance their learning through critical thinking. The Study Guide is designed to assist students in mastering the content presented in the text, developing problem-solving skills, and applying their knowledge to nursing practice.

Each chapter in the Study Guide includes questions that will assist students to meet the objectives of each corresponding textbook chapter. Because most students using this Study Guide will also be preparing to pass the nursing examination (NCLEX), we have primarily used a multiple-choice format. Features to help students learn and retain pediatric terminology are included in each chapter. A Critical Thinking section is also included for each chapter, with questions designed to help students analyze the chapter's content and address their own attitudes about pediatric nursing practice. Case Studies are used in many of the Critical Thinking sections to give students experience in addressing specific practice issues. All case presentations are fictitious but designed to address situations frequently encountered by the nurse in practice.

HOW TO USE THE STUDY GUIDE

We intend for students to use this Study Guide as they study a chapter in the textbook, processing the material chapter by chapter and section by section. For this reason, we chose to present the questions in an order that generally follows the textbook's content. Students will find the answers to the questions for each chapter at the end of the Study Guide. Page numbers from the textbook have been included to facilitate finding content related to the answers.

It is our hope that this Study Guide will function as both an aid to learning and a means for measuring progress in the mastery of pediatric nursing practice.

David Wilson
Linda Sawyer McCampbell

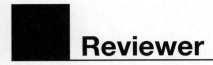

Reviewer

Beth Hopper
Lead Practical Nursing Instructor
Part-time PN class
Tennessee College of Applied Technology
Paris, Tennessee

Contents

Perspectives of Pediatric Nursing

1. According to *Healthy People 2020*, strategies that address leading health indicators for the nation would include all of the following areas *except:*
   a. decreasing tobacco use.
   b. increasing innovative treatments for cancer.
   c. decreasing substance abuse.
   d. increasing immunization rates.

2. Obesity in children and adolescents is defined as:
   a. BMI $\geq$ 90th percentile for age and height
   b. BMI $\leq$ 90th percentile for age and gender
   c. BMI $\geq$ 95th percentile for age and height
   d. BMI $\geq$ 95th percentile for age and gender

3. Mental health problems in children:
   a. affect 1 in 20 adolescents.
   b. make the children less likely to drop out of school than those with other disabilities.
   c. include attention deficit/hyperactivity disorder (ADHD).
   d. are more common in children living in large urban centers.

4. Which one of the following statements is true about infant mortality in the United States?
   a. There has been a recent dramatic increase in infant mortality in the United States.
   b. The United States is currently a world leader in reducing infant mortality.
   c. In 2001 the United States ranked last in infant mortality rate among nations with similar-sized populations.
   d. The United States has lower infant mortality rates than most other developed countries.

5. The major determinant of neonatal death in technologically developed countries is:
   a. birth weight.
   b. short gestation.
   c. long gestation.
   d. human immunodeficiency virus (HIV) infection.

6. Which of the following accounts for the most deaths in infants under 1 year of age?
   a. Pneumonia and influenza
   b. Infections specific to the perinatal period
   c. Accidental injuries
   d. Congenital anomalies

7. Infant mortality decreased significantly in the 1990s for which of the following?
   a. Low birth weight
   b. Congenital heart defects
   c. Human immunodeficiency virus (HIV) infection
   d. Sudden infant death syndrome (SIDS)

8. Which of the following differences is seen when infant death rates are categorized according to race?
   a. Disparities among races have continued to increase dramatically in the United States.
   b. Infant mortality for Hispanic infants is much higher than for any other group.
   c. Infant mortality for African-Americans is twice the rate of Caucasians.
   d. Infant mortality for Caucasian infants is the same as for other races.

9. After a child reaches the age of 1 year, the leading cause of death is from:
   a. human immunodeficiency virus (HIV).
   b. congenital anomalies.
   c. unintentional injuries.
   d. heart disease.

10. Children 12 years of age and older who are victims of homicide tend to be killed by:
    a. firearms.
    b. family members.
    c. stabbing.
    d. poor safety devices on firearms.

11. The disease that continues to be a leading cause of death in all age-groups of children is:
    a. type 1 diabetes mellitus.
    b. acquired immunodeficiency syndrome (AIDS).
    c. cancer.
    d. infectious disease.

12. Fifty percent of all acute conditions of childhood can be accounted for by:
    a. injuries and accidents.
    b. bacterial infections.
    c. parasitic disease.
    d. respiratory illness.

13. Identify one major category of disease that children tend to contract in infancy and early childhood.

14. List three factors that contribute to increasing morbidity of any disorder in children.

15. Another term for "the new morbidity" is:
    a. pediatric social illness.
    b. pediatric noncompliance.
    c. learning disorder.
    d. autism spectrum disorder.

16. Which one of the following statements about injuries in childhood is *false*?
    a. Developmental stage partially determines the prevalence of injuries at a given age.
    b. Most fatal injuries occur in children under the age of 9 years.
    c. Developmental stage helps to direct preventive measures.
    d. Children ages 5 to 9 years are at greatest risk for bicycle fatalities.

17. List three strategies that may be used to prevent fatal accidents in children.

18. The incidence of accidental drowning is highest in both boys and girls in what age-group?
    a. Less than 1 year
    b. 1 to 4 years
    c. 5 to 14 years
    d. 15 to 24 years

19. The current trend toward evidence-based practice involves:
    a. questioning whether a better approach exists.
    b. analyzing published clinical research.
    c. increased emphasis on measurable outcomes.
    d. a, b, and c are correct.

20. _____ _____ refers to the best approach to prevention that uses teaching and counseling of parents and others about developmental expectations and that alerts parents to the issues that are most likely to arise at a given age.

21. Describe the concept of atraumatic care and list the three principles that provide a framework for its implementation.

22. Two basic concepts in the philosophy of family-centered pediatric nursing care are:
    a. enabling and empowerment.
    b. empowerment and bias.
    c. enabling and curing.
    d. empowerment and self-control.

23. The role of the nurse in the parent-professional partnership is to:
    a. decide what is most important for the family.
    b. decide what is most important for the child.
    c. strengthen the family's ability to nurture.
    d. manipulate the available resources.

24. An example of atraumatic care would be to:
    a. eliminate all traumatic procedures.
    b. restrict visiting hours to adults only.
    c. allow parents to "room in" with the child.
    d. remove parents from the room during painful procedures.

25. _____ _____ _____ involves questioning why something is effective and whether a better approach exists. The concept also involves analyzing and translating published clinical research into the everyday practice of nursing.

26. As the movement for providing care based on evidence continues, nurses will be using methods to evaluate research such as:
    a. Agency for Health Care Policy and Research (AHCPR) guidelines in place of guidelines developed locally.
    b. guidelines that are based on traditional practice.
    c. the GRADE criteria.
    d. guidelines that reflect current research but decrease job satisfaction.

27. Match each role of the pediatric nurse with its description.

    a. Family advocacy and caring
    b. Disease prevention and health promotion
    c. Health teaching
    d. Support
    e. Counseling
    f. Therapeutic relationship
    g. Coordination and collaboration
    h. Ethical decision making
    i. Research and evidence-based practice

    _____ A mutual exchange of ideas and opinions

    _____ Health maintenance strategies

    _____ Working together as a member of the health team

    _____ Establishing relationships with children and families yet remaining separate

    _____ Systematically recording and analyzing observations

3

Copyright © 2015 by Mosby, an imprint of Elsevier Inc. All rights reserved.
Copyright © 2011, 2007, 2003 by Mosby, Inc., an affiliate of Elsevier Inc. All rights reserved.

Chapter **1** **Perspectives of Pediatric Nursing**

_____ Attention to emotional needs (listening, physical presence)

_____ Transmitting information

_____ Using patient, family, and societal values in care

_____ Acting in the child's best interest

CRITICAL THINKING—CASE STUDY

Marisa Gutierrez arrives with her infant, Sara, in the well-baby clinic. Sara, who is 15 months old, is the youngest of three children. Her mother has brought her to the clinic for well-child care. Sara's two brothers, who are 7 and 8 years old, have come as well. As the nurse interviews the mother, Sara explores the examination room. She reaches for her older brothers' coins and puts one in her mouth.

28. After organizing the data into similar categories, the nurse correctly makes which one of the following decisions?
    a. No dysfunctional health problems are evident.
    b. High risk for dysfunctional health problems exists.
    c. Actual dysfunctional health problems are evident.
    d. Potential complications are evident.

29. The nurse then identifies a possible human response pattern to further classify the data. Which one of the following functional health patterns would be best for the nurse to select?
    a. Role-relationship pattern
    b. Nutritional-metabolic pattern
    c. Coping–stress tolerance pattern
    d. Self-perception/self-concept pattern

30. Based on the data collected, which one of the following nursing diagnoses would be most appropriate?
    a. Altered Family Process
    b. Altered Family Coping
    c. Altered Individual Coping
    d. Altered Parenting

31. Which one of the following patient outcomes is individualized for Sara?
    a. Sara will receive her immunizations on time.
    b. Sara will demonstrate adherence to the nurse's recommendations.
    c. Marisa Gutierrez will verbalize the need to keep small objects away from Sara to avoid aspiration.
    d. Sara's brothers will verbalize the need to stop playing with small objects.

32. During the evaluation phase, which one of the following responses by Sara's mother would indicate that the expected outcomes have been met?
    a. "I will have to go through all of the boys' things when we get home to be sure there aren't any other small objects that could hurt Sara."
    b. "I had forgotten how curious babies are. It has been many years since the boys were babies, and they didn't have an older child's toys around."
    c. "I will have to start to discipline Sara now so that she knows not to play with the older children's belongings."
    d. "I am afraid she cannot receive her immunizations. She had a fever after her last one."

33. At Sara's next well-baby visit, what information will be most important to document in the chart?
    a. Written evidence of progress toward outcomes
    b. The standard plan of care
    c. Broad-based goals
    d. Interventions applicable to patients like Sara

34. List three patient-centered outcome measures that may be applicable to an acutely ill, hospitalized child.

2 Social, Cultural, Religious, and Family Influences on Child Health Promotion

1. Match each term with its description or characteristics.

   a. Family
   b. Family structure
   c. Consanguineous
   d. Nuclear family
   e. Discipline
   f. Limit-setting
   g. Time-out

   h. Divided or split custody
   i. Joint custody
   j. Family function
   k. Adoption
   l. Blended family
   m. Household
   n. Family of origin

   o. Open family
   p. Closed family
   q. Behavior modification
   r. Affinal
   s. Foster care

   _____ Establishment of the rules or guidelines for behavior

   _____ Marital relationships

   _____ Interaction of family members

   _____ Persons sharing a common dwelling

   _____ A group of people, living together or in close contact, who take care of one another and provide guidance for their dependent members

   _____ Blood relationships

   _____ A system of rules governing conduct

   _____ Family situation in which each parent is awarded custody of one or more of the children, thereby separating siblings

   _____ Composed of two parents and their children

   _____ Family unit into which a person is born

   _____ Composition of the family

   _____ Refinement of the practice of "sending the child to his or her room"; based on the premise of removing the reinforcer and using the strategy of unrelated consequences

   _____ Accepting of new ideas, resources, and opportunities

   _____ Family situation in which the children reside with one parent, although both parents act as legal guardians and both participate in childrearing

   _____ Resists input; views change as threatening and suspicious

   _____ Placement in an approved living situation away from the family of origin

   _____ Establishment of a legal relationship of parent and child between persons not related by birth

   _____ Family situation that includes at least one stepparent, stepsibling, or half-sibling.

   _____ Practice based on the belief that behavior, if rewarded, will be repeated and behavior not rewarded will be eliminated

2. Which one of the following is *not* a correct definition of the term *family* as it is viewed today?
   a. The family is what the patient considers it to be.
   b. The family may be related or unrelated.
   c. The family is always related by legal ties or genetic relationships, and members live in the same household.
   d. The family members share a sense of belonging to their own family.

3. Match each family theory with its description. (Some theories may be used more than once.)

    a. Family systems theory
    b. Family stress theory
    c. Developmental theory

_____ Crisis intervention strategies are used, with the focus on helping members cope with the challenging event.

_____ Continual interaction occurs between family members and the environment.

_____ Focus is on the interactions of family members rather than on an individual member. A problem or dysfunction is not viewed as lying in any one family member but rather in the interactions within the family.

_____ Concepts of basic attributes, resources, perception, and coping behaviors or strategies are used in assessing family crisis management.

_____ Changes in the family over time are addressed, based on the predictable changes in the structure, function, and roles of the family, with the age of the oldest child as the marker for stage transition.

_____ The family and each individual member must achieve developmental tasks as part of each family life cycle stage.

4. In working with children, nurses include family members in the care plan. Which of the following statements does the nurse recognize as *false* when planning nursing interventions for the family?
    a. A complete family assessment is needed to discover family dynamics, family strengths, and family weaknesses.
    b. There is no expectation for parents to participate in their child's care when using the systems theory.
    c. The intervention used with families depends on the nurse's view of the theoretic model of the family.
    d. The level of assistance a family needs depends on the type of crisis, factors affecting family adjustment, and the family's level of functioning.

5. Debbie is 2 years old and lives with her brother, Mark, her sister, Mary, and her mother. Her father and mother recently divorced, and now her father lives 1 hour away. Debbie sees her father once a month for a day's visit. Her mother retains custody of Debbie. Debbie's grandparents live in a different state, but she visits them each year. Debbie's family represents which one of the following?
    a. Binuclear family
    b. Extended family
    c. Single-parent family
    d. Blended family

6. Describe how knowledge of family characteristics that help families function effectively can be utilized by the nurse.

7. Identify the following statements as true or false.

_____ Roles are learned through the socialization process.

_____ Role structuring initially takes place within the school system as the child is introduced to direct and indirect pressures forcing the child into desired patterns of behavior.

_____ All families have strengths and vulnerabilities.

_____ Each family has its own standards for interaction within and outside the family.

_____ Role definitions are changing as a result of the changing economy and increased opportunities for women. Marital roles, however, are still most stereotyped among the middle classes.

_____ One quality of a strong family is the flexibility and adaptability of the roles necessary to obtain resources needed for the family.

8. Parenting practices differ in small and large families. Which one of the following characteristics is *not* found in small families?
   a. Emphasis is placed on the individual development of the child, with constant pressure to measure up to family expectations.
   b. Adolescents identify more strongly with their parents and rely more on their parents for advice.
   c. Emphasis is placed more on the group and less on the individual.
   d. Children's development and achievement are measured against those of children in the same neighborhood and social class.

9. Limit setting and discipline are positive, necessary components of childrearing. Which one of the following *best* describes how these functions help children?
   a. Reduce the need for children to have limits set
   b. Support children's ability to test their limits of control
   c. Allow unrestricted freedom to ensure children's growth potential
   d. Reassure children that they are able to protect themselves from harm

10. Match each parenting style with its description.

    a. Authoritarian
    b. Permissive
    c. Authoritative

    _____ Allows children to regulate their own activity; sees the parenting role as a resource rather than a role model

    _____ Establishes rules, regulations, and standards of conduct for children that are to be followed without question

    _____ Respects each child's individuality; directs the child's behavior by emphasizing the reason for rules

11. Child misbehavior requires parental implementation of appropriate disciplinary action. Identify which one of the following would *not* be an appropriate guideline for implementing discipline.
    a. Focus on the child and the misbehavior by using "you" messages rather than "I" messages.
    b. Maintain consistency with disciplinary action.
    c. Make sure all caregivers maintain unity by agreeing on the plan and being familiar with details before implementation.
    d. Maintain flexibility by planning disciplinary actions appropriate to the child's age, temperament, and severity of misbehavior.

12. Which one of the following is a *correct* interpretation in the use of reasoning as a form of discipline?
    a. Used for older children when moral issues are involved.
    b. Used for younger children to "see the other side" of an issue.
    c. Used only in combination with scolding and criticism.
    d. Used to allow children to obtain lengthy explanations and a greater degree of attention from parents.

13. Which one of the following is *not* a description of the use of time-out as a discipline?
    a. Allows the reinforcer to be maintained.
    b. Involves no physical punishment.
    c. Offers both parents and child "cooling off" time.
    d. Facilitates the parent's ability to consistently apply the punishment.

14. Johnny spills his milk on the living room rug. His mother smacks him on the bottom and says, "You are a messy, bad boy, Johnny." Which of the following discipline strategies are used?
    i. Consequence
    ii. Corporal punishment
    iii. Scolding
    iv. Behavior modification
    v. Ignoring

    a. i, ii, and iii
    b. ii and iii
    c. iii and v
    d. ii, iii, and iv

15. Mike and Beverly Parker are adopting a 3-year-old girl from Russia. They have approached you for preadoptive counseling. What would you include in the counseling?
    a. Provide information on appropriate referral agencies that can help with the adoptive process and support groups.
    b. Reassure them that because they are adopting the child at an early age, the child is less likely to remember previous parenting persons.
    c. Reassure them that because they are adopting, they will have greater sources of support and preparation than biologic parents.
    d. Instruct them on how to form an early parent-infant attachment that will eliminate difficulties.

16. Areas of concern for parents of adoptive children include:
    a. the initial attachment process.
    b. telling the children that they are adopted.
    c. identity formation of children during adolescence.
    d. all of the above.

17. Which of the following statements about adoption is true?
    a. Adoptive children from racial backgrounds different from that of the family should be treated no differently from biologic children.
    b. The task of telling children that they are adopted should follow clear-cut timing guidelines.
    c. The sooner infants enter their adoptive home, the better the chances of parent-infant attachment.
    d. Older children display fewer behavioral changes after adoption disclosure than do younger children.

18. Identify the following statements about the impact of divorce on children as true or false.

    _____ Research has shown that children of divorce suffer no lasting psychologic and social difficulties.

    _____ Divorce constitutes a major disruption for children of all ages, and all children suffer stress second only to the stress produced by the death of a parent.

    _____ Children of divorce cope better with their feelings of abandonment when there is continuing conflict between parents.

    _____ Preschoolers assume themselves to be the cause of the divorce and interpret the separation as punishment.

    _____ Positive outcomes of divorce include a successful postdivorce family that can improve the quality of life for both adults and children.

    _____ Adolescents have feelings of anxiety, may withdraw from family and friends, and may have a disturbed concept of sexuality.

    _____ Even when a divorce is amicable and open, children recall parental separation with the same emotions felt by victims of a natural disaster: loss, grief, and vulnerability to forces beyond their control.

    _____ Child characteristics such as age or sex are more crucial to the child's well-being during divorce than are family characteristics.

19. Which one of the following is *not* considered important by parents when telling their children about the decision to divorce?
    a. Initial disclosure should include both parents and siblings.
    b. Time should be allowed for discussion with each child individually.
    c. The initial disclosure should be kept simple, and reasons for divorce should not be included.
    d. Parents should physically hold or touch their child to provide feelings of warmth and reassurance.

20. Which of the following describes joint legal custody?
    a. Each parent is awarded custody of one or more of the children.
    b. The parents alternate the physical care and control of the children on an agreed-on basis while maintaining shared parenting responsibilities legally.
    c. The children reside with one parent but both parents are the legal guardians and both participate in childrearing.
    d. The children reside with the grandparents while both parents assume legal guardianship.

21. Single parenting, step-parenting, and dual-earner family parenting add stress to the parental role. Match each family type with an expected stressor or concern.

    a. Single parenting
    b. Step-parenting
    c. Dual-earner family parenting

    _____ Shortages of money, time, and energy are major concerns.

    _____ Overload is a common source of stress, and social activities are significantly curtailed, with time demands and scheduling seen as major problems.

    _____ Power conflicts; complexity of forming new lifestyles and interaction patterns.

22. Match each term with its definition or description.

    a. Cultural diffusion
    b. Race
    c. Ethnicity
    d. Ecological framework
    e. Ethnocentrism
    f. Social class
    g. Peer group influences

    h. Social roles
    i. Subculture influences
    j. Absolute standard of poverty
    k. Physical poverty
    l. Invisible poverty
    m. Relative standard of poverty

    _____ Delineates a basic set of resources needed for adequate existence

    _____ Groups people by their shared common characteristics or traditions

    _____ School is the center; standards of the larger group are disseminated into the community

    _____ Individuals adapt in response to changes in their surrounding environments

    _____ Children must accept and conform to their values to be part of the group

    _____ Relates to the family's economic and educational levels and their ability to access resources needed to thrive in daily life

    _____ Refers to a lack of money or material resources; for example, insufficient clothing, poor sanitation, and deteriorating housing

    _____ Ethnicity, social class, minority group membership, religion/spirituality, schools, communities and peer groups

    _____ Groups people by their outward, physical appearance

    _____ Cultural creations that define patterns of behavior for persons in a variety of social positions

    _____ Refers to social and cultural deprivation; for example, limited employment opportunities; inferior educational opportunities; lack of, or inferior, medical services or health care facilities; and absence of public services

_____ Reflects the median standard of living in a society; refers to childhood poverty in the United States

_____ Emotional attitude that one's values, beliefs, and perceptions are the correct ones and that the group's ways of living and behaving are the best

23. When children enter school:
   a. parents no longer exert the major influence on them.
   b. teachers have the most significant psychological impact on children's development and socializations within the community.
   c. the school becomes the center for establishing all rules and regulations.
   d. the school serves as a major source of socialization for the child.

24. A. List four categories of external assets that youths should receive from their community: _____

_____

   B. List the four categories of internal assets: _____

25. When considering the impact of culture on the pediatric patient, the nurse recognizes that culture:
   a. is synonymous with race.
   b. affects the development of health beliefs.
   c. refers to a group of people with similar physical characteristics.
   d. refers to the universal manner and sequence of growth and development.

26. Which of the following is a fast-expanding minority group in the United States and in the 2010 census made up over 16% of the population?
   a. Spanish/Hispanic
   b. African-American
   c. Asian
   d. Native American

27. To integrate spiritual care into practice, the nurse should:
   a. demonstrate respect.
   b. support visitation of spiritual leaders.
   c. listen to ensure understanding.
   d. do all of the above.

28. Which one of the following statements about mass media is true?
   a. Clear evidence documents a relationship between television viewing and increased risk behaviors in adolescents.
   b. Educational television programming teaches the habits of mind to be a good leader.
   c. Reading ability and intelligence are linked to the numbers and types of comic books read.
   d. From a public health perspective, media contributes to 10% to 20% of health problems in the United States.

29. Match each term as it relates to mass media.

   a. displacement effect
   b. social learning theory
   c. script theory
   d. super-peer

   _____ Emphasizes learning through observation and imitation

   _____ Describes media as an extreme source of pressure on youth to participate in what is shown to be normal behavior

   _____ Views media as providing youth with directions for how to behave in new situations

   _____ Time spent interacting with media competes with time that could be spent in other activities

30. To provide culturally sensitive care to children and their families, the nurse should:
   a. disregard one's own cultural values.
   b. identify behavior that is abnormal.
   c. recognize characteristic behaviors of certain cultures.
   d. rely on one's own feelings and experiences for guidance.

31. Which of the following is *not* included in cultural humility?
    a. Lifelong commitment to self-reflection and critique
    b. Addressing the power imbalances in the nurse-patient relationship
    c. Developing mutually beneficial partnerships with the community
    d. Conforming to cultural norms to provide security and encourage change

32. Evil eye is an example of an influence that is considered:
    a. a supernatural force.
    b. a natural force.
    c. an imbalance of the forces.
    d. an imbalance of the four humors.

33. Chi is:
    a. imbalance of forces.
    b. belief that illness is a weakness but not necessarily physical.
    c. believed to cause fatigue, low energy, and a variety of ailments.
    d. imbalance of the four humors (phlegm, blood, black bile, and yellow bile).

34. To understand and deal effectively with families in a multicultural community, nurses should:
    a. be aware of their own attitudes and values.
    b. learn about different cultural beliefs to manipulate them.
    c. learn how to change longstanding health beliefs.
    d. recognize that all cultures are very similar to one another.

35. The following terms are related to folk medicine practices that may be harmful. Match each term with its definition.

    a. Coining
    b. Forced kneeling
    c. Female genital mutilation (female circumcision)
    d. Topical garlic application
    e. Greta, azarcon, paylooah, surma

    _____ Traditional remedies that contain lead

    _____ Removal of, or injury to, any part of the female genital organ

    _____ Child discipline measure of some Caribbean groups

    _____ A practice of Yemenite Jews; applied to the wrist to treat infectious disease; can result in blister or burns

    _____ Vietnamese practice; may produce welt-like lesions on the child's back

CRITICAL THINKING—CASE STUDY

Ester and Roberto Garcia are the proud new parents of twin boys, Timothy and Thomas. Ester and Roberto have been married less than 1 year. Ester is 17 years old and plans to return to finish school next year. Roberto finished high school and works with his father in a local auto repair shop. He is taking a week off from work to help Ester at home with the boys. Neither Ester nor Roberto attended child parenting classes. You are making a home visit to the couple on the day after they have brought Timothy and Thomas home from the hospital. As you arrive at the house, you see that both boys are crying. Ester is trying to give Timothy his bath while Roberto is busy trying to get Thomas to take his formula. Both new parents appear tired, and Roberto admits they have been up all night with the infants and that either Timothy or Thomas seems to be crying "all the time" and that "something must be terribly wrong with them."

36. As you begin your assessment of the family, you know that the Garcias are in stage II, families with infants, according to Duvall's developmental stages of the family. Which one of the following is a developmental task of this stage?
    a. Reestablishing couple identity
    b. Socializing children
    c. Making decisions regarding parenthood
    d. Accommodating to parenting role

37. Which of the following is a *priority* nursing diagnosis for this family?
    a. Altered Family Process related to gain of family members
    b. Altered Growth and Development related to inadequate caretaking
    c. Fear related to new parental role
    d. High Risk for Injury related to unsafe environment

38. As the nurse developing the plan for this new family, you choose which of the following as the *priority* intervention?
    a. Teach the parents about Duvall's developmental stages, explaining that what they are experiencing is a normal transition into parenthood.
    b. Reassure the parents that you will examine both infants but that they appear to be healthy and that the parents are doing a good job.
    c. Take over the feeding and bathing of the infants, explaining to the parents the necessity of child parenting classes.
    d. Check the infant supplies and environment to make sure the home has been made safe for children.

39. Both Thomas and Timothy are now sleeping, and you have completed your family assessment with Roberto and Ester. As a nurse, you decide to use the family stress theory to promote adaptation to the family's new role. Which of the following is *not* a capability the family can use to manage the crisis?
    a. Basic attributes of the family
    b. Resources within the family
    c. The family's perception of the situation
    d. Closed boundary within the family system

40. Identify a long-term goal for the Garcia family, and discuss nursing interventions that will foster achievement of this long-term goal.

41. Compare and contrast the following types of consequences and give an example of a discipline technique for each type.
    a. Natural

    b. Logical

    c. Unrelated

42. Discuss the use of corporal punishment and the concerns of using this form of discipline to stop or decrease certain behaviors.

3 Hereditary Influences on Health Promotion of the Child and Family

1. The following terms are related to genetic influences on health. Match each term with its definition or description.

a. Gene
b. Fluorescence in situ hybridization
c. Major structural abnormalities
d. Teratogens
e. Syndrome
f. Association
g. Congenital anomalies
h. Cytogenetics

i. Structural chromosome abnormalities
j. Sequence
k. Euploid cell
l. Monosomy
m. Trisomy
n. Mitosis
o. Phenotype

p. Nondisjunction
q. Alleles
r. Aneuploidy
s. Transcription
t. Contiguous gene syndromes
u. Mutation
v. Variable expression

_____ Malformations that may result from genetic and/or prenatal environmental causes, resulting in serious medical, surgical, or quality-of-life consequences.

_____ A recognized pattern of malformations resulting from a single specific cause (e.g., Down syndrome or fetal alcohol syndrome).

_____ A segment of nucleic acid that contains genetic information necessary to control a certain function, such as the synthesis of a polypeptide. This segment is often referred to as a site, or locus, on a chromosome.

_____ A nonrandom pattern of malformations for which a cause has not been determined, such as VACTERL (vertebral defects, anal atresia, cardiac defect, tracheoesophageal, and renal and limb defects).

_____ Birth defects; occur in 2% to 4% of all live-born children; often classified as deformations, disruptions, dyplasias, or malformations; deviations from that which is normal or typical; examples are Down syndrome, fetal alcohol syndrome.

_____ Chromosomal alterations resulting from breakage, deletion, or translocation and rearrangement of some of the genes of a chromosome.

_____ A cell with a chromosome number that is a multiple of 23.

_____ The study of chromosome disorders, started in 1952 with Lejeune's discovery of the genetic basis of Down syndrome. In recent times, molecular-based knowledge and technologies have been greatly accelerated by the Human Genome Project, which is rapidly identifying genes and DNA variations associated with disease.

_____ Failure of homologous chromosomes or chromatids to separate properly during anaphase meiosis I and II, or mitosis, resulting in daughter cells with unequal chromosome numbers.

_____ Abnormal chromosome pattern; total number of chromosomes is not a multiple of the haploid number (n = 23); for example, 45 or 47 chromosomes.

_____ FISH; process in which chromosomes or portions of chromosomes are "painted" with fluorescent molecules; useful for identifying chromosomal microdeletions.

_____ Aneuploid condition; presence of an extra chromosome added to a pair; results in 47 chromosomes per cell; for example, Down syndrome.

_____ Disorders characterized by a microdeletion or microduplication of smaller chromosome segments, which may require special analysis techniques or molecular testing to detect.

_____ The aneuploid condition of having a chromosome represented by a single copy in a somatic cell, that is, the absence of a chromosome from a given pair.

_____ Type of equational cell division in which the resulting daughter cells have the same number of chromosomes as each other and the mother cell.

_____ One version of a gene at a given location (locus) along a chromosome.

_____ Differences in the extent and/or severity of manifestations of genetic diseases.

_____ The process by which genetic information is copied from DNA to RNA.

_____ Any observable or measurable expression of gene function in an individual. For instance, eye color and hemoglobin type expressions of specific genes.

_____ Structural or chemical alteration in genetic material that persists and is transmitted to future generations.

_____ Agents that cause birth defects when present in the prenatal environment.

_____ When a single anomaly leads to a cascade of additional defects with a predictable pattern; an example is Pierre Robin.

2. Match the following types of hereditary conditions with the appropriate description.

a. Phenylketonuria
b. Prader-Willi syndrome
c. Angelman syndrome

d. Turner syndrome
e. Klinefelter syndrome
f. Fragile X syndrome

_____ Children with this condition exhibit ovarian dysgenesis with an absence of secondary sex characteristics and infertility is common; children may have behavioral problems.

_____ The most common cause of inherited cognitive impairment.

_____ A disorder that includes severe cognitive impairment, characteristic facies, abnormal (puppetlike) gait, and paroxysms of inappropriate laughter. Children with this syndrome are usually nonverbal, although they may vocalize.

_____ A single-gene disorder resulting from the absence of an amino acid that metabolizes phenylalanine.

_____ A disorder of decreased masculinization characterized by gynecomastia, hypogonadism, and long limbs; mental development is normal in most cases.

_____ Characterized by central hypotonia, cognitive dysfunction, dysmorphic appearance, behavioral disturbances, hypothalamic hypogonadism, short stature, obesity, abnormally low body temperature, an increased tolerance to pain, and diminished salivation.

3. Trisomy 21, or Down syndrome, is an example of a(n):
   a. congenital chromosomal association.
   b. sex chromosomal abnormality.
   c. autoimmune aberration.
   d. autosome aneuploidy.

4. All of the following chromosomal disorders are considered sex chromosomal abnormalities *except*:
   a. Turner syndrome.
   b. Klinefelter syndrome.
   c. cri du chat syndrome.
   d. triple X syndrome.

5. Lyonization refers to:
   a. X inactivation in females during embryonic development.
   b. children with shorter stature and poor coordination.
   c. chromosome abnormalities that are easily identified at birth.
   d. chromosome abnormalities that result in severe disabilities.

6. Match each disorder with its pattern of inheritance. (Inheritance patterns may be used more than once.)

   a. Autosomal dominant
   b. Autosomal recessive
   c. Sex-linked (dominant or recessive)

   _____ Xeroderma

   _____ Tay-Sachs disease

   _____ Gardner syndrome

   _____ Neurofibromatosis

   _____ Duchenne muscular dystrophy

   _____ Adenosine deaminase deficiency

   _____ Hemophilia A

   _____ Fragile X syndrome

   _____ Ocular albinism type 1

   _____ Achondroplasia

   _____ Cystic fibrosis

   _____ Galactosemia

   _____ Friedreich ataxia

   _____ Marfan syndrome

   _____ Myotonic dystrophy

   _____ Huntington disease

   _____ Phenylketonuria

   _____ Thalassemia

7. A disease or defect encountered frequently in the population without a clear-cut inheritance pattern is classified as:
   a. a mutation.
   b. a mosaicism.
   c. a uniparental disomy.
   d. multifactorial.

8. Which one of the following disorders is considered to be teratogenic?
   a. Type 1 diabetes mellitus
   b. Rheumatoid arthritis
   c. Fetal alcohol syndrome
   d. Myasthenia gravis

9. One common use of fetal surgery that has been controversial is the treatment of:
   a. ambiguous genitalia.
   b. urinary tract abnormalities.
   c. facial and limb deformities.
   d. pyloric stenosis.

10. The deleterious effects of phenylketonuria are expressed with the ingestion of:
    a. milk.
    b. hormones.
    c. gluten.
    d. vitamin supplement.

11. The *Essential Nursing Competencies and Curricula Guidelines for Genetics and Genomics* delineates that the registered nurse:
   a. integrate genetic and genomic knowledge into assessment and planning.
   b. identify clients who may benefit from specific genetic and genomic information.
   c. interpret selective genetic and genomic information for clients.
   d. perform all of the above.

12. Careful counseling is necessary when screening an individual for carrier status of hereditary disorders (e.g., cystic fibrosis) because:
   a. mass screening for these disorders is widely conducted.
   b. of possible ethical dilemmas.
   c. this type of screening is expensive.
   d. the emotional threat for the child is always devastating.

13. Which one of the following statements is *not* a part of the controversial aspect of mass genetic screening programs?
   a. Health professionals sometimes lack knowledge about the purpose of the testing.
   b. The public cost of testing does not always outweigh the benefits.
   c. Technology is advancing for routine mass screenings of numerous genetic disorders.
   d. The psychologic implications of the carrier status may not be handled properly.

14. Match each type of prenatal genetic test with its purpose.

   a. Biochemical maternal serum testing   c. Amniocentesis
   b. Ultrasonography   d. Chorionic villi sampling

   _____ To perform chromosomal and biochemical analysis

   _____ To estimate gestational age and identify structural abnormalities

   _____ To perform chromosomal analysis at the earliest possible point during pregnancy

   _____ To screen for chromosome anomalies (aneuploidy) and neural tube defects

15. Preimplantation genetic diagnosis has been used for parents at risk for having a child with:
   a. Down syndrome.
   b. a neural tube defect.
   c. a congenital heart defect.
   d. cystic fibrosis.

16. Which of the following actions is *not* considered an appropriate nursing responsibility in genetic counseling?
   a. Choose the best course of action for the family.
   b. Identify families who would benefit from genetic evaluation.
   c. Become familiar with community resources for genetic evaluation.
   d. Learn basic genetic principles.

17. The most efficient genetic counseling service provided by a group of genetic screening specialists may:
   a. predict the outcome of the disease.
   b. take less than 2 hours.
   c. evaluate the affected child only.
   d. be inaccessible to the people who need it most.

18. *Proband* is the term used in genetic counseling to mean the:
   a. affected person.
   b. genetic history.
   c. clinical manifestations.
   d. mode of inheritance.

19. When teaching families about genetic risks and probabilities, the nurse may need to:
    a. make specific recommendations.
    b. use the example of games such as flipping coins and horse racing.
    c. realize that most people have a basic understanding of biology.
    d. recognize that each pregnancy's probabilities build on the previous pregnancy's probabilities.

20. Which one of the following assessment findings should alert the nurse to the need for genetic counseling?
    a. Individuals with a family history of tuberculosis
    b. Parents who had an infant born at 42 weeks' gestation
    c. Couples with a history of infertility
    d. Pregnant adolescents

21. Which one of the following assessment findings in an infant would indicate to the nurse that there is a need for genetic referral?
    a. Vernix caseosa
    b. Acrocyanosis
    c. Mongolian spots
    d. Unusual breath odor

22. In a drawing of a pedigree genogram for genetic purposes, which one of the following facts is *least* significant?
    a. The proband's paternal grandmother had two stillbirth pregnancies.
    b. The proband's sibling died as an infant in a motor vehicle accident.
    c. The proband's paternal grandfather was a carrier for sickle cell disease.
    d. The proband's half-brother carries the sickle cell trait.

23. In regard to genetic counseling, which one of the following statements is *false*?
    a. Families have a tendency to be more ashamed of a hereditary disorder than other illnesses.
    b. The nurse's role in genetic counseling involves sympathy and supportive listening.
    c. The nurse ensures that patients have accurate and complete information to make decisions.
    d. Once the family understands the situation intellectually, they will be able to cope.

CRITICAL THINKING CASE STUDY

Mr. and Mrs. Jones are waiting in the obstetrician's office for a routine prenatal checkup. They are Roman Catholic and do not view abortion as a feasible option. The obstetrician has recommended a screening test to rule out neural tube defects. Mrs. Jones does not see any benefit from this testing procedure and does not want to undergo the procedure.
    Items 24 to 27 relate to this case study.

24. Which one of the following factors is the *least* important consideration during the assessment phase of this visit?
    a. The nurse is not Roman Catholic.
    b. The test is a venipuncture and carries little risk.
    c. Most couples receive normal results from prenatal tests.
    d. Results of the tests will be provided before the delivery date.

25. Which one of the following considerations should the nurse deal with first?
    a. The couple believes that testing is used to identify anomalies in order to terminate a pregnancy.
    b. The couple's clear-cut beliefs about pregnancy termination are different from the reality of raising a child with a disability.
    c. The nurse believes that pregnancy termination for fetal abnormalities is often the best option.
    d. The nurse believes that raising a child with a terminal illness is extremely difficult.

26. Which one of the following goals is most appropriate for the nurse in this situation?
    a. To provide nonjudgmental supportive counseling
    b. To help Mr. and Mrs. Jones make their decision
    c. To provide follow-up care to the couple
    d. To educate the couple about neural tube defects

27. Which of the following statements by Mrs. Jones indicates that the nurse's goal was met?
    a. "I had no idea what was involved in raising a disabled child."
    b. "Your ideas have been very helpful. I think one of them will work."
    c. "We will discuss this and call you tomorrow with our decision."
    d. "I had no idea what neural tube defects were."

28. When teaching the parents of the newborn about testing for phenylketonuria, the nurse should include which one of the following key points?
    a. The test is performed only on infants expected to have the disorder.
    b. The test is performed on cord blood.
    c. The test is not reliable if the blood sample is taken after the infant has ingested a source of protein.
    d. The test should be performed on all newborns before they leave the hospital, and a repeat blood specimen should be obtained by 2 weeks of age if the first test was taken within the first 24 hours of life.

29. Dietary instructions for the parents of a child with phenylketonuria include which of the following?
    i. Maintain a low-phenylalanine diet through adulthood.
    ii. Increase intake of high-protein foods such as meat and dairy products.
    iii. Measure vegetables, fruits, juices, breads, and starches.
    iv. Illness and growth spurts will increase the need for phenylalanine.
    v. Introduce solid foods such as cereal, fruits, and vegetables during infancy as usual.
    vi. Use soy formula during infancy.

    a. i, ii, iii, and iv
    b. i, iii, iv, v, and vi
    c. iii, iv, and v
    d. i, iii, iv, and v

30. In educating the parents of a newborn with galactosemia, the nurse includes which one of the following in the plan?
    a. All food labels should be read carefully for the presence of lactose.
    b. Once the diagnosis is made and the diet is altered, little follow-up of these infants is necessary.
    c. Breast milk is acceptable for infants with galactosemia.
    d. Signs of visual impairment are unlikely in children with this disorder.

4 Communication, Physical, and Developmental Assessment

1. Match each term with its definition or description.

   a. Interview process
   b. Listening
   c. Sympathy
   d. Egocentric
   e. First-degree relatives

   f. Triage
   g. Empathy
   h. Growth charts
   i. Anthropometry
   j. Orthostatic hypotension

   k. Skinfold thickness
   l. Arm circumference
   m. BMI
   n. Indirect history taking
   o. Information overload

   _____ Seeing things only in relation to oneself and one's own point of view

   _____ An essential parameter of nutritional status; the measurement of height, weight, head circumference, proportions, skinfold thickness, and arm circumference

   _____ The capacity to understand what another person is experiencing from within that person's frame of reference

   _____ Requires child's weight and height in order to determine

   _____ Receives too much information

   _____ Not therapeutic in the helping relationship because it leads to feelings of emotional overinvolvement and possible professional burnout

   _____ Most important component of effective communication

   _____ Parents, siblings, grandparents, and immediate aunts and uncles

   _____ Measurement of body fat

   _____ Specific form of goal-directed communication

   _____ Uses a series of percentile curves to demonstrate the distribution of body measurements in children

   _____ Patient or parent completes questionnaire

   _____ Indirect measurement of muscle mass

   _____ Involves assessing symptoms and forming clinical judgment for further medical care

   _____ Often manifests as dizziness or syncope

2. Which of the following would negatively affect the communication process between the nurse and the patient?
   a. The nurse allows the child to express his or her concerns and fears.
   b. The nurse includes the child, as well as the parents, in the communication process.
   c. The nurse uses verbal and nonverbal communication to reflect approval of the patient's statement.
   d. The nurse uses a slow, even, steady voice to convey instruction.

3. Mrs. Green has brought her daughter Karen to the clinic where you work as a nurse. Karen, age 12 years, is a new patient and needs a physical examination so that she can play volleyball. Which of the following techniques would *not* be helpful to establish effective communication during the interview process?
   a. You introduce yourself and ask the name of all family members present.
   b. After the introduction, you are careful to direct questions about Karen to Mrs. Green, since she is the best source of information.
   c. After the introduction and explanation of your role, you begin the interview by saying to Karen, "Tell me about your volleyball team."
   d. You choose to conduct the interview in a quiet area with few distractions.

4. The nurse says to 15-year-old Monique, "Tell me about your cough." This is an example of which type of communication technique?
   a. Direct
   b. Open ended
   c. Reflective
   d. Closed

5. While conducting an assessment of the child, the nurse communicates with the child's family. Which one of the following does the nurse recognize as *not* productive in obtaining information?
   a. Obtaining verbal and nonverbal input from the child
   b. Observing the relationship between parents and child
   c. Using broad, open-ended questions
   d. Avoiding the use of guiding statements to direct the focus of the interview

6. The receptionist at the clinic where you are employed as a nurse has forwarded a call to you from Mrs. Garcia, mother of 4-year-old Maria. Mrs. Garcia tells you that Maria has had a fever all morning of around 37.8° C (100° F) and that she now has diarrhea and vomiting. As you provide triage by phone, which one of the following actions is appropriate?
   a. Reassure Mrs. Garcia that Maria is not very sick and will be fine in a day or two.
   b. Confer with the practitioner at once.
   c. Wait to document in Maria's medical record until she comes in for a visit.
   d. Offer advice for home care and instruct Mrs. Garcia to call or come to the clinic if Maria's symptoms do not improve.

7. _____ is the capacity to understand what another person is feeling by experiencing the situation from that person's frame of reference.
   a. Sympathy
   b. Empathy
   c. Reassurance
   d. Encouragement

8. The nurse is conducting an interview with 8-year-old Jesus and his mother, Mrs. Lopez. Mrs. Lopez is worried because Jesus has been acting up at home and at school and disrupting everyone. An interpreter has been requested, since the mother speaks little English. When using an interpreter for communication with Mrs. Lopez, the nurse realizes that:
   a. the interpreter will have little to do because Jesus can interpret for his mother.
   b. when the interpreter and Mrs. Lopez speak for a long period, it will be necessary to interrupt to refocus the interview.
   c. the nurse needs to communicate directly with Mrs. Lopez and ignore the interpreter.
   d. the nurse needs to pose questions to elicit only one answer at a time from Mrs. Lopez.

9. Identify whether the following statements are true or false when planning how to communicate effectively with children.

   _____ Nonverbal components of the communication process do not convey significant messages.

   _____ Children are alert to their surroundings and attach meaning to gestures.

   _____ Actively attempting to make friends with children before they have had an opportunity to evaluate an unfamiliar person will increase their anxiety.

   _____ The nurse should assume a position that is at eye level with the child.

   _____ Communication through transition objects, such as dolls or stuffed animals, delays the child's response to verbal communication offered by the nurse.

10. To effectively provide anticipatory guidance to the family, the nurse should:
   a. provide information to deal with each problem as it develops.
   b. provide teaching and interventions based on needs identified by the professional.
   c. be suspicious of the parent's ability to deal effectively with the child's needs.
   d. assist the parents in building competence in their parenting abilities.

11. Communication with children must reflect their developmental thought process. Match each developmental stage with the communication guidelines important at that stage. (Stages may be used more than once.)

a. Infancy
b. Early childhood
c. School-age years
d. Adolescence

_____ Focus communication on the child; experiences of others are of no interest to children in this stage.

_____ Children in this stage primarily use and respond to nonverbal communication.

_____ Children in this stage interpret words literally and are unable to separate fact from fantasy.

_____ Children in this stage require explanations and reasons why procedures are being done to them.

_____ Children in this stage have a heightened concern about body integrity, being overly sensitive to any activity that constitutes a threat to it.

_____ Children in this stage are often interviewed first, before their parents.

12. Which one of the following best describes the appropriate use of play as a communication technique with children?
   a. Small infants have little response to activities that focus on repetitive actions like patting and stroking.
   b. Few clues about intellectual or social developmental progress are obtained from the observation of children's play behaviors.
   c. Therapeutic play has little value in reduction of trauma from illness or hospitalization.
   d. Play sessions serve as assessment tools for determining children's awareness and perception of illness.

13. Several creative communication techniques may be used with children. Identify which technique is being used in each of the following examples.

a. _____ The nurse shows Tina a picture of a child having an intravenous infusion started and asks Tina to describe the scene.

b. _____ The nurse says to Tina, "I am concerned about how the medicine treatments are going because I want you to feel better."

c. _____ The nurse reads Tina a story from a book and asks her to retell the story.

d. _____ The nurse provides Tina with crayons and paper and asks her to draw a picture of her family.

e. _____ The nurse gives Tina a doll and a stethoscope and allows her to listen to the doll's heart.

14. A complete pediatric health history includes 10 expected components. List these components.

15. In eliciting the chief complaint, the nurse identifies which one of the following techniques as *not* appropriate?
   a. Limiting the chief complaint to a brief statement restricted to one or two symptoms
   b. Using labeling-type questions such as "How are you sick?" to facilitate information exchange
   c. Recording the chief complaint in the child's or parent's own words
   d. Using open-ended neutral questions to elicit information

16. Read the following entry from a pediatric health history: "Nausea and vomiting for 3 days. Started with abdominal cramping after eating hamburger at home. No pain or cramping at present. Unable to keep any food down but able to drink clear liquids without vomiting. No temperature elevation, no diarrhea." This entry represents which component of the health history?
   a. Chief complaint
   b. Past history
   c. Present illness
   d. Review of systems

17. Which one of the following is *not* part of the past history to be included in a pediatric health history?
    a. Symptom analysis
    b. Allergies
    c. Birth history
    d. Current medications

18. What are the most important previous growth patterns to record when completing a child's history of growth and development?

19. What are the most important developmental milestones to record when completing the child's health history?

20. The nurse knows that the best description of the sexual history for a pediatric health history:
    a. includes a discussion of the patient's plans for future children.
    b. allows the patient to introduce sexual activity history.
    c. includes discussion of contraception methods only when the patient discloses current sexual activity.
    d. alerts the nurse to the need for sexually transmitted infection screening.

21. List the five assessment components to be evaluated in the analysis of the symptom of pain.

22. Indications for the nurse to conduct a comprehensive family assessment include which of the following?
    i. Children with developmental delays
    ii. Children with history of repeated accidental injuries
    iii. Children with behavioral problems
    iv. Children receiving comprehensive well-child care

    a. i, ii, iii, and iv
    b. ii, iii, and iv
    c. i, ii, and iii
    d. ii and iii

23. Assessment of family interactions and roles, decision making and problem solving, communication, and expression of feelings and individuality is known as assessment of:
    a. family structure.
    b. family function.
    c. family composition.
    d. home and community environment.

24. Describe four principal areas of concern the nurse should focus on when assessing family structure.

25. The dietary history of a pediatric patient includes:
    a. a 12-hour dietary intake recall.
    b. a more specific, detailed history for the older child.
    c. financial and cultural factors that influence food selection.
    d. criticism of parents' allowance of nonessential foods.

26. In pediatric examinations, the normal sequence of head-to-toe direction is often altered to accommodate the patient's developmental needs. The nurse identifies which of the following goals as *least* likely to guide the examination process?
    a. Minimizing the stress and anxiety associated with the assessment of body parts.
    b. Recording the findings according to the normal sequence.
    c. Fostering a trusting nurse-child relationship.
    d. Preserving the essential security of the parent-child relationship.

27. Mr. Alls brings his 12-month-old son, Keith, in for his regular well-infant examination. The nurse knows that the best approach to the physical examination for this patient will be to:
    a. have the infant sit in the parent's lap to complete as much of the examination as possible.
    b. place the infant on the examination table with parent out of view.
    c. perform examination in head-to-toe direction.
    d. completely undress Keith and leave him undressed during the examination.

28. Behavior that signals the child's readiness to cooperate during the physical examination does *not* include:
    a. talking to the nurse.
    b. making eye contact with the nurse.
    c. allowing physical touching.
    d. sitting on the parent's lap or playing with a doll.

29. The assessment method that the nurse expects to provide the most reliable evaluation about the physical growth pattern of a preschool-age child is:
    a. recording height and weight measurements of the child and comparing growth measurements over time.
    b. keeping a flow sheet for height, weight, and head circumference increases.
    c. obtaining a history of sibling growth patterns.
    d. measuring the height, weight, and head circumference of the child.

30. Describe how to measure recumbent length in a 14-month-old child.

31. Which one of the following findings for growth is cause for potential concern and should be followed closely?
    a. Height and weight fall above the 5th percentile on the growth chart.
    b. Height and weight fall below the 5th percentile on the growth chart.
    c. Height and weight fall below the 95th percentile on the growth chart.
    d. Height and weight fall within the 50th percentile on the growth chart.

32. Head circumference is:
    a. measured in all children up to the age of 24 months.
    b. equal to chest circumferences at about 1 to 2 years of age.
    c. about 8 to 9 cm smaller than chest circumference during childhood.
    d. measured slightly below the eyebrows and pinna of the ears.

33. In infants and young children, the _____ pulse should be taken because it is the most reliable. This pulse should be counted for _____ because of the possibility of irregularities in rhythm. When counting respirations in infants, observe the _____ movements and count for _____ because their movements are irregular.

34. Which of the following statements about temperature measurement in children is true?
    a. Rectal site is preferred in children under 1 month of age.
    b. Tympanic artery thermometry for children older than 2 years of age and temporal artery thermometry in all age groups is recommended.
    c. Ear (tympanic) temperature is a precise measurement of core body measurement.
    d. Oral temperature is a better indicator of rapid changes in core body temperature and accuracy and is the preferred method when the patient is under 5 years of age.

35. The nurse should obtain the vital signs of an infant in what order?
    a. Measure temperature, then count the pulse, and then count respirations.
    b. Count the pulse, then count respirations, and then measure the temperature.
    c. Count respirations, then count the pulse, and then measure the temperature.
    d. Measure the temperature, then count respirations, and then count the pulse.

36. Which one of the following findings should the nurse recognize as normal when measuring the vital signs of a 5-year-old child?
    a. Femoral pulses graded at +1
    b. Oral temperature of 100.9° F
    c. Blood pressure of 101/61
    d. Respiratory rate of 30 breaths/min

37. The nurse should eliminate which of the following observations when recording the general appearance of the child?
    a. Impression of child's nutritional status
    b. Behavior, interactions with parents
    c. Hygiene, cleanliness
    d. Vital signs

38. Match each term with its description or associated assessment findings. (Terms may be used more than once.)

a. Cyanosis
b. Pallor
c. Erythema
d. Ecchymosis
e. Petechiae
f. Jaundice
g. Craniosynostosis
h. Tissue turgor

i. Barrel chest
j. Pigeon chest
k. Capillary refill time
l. Wry neck, or torticollis
m. Opisthotonos
n. Genu valgum
o. Genu varum
p. Gynecomastia

q. Wheezes
r. Crackles
s. Innocent murmur
t. Functional murmur
u. Organic murmur
v. Polydactyly
w. Syndactyly

_____ Appears in dark-skinned patients as ashen-gray lips and tongue

_____ Appears in light-skinned patients as purplish to yellow-green areas

_____ May be a sign of anemia, chronic disease, edema, or shock

_____ Fusion of digits

_____ Redness of the skin that may be the result of infection, local inflammation, or increased temperature due to climatic conditions

_____ Large, diffuse areas, usually blue or black and the result of injury

_____ Small, distinct, pinpoint hemorrhages

_____ Yellow staining of the skin usually caused by bile pigments

_____ Time it takes for the blanched area to return to its original color; used to test for circulation and hydration

_____ Extra digit

_____ Injury to the sternocleidomastoid muscle with subsequent holding of the head to one side with the chin pointing toward the opposite side

_____ Hyperextension of the head

_____ Round chest

_____ Sternum that protrudes outward

_____ Premature closure of the sutures of the head

_____ Amount of elasticity to the skin

_____ Breast enlargement

_____ Lateral bowing of the tibia

_____ Stance in which knees are close together but feet are spread apart; "knock-knee"

_____ Result of the passage of air through narrowed passageways in the lungs

_____ Result of the passage of air through fluid or moisture in the lungs

_____ No anatomic or physiologic abnormality exists

_____ A cardiac defect with or without a physiologic abnormality exists

_____ No anatomic cardiac defect exists, but a physiologic abnormality such as anemia is present

39. You are assessing skin turgor in 10-month-old Ryan. You grasp the skin on the abdomen between the thumb and index finger, pull it taut, and quickly release it. The tissue remains suspended, or tented, for a few seconds and then slowly falls back on the abdomen. Which of the following conclusions can you correctly assume?
   a. The tissue shows normal elasticity.
   b. The child is properly hydrated.
   c. The assessment was done incorrectly.
   d. The child has poor skin turgor.

40. You are assessing 7-year-old Mary's lymph nodes. Using the distal portions of your fingers, you press gently but firmly in a circular motion along the occipital and postauricular node areas. You record the findings as "tender, enlarged, warm lymph nodes." Which of the following is true?
   a. Your findings are within normal limits for Mary's age.
   b. Your assessment technique was incorrect and should be repeated.
   c. Your findings suggest infection or inflammation in the scalp area or external ear canal.
   d. Your recording of the information is complete because it includes temperature and tenderness.

41. Which of the following assessment findings of the head and neck does *not* require a referral?
   a. Head lag before 6 months of age
   b. Hyperextension of the head with pain on flexion
   c. Palpable thyroid gland, including isthmus and lobes
   d. Closure of the anterior fontanel at the age of 9 months

42. Normal findings on examination of the pupils may be recorded as PERRLA, which means:

43. Match each term with its description.

   a. Palpebral conjunctiva
   b. Testing eyes for reaction to light
   c. Testing eyes for accommodation
   d. Permanent eye color
   e. Strabismus

   f. Amblyopia
   g. Testing eyes for malalignment
   h. Testing light perception
   i. Testing peripheral vision

   _____ Usually established by age 6 to 12 months

   _____ Corneal light reflex test and cover test

   _____ Performed by having the child look at a shiny object—first at a distance, then closer to the eyes; pupils should constrict as the object is brought near the eyes

   _____ One eye deviating from point of fixation

   _____ Performed by quickly shining a light source toward the eye and removing it; pupils constrict and then dilate

   _____ Type of blindness resulting from uncorrected "lazy" eye

   _____ Performed by having child fixate on a finger directly in front of the eyes and then moving it from the child's field of vision

_____ Inside lining of the eyelids

_____ Performed by shining light in the eyes and noting responses; used in newborns to test visual acuity

44. Which one of the following is an expected finding in the child's eye examination?
    a. Opaque red reflex of the eye
    b. Ophthalmoscopic examination revealing that veins are darker and about one-fourth larger than the arteries
    c. Strabismus in the 12-month-old infant
    d. A 5-year-old child who reads the Snellen eye chart at the 20/40 level

45. Match each type of eye chart with the procedure used for that chart.

    a. Snellen chart
    b. Tumbling chart
    c. HOTV chart

    _____ To "pass" a line, child must correctly identify four out of six letters on the line; used for children who can read letters.

    _____ Child is asked to point in the direction the letter is facing.

    _____ Child is asked to point to the correct letter on a board held in the hands.

46. Which of the following children meet(s) referral criteria?
    a. Jason, age 14 years, who identified fewer than four out of six correct letters with his right eye and five out of six correct with his left eye during visual acuity testing
    b. Sandra, age 3 years, who demonstrated eye movement with the unilateral cover test
    c. Tommy, age 4 years, who demonstrated a two-line difference between eyes on his visual acuity testing
    d. All of the above

47. When assessing the ear of a 2-year-old child, the nurse should:
    a. expect cerumen in the external ear canal.
    b. use the smallest speculum to prevent trauma to the ear.
    c. pull the pinna up and back to visualize the canal better.
    d. pull the pinna down and back to visualize the canal better.

48. The nurse is performing an otoscopic examination on 14-month-old Justin. Which one of the following is recognized as an abnormal finding?
    a. The umbo, tip of the malleus, appears as a round, opaque, concave spot near the center of the drum.
    b. Light reflex is pointing away from the face.
    c. Tympanic membrane is translucent, light pearly pink or gray.
    d. Tympanic membrane is dull, nontransparent.

49. The nurse is assessing the mouth and throat of 7-month-old Alex. Which of the following is recognized as a normal finding?
    a. Membranes are bright pink, smooth, and glistening.
    b. White curdy plaques are located on the tongue.
    c. Redness and puffiness are present along the gum line.
    d. Tip of the tongue extends to the gum line.

50. When assessing 4-year-old Gail's chest, the nurse should expect:
    a. movement of the chest wall to be symmetric bilaterally and coordinated with breathing.
    b. respiratory movements to be chiefly thoracic.
    c. anteroposterior diameter to be equal to the transverse diameter.
    d. retraction of the muscles between the ribs on respiratory movement.

51. On auscultation of 8-year-old Tammie's lung fields, the nurse hears inspiratory sounds that are louder, longer, and higher pitched than on expiration. These sounds are heard over the chest, except over the scapula and sternum. These sounds are:
    a. bronchovesicular breath sounds.
    b. vesicular breath sounds.
    c. bronchial breath sounds.
    d. adventitious breath sounds.

52. On palpation of 3-year-old Jennifer's apical impulse, where would the nurse expect to place the fingers?
    a. At the left midclavicular line and fourth intercostal space
    b. Lateral to the left midclavicular line and fifth intercostal space
    c. Over the pulmonic valve
    d. Over the aortic valve

53. When listening over the aortic area of the heart, the nurse should place the stethoscope where?
    a. Second right intercostal space, close to sternum
    b. Second left intercostal space, close to sternum
    c. Fifth left intercostal space, close to sternum
    d. Fifth right intercostal space, left midclavicular line

54. Examination of the abdomen is performed correctly by the nurse in what order?
    a. Inspection, palpation, and auscultation
    b. Inspection, auscultation, and palpation
    c. Palpation, auscultation, and inspection
    d. Auscultation, inspection, and palpation

55. When examining a child's genitalia, the nurse should:
    a. conduct this examination first so that the child will not be as apprehensive.
    b. ask the parent to leave the room so that the young child will not be as shy.
    c. wait until the end of the examination before discussing findings with the parent and child.
    d. understand that this examination may provoke anxiety in the child.

56. In performing an examination for scoliosis, the nurse understands that which one of the following is an incorrect method?
    a. The child should be examined only in his or her underpants (and a bra if an older girl).
    b. The child should stand erect, with the nurse observing from behind.
    c. The child should squat down with hands extended forward so the nurse can observe for asymmetry of the shoulder blades.
    d. The child should bend forward with the back parallel to the floor so that the nurse can observe from the side.

57. Identify the following physical findings as normal or abnormal (needing additional evaluation).

    a. _____ Asymmetric bowlegs before the age of 2 years

    b. _____ Knock-knee accompanied by short stature in a 9-year-old child

    c. _____ Flat feet in an 18-month-old toddler

    d. _____ Broad-based gait in a 20-month-old toddler

    e. _____ Positive Babinski sign in a 9-month-old toddler

58. Name the six areas included in the neurologic examination.

59. Which of the following statements about developmental assessment is true?
   a. Screening procedures are designed to identify normal developmental levels.
   b. They provide a means of obtaining subjective measurements of present developmental function.
   c. The Denver-II is the most sensitive and specific method for testing age-appropriate development markers.
   d. The Ages & Stages Questionnaires are age-specific surveys asking parents about developmental skills common in daily life for their children.

CRITICAL THINKING—CASE STUDIES

Mrs. Brown brings her 11-year-old son, Kenny, for a physical at the clinic where you work as a nurse. She is concerned because Kenny comes home from school "very tired and only wants to watch television." Kenny's bedtime has not changed, he performs well in school, and his mother denies stress or problems within the home. On physical examination, you discover Kenny is above the 90th percentile for weight by 11.3 kg (25 lb).

60. To effectively establish a setting for communication, you enter the room, introduce yourself to Mrs. Brown and Kenny, and explain your role and the purpose of the interview. You include Kenny in the interaction as you ask his name and age and what he is expecting at his visit today. You next inform Mrs. Brown and Kenny that he is 25 lb overweight and that his diet and exercise plan must be "terrible" for Kenny to be in "such bad shape." Which aspect of effective communication have you, as a nurse, forgotten that will most significantly affect the exchange of information during this interview?
   a. Assurance of privacy and confidentiality
   b. Preliminary acquaintance
   c. Directing the focus away from the complaint of fatigue to one of obesity
   d. Injecting your own attitudes and feelings into the interview

61. Based on the information provided in the case study, you can correctly record which of the following?
   a. Chief complaint
   b. Present illness
   c. Past medical history
   d. Symptom analysis

62. Mrs. Brown, Kenny, and you agree to the need to conduct a more intensive nutritional assessment. Which one of the following ways to record Kenny's dietary intake would you suggest as most reliable in providing needed information to assess his dietary habits?
   a. 12-hour recall
   b. 24-hour recall
   c. Food diary for 3-day period
   d. Food frequency questionnaire

63. During the physical examination, which of the following physical findings could be consistent with excess carbohydrate nutrition?
   a. Caries
   b. Skin elastic and firm
   c. Hair stringy, friable, dull, and dry
   d. Enlarged thyroid

64. The physical examination has been completed and reflects that, other than his obesity, Kenny is in excellent physical health with normal blood counts. The completed nutritional assessment reflects that Mrs. Brown has little knowledge about proper nutrition and that Kenny has a large intake of "junk" foods high in fat and calories but low in nutrients. Based on the data collected, which of the following nursing diagnoses are most appropriate?
   i. Altered Family Process related to parent's knowledge deficit
   ii. Altered Family Coping related to family's inability to purchase needed foods
   iii. Altered Family Coping related to fatigue from poor dietary habits
   iv. Altered Nutrition: More Than Body Requirements, related to eating practices
   v. Altered Nutrition: More Than Body Requirements, related to knowledge deficit of parent

   a. i, ii, and iv
   b. iii and iv
   c. iii, iv, and v
   d. iv and v

28

Mary, a 13-year-old, has come to the clinic with her mother. She is complaining of right-sided abdominal pain of 24 hours' duration. Mary tells you, the nurse, that she has had some nausea and vomiting but no diarrhea. Her appetite is depressed and she feels hot and feverish. She has taken acetaminophen for pain but with little relief. A complete blood count has been ordered and results are pending.

65. You are preparing Mary for a physical examination. You know that during the examination, Mary, as an adolescent, will likely:
    a. prefer her parents to be present during the entire examination.
    b. wish to undress in private and feel more comfortable when provided with a gown.
    c. prefer that traumatic procedures such as ear and mouth examinations be performed last.
    d. need to have heart and lungs auscultated first.

66. You complete the physical examination and determine that which one of the following is an abnormal finding?
    a. Bowel sounds are stimulated by stroking the abdominal surface with the fingernail.
    b. Mary has no abdominal discomfort when she is supine with the legs flexed at the hips and knees.
    c. Mary's eyes are open during palpation of the abdomen.
    d. When the nurse presses firmly over the area distal to the right side of the abdomen and quickly releases this pressure, pain is intensified in the lower right side.

67. Which one of the following organs is located in the lower right quadrant of the abdomen?
    a. Bladder
    b. Liver
    c. Ovaries
    d. Appendix

68. Mary's mother is apprehensive about her daughter's condition and asks you whether "it is serious." Which one of the following is your best response?
    a. "Mary has appendicitis and will need to have surgery immediately."
    b. "You will have to ask the doctor about her condition."
    c. "Mary has some abdominal pain that is not normal. We are watching her very carefully and will be able to tell you more when the laboratory tests are completed."
    d. "Mary should be able to go home as soon as the doctor finishes with the examination and the laboratory tests are completed."

69. While inspecting the abdomen, you should recognize which one of the following as a normal finding?
    a. Peristaltic waves
    b. Silvery, whitish lines when the skin is stretched out
    c. Bulging at the umbilicus
    d. Protruding abdomen with skin pulled tight

Gerald, age 16, has been complaining to the school nurse of chest pain during physical education class at school. The nurse is performing an assessment of the heart.

70. _____ is the sound caused by the closure of the tricuspid and mitral valves. It is heard loudest at the _____ of the heart. _____ is the sound heard as a result of the closure of the pulmonic and aortic valves. It is heard loudest at the _____ of the heart.

71. During auscultation of S_2, a split is heard that does not change during inspiration. Based on this, the nurse should suspect:
    a. a normal finding referred to as physiologic splitting.
    b. mitral valve prolapse.
    c. that no anatomic cardiac defect exists, but that a physiologic abnormality such as anemia is likely to be present.
    d. fixed splitting, which can be a diagnostic sign of atrial septal defect.

5 Pain Assessment and Management in Children

1. The inconsistency of pain management in children is related to four practices. List them.

2. The Pediatric Initiative on Methods, Measurements, and Pain Assessment in Clinical Trials (PedIMMPACT):
   a. is easy to use but less reliable than other methods.
   b. is used to assess pain in children including pain intensity, global judgment of satisfaction with treatment, symptoms and adverse events, physical recovery, and emotional response.
   c. is used for children up to 4 years of age.
   d. is used to understand the pain intensity experienced by the child along with types of discomfort.

3. Behavioral pain measures:
   a. are used most often with school-aged children.
   b. are less effective and more time consuming when used in conjunction with a subject self-report measure.
   c. are most reliable when measuring recurrent or chronic pain.
   d. are most reliable when measuring short, sharp procedural pain.

4. In regard to behavioral and physiologic responses to pain, children:
   a. remain consistent from age to age.
   b. vary widely in their responses.
   c. exhibit typical behaviors at each development stage.
   d. are unaffected by temperament.

5. Which one of the following characteristics is most likely to be exhibited by an adolescent who is in pain?
   a. Decreased verbal expression and withdrawal
   b. Requests to terminate the procedure
   c. Verbal expression such as "You're hurting me!"
   d. Facial expression of pain and anger

6. Which one of the following behavioral pain measures includes five categories of behavior and uses a scoring system to quantify pain behaviors, with 0 being no pain behaviors and 10 being the most possible pain behaviors?
   a. FLACC Pain Assessment Tool (Facial expression, Leg movement, Activity, Cry, and Consolability)
   b. Children's Hospital of Eastern Ontario Pain Scale (CHEOPS)
   c. COMFORT Scale
   d. All of the above

7. Which one of the following pain assessment scales was developed with input from recovery room nurses, includes six categories of behaviors, and uses a scoring system to quantify pain behavior?
   a. FLACC Pain Assessment Tool (Facial expression, Leg movement, Activity, Cry, and Consolability)
   b. Children's Hospital of Eastern Ontario Pain Scale (CHEOPS)
   c. COMFORT Scale
   d. All of the above

8. The Wong-Baker FACES Pain Rating Scale:
   a. is easy to use but less reliable than other methods.
   b. is a rating of how children are feeling.
   c. has a coding system from 0.4 to 0.97.
   d. consists of six cartoon faces.

9. The Numeric Rating Scale:
   a. consists of six culturally specific photographs of faces.
   b. uses a straight line.
   c. uses descriptive words.
   d. is harder to use but more reliable than other methods.

10. The Visual Analog Scale (VAS):
    a. requires a higher degree of abstract thought.
    b. is recommended for children who understand the value of numbers.
    c. does not offer an option for "no pain."
    d. is recommended for children under 3 years of age.

11. The Adolescent Pediatric Pain Tool (APPT):
    a. is used in children over 6 years of age.
    b. is grouped by sensory, affective, and evaluative qualities.
    c. uses a straight line.
    d. uses the scale of 0 to 10 to rate the degree of pain.

12. The Pediatric Pain Questionnaire:
    a. is useful in infants.
    b. is used to assess patient and parental pain perceptions.
    c. consists of a series of four questions related to pain assessment.
    d. is completed jointly by the physician, child, and family.

13. The Functional Disability Inventory (FDI):
    a. is used to evaluate depression in children with chronic pain.
    b. is used to evaluate the influence of acute pain on physical functioning.
    c. is used to assess the child's ability to perform everyday physical activities.
    d. has both child and parent versions.

14. List the five indicators used in the CRIES pain assessment tool:

    C:

    R:

    I:

    E:

    S:

15. The Non-Communicating Children's pain Checklist (NCCPC):
    a. is designed specifically to be used with all children ages 3 to 18.
    b. uses facial pictures so the child can point to the one that best describes his/her pain.
    c. has a scale that discriminates between periods of pain and calm and can predict behavior during subsequent episodes of pain.
    d. consists of 8 subscales that are scored based on the number of times the items are observed over 30 minutes.

16. In assessing pain in children with chronic illness and complex pain, the nurse understands that:
    a. the most important aspect is the relationship that develops between the child and the family.
    b. the most important aspect is the relationship that develops between the family and the nurse.
    c. the assessment should occur when the child is in pain.
    d. the assessment should occur when the child is pain free.

17. Which one of the following statements is true in regard to nonpharmacologic pain management?
    a. When used properly, nonpharmacologic measures are a good substitute for analgesics.
    b. Nurses and physicians are generally well educated about nonpharmacologic approaches to pain management.
    c. Nonpharmacologic approaches to pain management are not effective with children.
    d. Whenever possible, nonpharmacologic and pharmacologic measures should be combined to manage pain.

18. Identify three specific nonpharmacologic strategies that can be used to manage pain.

19. Which one of the following has been shown to have calming and pain-relieving effects when used with invasive procedures in neonates?
    a. Allowing parent to hold neonate during procedure
    b. Allowing neonate quiet time in the bassinet before the procedure
    c. Administering concentrated sucrose with or without nonnutritive sucking before procedure
    d. Using relaxation techniques during the procedure

20. Which one of the following is an acute manifestation of pain in the neonate?
    a. Increased transcutaneous oxygen saturation
    b. Increased heart rate, rapid and shallow respirations
    c. Decreased muscle tone and increased vagal nerve tone
    d. Increased skin dryness, decreased blood pressure, hyperglycemia

21. Infants and children experience a substantial amount of pain due to routine immunization. Based on current research, which of the following statements is *false*?
    a. The child should be positioned upright, either sitting or being held by the caregiver during the immunizations.
    b. The caregiver and the nurse should use verbal reassurance, empathy, and apology during the immunizations.
    c. The nurse should administer the least painful vaccine first when administering multiple vaccines.
    d. The nurse should administer the vaccines rapidly and without aspiration.

22. List the five classes of complementary and alternative medicine therapies.

23. The two-step approach for pain management:
    a. is used with children older than 3 years of age.
    b. always starts with administration of a nonopioid.
    c. consists of a choice of category of analgesic medications according to the level of pain.
    d. always starts with the administration of morphine as the drug of choice.

24. Nonopioids:
    a. are used for moderate to severe pain.
    b. have the same effect on pain as morphine.
    c. have little antipyretic actions.
    d. take about 1 hour for effect.

25. Which one of the following opioids is considered the gold standard for severe pain management?
    a. Hydromorphone
    b. Gentanyl
    c. Oxycodone
    d. Morphine

26. When choosing the pain medication dose for use in children:
    a. use the weight and height to determine exact dosing.
    b. younger than 6 months of age and not mechanically ventilated, use one fourth to one third the recommended starting dose of opioids for older children.
    c. use smaller doses because tolerance develops slowly.
    d. increase the dose for moderate pain by 75% if pain relief is inadequate.

27. Children older than 6 months of age:
    a. metabolize drugs more rapidly than do adults.
    b. metabolize drugs less rapidly than do adults.
    c. require smaller doses of opioids to achieve the same analgesic effect.
    d. have greater pain relief when the nonopioid dosage is past the ceiling effect.

28. Describe the three typical methods of drug administration used with patient-controlled analgesia.

29. When patient-controlled analgesia (PCA) is used with children, the:
    a. drug of choice is meperidine.
    b. patient should control the dosing.
    c. nurse should control the dosing.
    d. drug of choice is morphine.

30. When using epidural analgesia to manage pain, the nurse knows that:
    a. analgesia results from the drug's effect on the brain.
    b. respiratory depression is fast to develop, usually 1 to 2 hours after administration.
    c. the epidural spaces at the lumbar and caudal level are used most often.
    d. securing the catheter with an occlusive dressing does little to prevent infection.

31. The transdermal patch Duragesic may be used:
    a. in infants for acute pain management.
    b. for patients who are opioid tolerant.
    c. as a safe and effective medication for children of all ages.
    d. to provide prolonged pain relief for more than 96 hours.

32. Which one of the following methods of analgesic drug administration is a liquid gel that provides anesthesia to nonintact skin in about 15 minutes?
    a. Midazolam
    b. EMLA (eutectic mixture of local anesthetics)
    c. LAT (lidocaine-adrenaline-tetracaine)
    d. Numby Stuff

33. The anesthetic EMLA is used:
    a. before invasive procedures.
    b. as preoperative oral sedation.
    c. for chronic cancer pain.
    d. postoperatively.

34. To manage opioid-induced respiratory depression in patients receiving opioids by continuous infusion, the nurse should:
    a. increase the infusion 25%.
    b. allow the patient long periods of uninterrupted sleep.
    c. administer naloxone and discontinue the infusion.
    d. administer naloxone by slow intravenous push every 2 minutes until the effect is obtained.

35. For postoperative or cancer pain control, analgesics should be administered:
    a. whenever needed.
    b. around the clock.
    c. before the pain escalates.
    d. after the pain peaks.

36. The most common side effect of opioid therapy is:
    a. respiratory depression.
    b. pruritus.
    c. nausea and vomiting.
    d. constipation.

37. Treatment of tolerance to opioid therapy includes:
    a. discontinuing the drug.
    b. decreasing the dose.
    c. increasing the dose.
    d. increasing the duration between doses.

38. Which of the following terms describes a physiologic state in which abrupt cessation of an opioid results in a withdrawal syndrome?
    a. Tolerance
    b. Physical dependence
    c. Addiction
    d. Pseudoaddiction

39. The mismanagement of infant pain is partially the result of misconceptions regarding _____ and _____.

40. Which of the following describes moderate sedation (previously termed *conscious sedation*)?
    a. Patient is not easily aroused and does not respond to verbal commands.
    b. Patient responds normally to verbal commands but may not respond to light tactile stimulation.
    c. Patient's cognitive function may be impaired.
    d. Patient is not able to maintain a patent airway independently.

41. Preemptive analgesia administered for postoperative pain:
    a. is associated with higher analgesic requirements.
    b. is administered immediately after surgery.
    c. increases analgesic requirements.
    d. decreases hospital stay.

42. The biggest challenge in management of burn pain is:
    a. providing analgesia without interfering with the patient's awareness during and after procedures.
    b. providing analgesia that allows safe sedation during and after procedures.
    c. adding additional medications that decrease anxiety without adversely affecting respirations.
    d. using psychologic interventions effectively.

43. The two main nonpharmacologic approaches to management of headache are:

44. Recurrent abdominal pain in children:
    a. occurs at least once per week.
    b. does not interfere with the child's normal activities.
    c. requires individualized management.
    d. requires the nurse to understand that because there is no organic cause for the pain, the reported pain is not a true pain.

45. Which one of the following can the nurse expect to be included in the care plan for controlling acute pain in sickle cell crisis?
    a. Administration of long-term oxygen
    b. Application of cold compresses
    c. Use of opioids started early in childhood and continued throughout adult life
    d. Relieving the pain completely as the goal of treatment of the acute episode

46. Identify the following statements about cancer pain in children as true or false.

    _____ Pain is the most prevalent symptom with cancer.

    _____ Cancer pain in children is rarely present before diagnosis.

    _____ A major source of pain in children with cancer is treatment related.

    _____ Oral mucositis occurs most often in patients undergoing bone marrow transplant, chemotherapy, and radiation.

    _____ Antihistamines, local anesthetics, and opioids provide long-lasting pain relief for lesions associated with oral mucositis.

    _____ Morphine administered as a continuous infusion may be necessary for pain until mucositis is resolved.

    _____ Postdural puncture headaches should be treated by administering nonopioid analgesics and keeping the patient supine for 1 hour.

CRITICAL THINKING—CASE STUDIES

Beverly is a 10-year-old child who is coming to the health clinic because she has been having recurrent headaches for more than 6 months. She is an honor student who loves to play the violin. Beverly lives at home with both her parents and her 13-year-old sister, Sharon, who is also an honor student.

Beverly's mother is with her during the interview and physical examination. Beverly describes the headaches as increasing in frequency and always occurring in the morning during her first-period advanced math class. She has been taking acetaminophen almost daily with only moderate relief. A physical examination done by the health care provider was within normal limits.

47. Describe interventions that could be helpful in assessing Beverly's headaches.

48. After reviewing information collected and talking with Beverly, her parents, and her math teacher, the nurse believes that the headaches could be related to Beverly pushing herself in math class. She is doing well in math class, however, and does not want to stop the advanced class. What interventions could be helpful for Beverly and her parents at this point to control her headaches?

Brian is a 5-year-old boy being readmitted to the hospital because of his cancer. He has been doing fairly well at home; he is eating and sleeping well. Brian's weight has increased to 25 kg (56 lb), and he is now 1.2 m (4 ft) tall. His mother is with him at the hospital and is his primary caregiver at home.

49. If Brian becomes neutropenic, the nurse knows to avoid which one of the following medications for pain?
    a. Acetaminophen
    b. Morphine
    c. All intramuscular medications
    d. Codeine

50. If Brian develops thrombocytopenia, the nurse knows to avoid which one of the following medications for pain?
    a. Acetaminophen
    b. Nonsteroidal antiinflammatory drugs
    c. Morphine
    d. Codeine

6 Childhood Communicable and Infectious Diseases

1. Match each term with its description.

   a. Hospital-acquired infection (HIA)
   b. Standard Precautions
   c. Transmission-Based Precautions
   d. Droplet Precautions
   e. Contact Precautions

   f. Airborne Precautions
   g. Universal Precautions
   h. Body substance isolation
   i. Direct contact transmission
   j. Indirect contact transmission

   _____ Designed to reduce the transmission of infectious agents that remain suspended in air or by dust particles containing the infectious agent

   _____ Designed for patients documented or suspected to be infected or colonized with highly transmissible or epidemiologically important pathogens for which interventions beyond Standard Precautions are needed to interrupt transmission in hospitals

   _____ Infections occur when there is interaction among patients, health care personnel, equipment, and bacteria.

   _____ Designed to reduce the risk for transmission of infectious agents that are spread when large particles generated during coughing, sneezing, or talking come into contact with the conjunctiva or the mucous membrane of the nose or mouth of a susceptible person; suctioning or bronchoscopy generates these particles

   _____ Designed to reduce the risk for transmission of microorganisms transmitted by direct or indirect contact

   _____ Interventions that synthesize the major features of universal (blood and body fluid) precautions and body substance isolation; involve the use of barrier protection; designed for the care of all patients to reduce the risk for transmission of microorganism from both recognized and unrecognized sources of infection

   _____ Designed to reduce the risk of transmission of pathogens from moist body substances

   _____ Blood and body fluid precautions designed to reduce the risk of transmission of blood-borne pathogens

   _____ Involves skin-to-skin contact and physical transfer of microorganisms to a susceptible host from an infected or colonized person

   _____ Involves contact of a susceptible host with a contaminated intermediate object, usually an inanimate object in the patient's environment

2. Standard Precautions involve the use of barrier protection to prevent contamination from:
   a. blood.
   b. body fluids.
   c. mucous membranes.
   d. all of the above.

3. In hospitals, which of the following is the most significant source of methicillin-resistant *Staphylococcus aureus* (MRSA) and the major mode of transport?
   a. Patient to patient via the hands of the health care provider
   b. Patients coming in direct contact with other patients
   c. Failure of hospital personnel to wear face masks when working with patients in an airborne infection isolation room
   d. Indirect contact transmission from hospital equipment

4. To prevent spread of contamination from one patient to another after procedures, the most important strategy the nurse can use is to:
   a. follow disease-specific infection control guidelines.
   b. wear vinyl gloves.
   c. avoid wearing nail polish.
   d. wash the hands routinely after each patient contact and after removing gloves.

5. In scheduling immunizations, the nurse knows which of the following is correct?
   a. The beginning primary immunization for infants begins at 2 months of age.
   b. Children who are born preterm receive only half the normal dose of each vaccine followed by the second half of the vaccine 2 weeks later.
   c. Children who begin primary immunization at the recommended age but fail to receive all the doses by the suggested age need to begin the series again.
   d. When there is doubt that the child will return for follow-up immunizations according to the optimum schedule, HBV vaccine (HepB), DTaP, IPV (poliovirus vaccine), MMR, varicella, and Hib vaccines can be administered simultaneously at separate injection sites.

6. Match each immunization term with its description.

   a. Natural immunity
   b. Acquired immunity
   c. Active immunity
   d. Passive immunity
   e. Attenuate

   f. Toxoid
   g. Antitoxin
   h. Immunoglobulin
   i. Herd immunity
   j. Monovalent vaccine

   k. Conjugate vaccine
   l. Combination vaccine
   m. Polyvalent vaccine
   n. Cocooning

   _____ Strategy of protecting infants from pertussis by vaccinating all persons who come in close contact with the infant

   _____ Multiple vaccines into one parenteral form

   _____ A carrier protein with proven immunologic potential combined with a less antigenic polysaccharide antigen to enhance the type and magnitude of the immune response; Hib

   _____ Designed to vaccinate against muliple antigens or organisms; meningococcal polysaccharide vaccine

   _____ Designed to vaccinate against a single antigen or organism

   _____ Innate resistance to infection

   _____ Occurs from exposue to the invading agent

   _____ Immune bodies are actively formed against specific antigens by having had the disease or by introducing the antigen into the individual

   _____ Temporary immunity obtained by tranfusing immunoglobulin or antitoxins from a person or animal that has been actively immunized against the antigen

   _____ Modified bacterial toxin that has been made nontoxic but retains its ability to stimulate the formation of antitoxin

   _____ To reduce the virulence of a pathogenic microorganism by treating it or cultivating it on a certain medium

   _____ A solution of antibodies derived from the serum of animals immunized with specific antigens and used to confer passive immunity

   _____ The majority of the population is vaccinated and the spread of disease is stopped without the rest of the population getting vaccinated.

   _____ A sterile solution containing antibodies from large pools of human blood plasma

7. The HBsAg negative mother of Daniella, a premature infant weighing 4 pounds and born 6 hours ago, asks, "Have you already given Daniella her hepatitis B vaccine?" What is your correct response?
   a. "Don't worry, we will give it before she leaves the hospital."
   b. "Daniella is sleeping right now. I will give it as soon as she wakes up."
   c. "Because Daniella only weighs 4 pounds, she will not receive her vaccine until she is 1 month of age."
   d. "Because Daniella is premature and weighs only 4 pounds, she will be given one vaccine dose now and then she will need another in 2 months."

8. The following statements are about hepatitis A illness or vaccination. Which one is correct?
   a. The illness has a gradual onset, with often dark urine and jaundice being the only symptoms.
   b. The vaccine is recommended for all children between the ages of 12 and 23 months.
   c. The vaccine consists of a series of 3 injections timed 2 months apart.
   d. The illness is spread by all body secretions.

9. When educating the public about diphtheria vaccine, the nurse recognizes which of the following as correct?
   i. Diphtheria vaccine is commonly administered in combination with tetanus and pertussis vaccines (DTaP) or DTaP and Hib vaccines for children under 7 years of age.
   ii. Diphtheria vaccine is administered with tetanus and acellular pertussin (Tdap) for children 11 years and older.
   iii. Diphtheria vaccine produces absolute immunity after 3 doses.
   iv. Several vaccines contain diphtheria toxoid (Hib, meningococcal, pneumococcal), which confers immunity to the disease.

   a. i, ii, iii, and iv
   b. i and ii
   c. i, ii, and iii
   d. iii and iv

10. Joey, a 14-year-old adolescent, has recently relocated from Mexico to the United States. While helping his dad do farm work, Joey suffered a laceration in the horse barn. Review of Joey's immunization record from Mexico shows that Joey has had 2 previous tetanus and diphtheria vaccine immunization shots, the last one being at the age of 6 years. Which of the following would the nurse in the emergency department *expect to* give at this time?
    a. Tdap
    b. DTaP
    c. Td booster
    d. Tetanus immunoglobulin (TIG) human and Tdap

11. For which of the following populations is pertussis vaccine currently recommended?
    i. All children from 6 weeks to the seventh birthday
    ii. Children ages 11 to 12 years who have completed the DTaP/DTP childhood series
    iii. A second booster for previously immunized adolescents and adults
    iv. Children ages 7 through 10 years who are not fully vaccinated for pertussis, (i.e., did not receive 5 doses of DTaP, or who received 4 doses of DTaP with the fourth dose being administered on or after the fourth birthday)
    v. Pregnant adolescents between 27 and 36 weeks' gestation, if not previously protected

    a. i, ii, iv, and v
    b. i, iii, and iv
    c. ii, iii, and v
    d. i, ii, iii, and iv

12. When administering the pertussis vaccine, the nurse recognizes which of the following as incorrect?
    a. Can be given any time during pregnancy
    b. Cannot be given to the postpartum mother who is breastfeeding
    c. The acellular pertussis vaccine, from the same manufacturer, is recommended for the first three immunizations and is given along with diphtheria and tetanus at 2, 4, and 6 months of age.
    d. Is recommended for health care workers having close contact with infants under the age of 12 months

13. Which of the following statements about polio vaccine and immunization is *not* correct?
    a. Inactivated poliovirus vaccine (IPV) is now recommended for routine childhood vaccination in the United States.
    b. Oral polio vaccine (OPV) has been associated with vaccine-associated polio paralysis.
    c. KINRIX contains DTaP, hepatitis B, and IPV and may be used only in children aged 4 years or older as the fourth dose.
    d. The combination vaccine PEDIARIX (containing DTaP, hepatitis B, and IPV) may be used as the primary immunization beginning at 2 months of age.

14. Measles immunization includes which of the following?
    a. Given at 12 to 15 months of age with a second dose given at age 4 to 6 years of age and revaccination at 11 to 12 years of age.
    b. Child vaccinated before 12 months of age should receive two additional doses beginning at 12 to 15 months and separated by at least 4 weeks.
    c. Revaccination of all individuals born after 1956 who have not received two doses of measles vaccine after 12 months of age.
    d. All of the above

15. Mumps immunization:
    a. is recommended for children ages 4 years of age or older.
    b. is typically given in combination with measles and rubella.
    c. can be administered to infants as young as 6 months of age.
    d. All of the above

16. Rubella vaccine administration:
    a. is given as protection for the unborn child rather than for the recipient of the immunization.
    b. is recommended for all children beginning at 4 to 6 years of age.
    c. is given to all pregnant women if not previously immunized.
    d. is not given to children whose mother is currently pregnant.

17. Which of the following statements about *Haemophilus influenzae* type b (Hib) vaccine is true?
    a. The vaccine protects against a number of infections including bacterial meningitis, epiglottitis, bacterial pneumonia, septic arthritis, and sepsis.
    b. The vaccine protects against the virus that produces influenza.
    c. Only two doses of Hib vaccine should be given to children 15 months of age or older who have not been previously vaccinated.
    d. Hiberix is a conjugate vaccine licensed for use in infants over the age of 2 months.

18. Which of the following statements about varicella vaccine is correct?
    a. Varicella vaccine is recommended for all children regardless of past disease history.
    b. A single dose of 0.5 ml of varicella vaccine should be given by deep intramuscular injection.
    c. The first dose of varicella vaccine is recommended for children ages 12 to 15 months, and to ensure adequate protection, a second varicella vaccination is recommended for children at 4 to 6 years of age.
    d. Varicella vaccine should not be administered simultaneously with MMR.

19. Bryan, age 6 months, is starting daycare as his mother is returning to work. Bryan has had no immunizations. Which of the following statements provided by the nurse to the mother is the most appropriate at this time?
    a. "Since Bryan has not started his immunizations for streptococcal pneumococci yet, it is best to wait until after he gets established at daycare before beginning his injections."
    b. "Streptococcal pneumococci are responsible for a number of bacterial infections that are especially problematic for children under 2 years of age who attend daycare. Bryan should start his series of pneumococcal vaccine right away."
    c. "Why has Bryan not received any immunizations? He is past due. Don't you care about his health?"
    d. "Pneumococcal vaccine (PCV13) is the only vaccine recommended for Bryan at this time."

20. Which of the following is not an influenza vaccine recommendation?
    a. The vaccine is administered in early fall before the flu season begins and is repeated yearly.
    b. Fluzone, a quadrivalent influenza vaccine, offers protection against type A and type B and is approved for vaccine use in children ages 6 months and older.
    c. Children with severe egg allergy history should not routinely receive the influenza vaccine.
    d. The live attenuated influenza vaccine (LAIV) form is recommended for children 2 to 4 years of age with a history of wheezing or asthma.

21. Meningococcal conjugate vaccines (MCV4) are not recommended for which of the following populations?
    a. Routinely for children ages 9 months to 10 years
    b. Children aged 2 years to 18 years who travel to or reside in countries where *N. meningitidis* is hyperendemic or epidemic
    c. Children and adolescents 11 to 12 years of age
    d. College freshmen living in dormitories

22. Which of the following statements about rotavirus disease or immunization against rotavirus is correct?
    a. Rotavirus is one of the leading causes of diarrhea in infants and young children.
    b. Rotavirus is one of the leading causes of otitis media in young children.
    c. One vaccine for rotavirus is RotaTeq, which is approved for children 32 weeks of age or older.
    d. Rotavirus vaccine usually causes only mild reaction, redness, and soreness at the site of injection.

23. Human papillomavirus (HPV) vaccine is recommended for all of the following populations *except*:
    a. female adolescents to prevent HPV-related cervical cancer.
    b. boys and men (9 to 26 years) to reduce the likelihood of genital warts.
    c. female preadolescents ages 7 to 9 years.
    d. female adolescents who are not sexually active.

24. Which one of the following techniques is recommended to provide atraumatic care for immunization administration to infants?
    a. Select a 25-mm needle to deposit vaccine deep into the muscle mass.
    b. Use an air bubble to clear the needle before injection.
    c. Use the deltoid muscle.
    d. Use the EMLA patch before administration.

25. When administering vaccines, a(n) _____ is considered a condition in a person that does increase the risk for a serious adverse reaction (e.g., not administering a live virus vaccine to a severely immune-compromised child.)

    When administering vaccines, a(n) _____ is a condition in a person that might increase the risk for a serious adverse reaction or that might compromise the ability of the vaccine to produce immunity.

26. The general contraindication for all immunizations is:
    a. minor illness such as common cold.
    b. breastfeeding.
    c. pregnancy.
    d. severe febrile illness.

27. The nurse is administering immunizations to 2-month-old Brian. Describe what should be documented on the medical record.

28. Match each communicable disease with its description or characteristics.
    a. Varicella
    b. Diphtheria
    c. Fifth disease
    d. Roseola
    e. Rubeola
    f. Mumps
    g. Pertussis
    h. Rubella

    i. Scarlet fever
    j. Poliomyelitis

    _____ Rash appears in three stages; stage I is erythema on face, chiefly on cheeks.

    _____ This condition has a rash that begins as macules, rapidly progressing to papules and then to vesicles, eventually breaking and forming crusts.

    _____ Tonsillar pharyngeal areas are covered with white or gray membrane; complications include myocarditis and neuritis.

    _____ Rash composed of rose-pink macules or maculopapules, appearing first on trunk, then spreading to neck, face, and extremities; rash is nonpruritic.

    _____ Cough occurs at night, and inspirations sound like crowing.

    _____ This condition results in earache that is aggravated by chewing.

_____ Rash appears 3 to 4 days after onset and maculopapular eruption on face with gradual spread downward; Koplik spots are present before the rash.

_____ Discrete pinkish red maculopapular rash appears on face and then spreads downward to neck, arms, trunk, and legs; greatest danger is teratogenic effect on fetus.

_____ Permanent paralysis may occur.

_____ Tonsils are enlarged, edematous, reddened, and covered with patches of exudate; rash is absent on face; desquamation occurs.

29. Primary prevention of communicable disease is best accomplished by:
    a. immunization.
    b. control of the disease spread.
    c. adequate water supply.
    d. implementing good hand-washing practices among hospital personnel.

30. Assessment of which of the following is *not* helpful in identifying potentially communicable diseases?
    a. Prodromal symptoms
    b. Immunization history
    c. Past medical history
    d. Family history

31. Certain groups of children are at risk for serious complications from communicable diseases. These children do *not* include which of the following groups?
    a. Children with an immunodeficiency or immunologic disorder
    b. Children receiving steroid therapy
    c. Children with leukemia
    d. Children who have recently undergone a surgical procedure

32. Name the two diseases caused by the varicella-zoster virus (VZV).

33. What antiviral agent is used to treat varicella infections in children at increased risk for complications associated with varicella?
    a. Varicella-zoster immune globulin
    b. Acyclovir
    c. Salicylates
    d. Steroids

34. The nurse knows, regarding pertussis, that:
    a. the incidence has decreased in infants younger than 6 months of age.
    b. a booster vaccine (Tdap) is now recommended for all children 11 to 18 years of age.
    c. treatment should begin as soon as exposure is confirmed and includes the antibiotic amoxicillin.
    d. the disease is not contagious, so close household members do not need treatment.

35. The American Academy of Pediatrics has recommended vitamin A supplements for certain pediatric patients with measles. Correct dosage of vitamin A and instructions to parents of these children include:
    i. single oral dose of 200,000 international units in children 1 year old.
    ii. single oral dose of 100,000 international units in children 6 to 12 months old.
    iii. dosage may be associated with vomiting and headache for a few hours.
    iv. safe storage of the drug to prevent accidental overdose.

    a. i, ii, iii, and iv
    b. i, ii, and iv
    c. i, iii, and iv
    d. ii and iv

36. The nurse is conducting an educational session for the parents of a child diagnosed with varicella. Which one of the following is *not* an appropriate comfort measure to include in this session?
    a. Use Aveeno bath treatment or oatmeal in bath water for added skin comfort.
    b. Use Caladryl lotion on rash to decrease itching.
    c. Use hot bath water to promote skin rash healing.
    d. Keep nails short and smooth to decrease chances of infection from scratching.

37. Which one of the following does the nurse recognize as contraindicated in providing comfort measures to children with communicable diseases?
    a. Use of acetaminophen or ibuprofen for control of elevated temperature in children with varicella.
    b. Use of diphenhydramine (Benadryl) or hydroxyzine (Atarax) for itching
    c. Use of aspirin to control elevated temperature and/or symptoms with varicella
    d. Use of lozenges and saline rinses in an 8-year-old child with sore throat

38. Clinical manifestations differentiate bacterial conjunctivitis from viral conjunctivitis. Which one of the following is present with bacterial conjunctivitis but not usually found with viral conjunctivitis?
    a. Child awakens with crusting of eyelids.
    b. Child has increase in watery drainage from eyes.
    c. Child has inflamed conjunctiva.
    d. Child has swollen eyelids.

39. When instructing the parents caring for an infant with conjunctivitis, the nurse will include which one of the following in the plan?
    a. Accumulated secretions are removed by wiping from outer canthus inward.
    b. Hydrogen peroxide placed on cotton swabs is helpful in removing crusts from eyelids.
    c. Compresses of warm tap water are kept in place on the eye to prevent crusting.
    d. Washcloth and towel used by the infant are kept separate and not used by others.

40. Identify the following statements about stomatitis as true or false.

    _____ Aphthous stomatitis may be associated with mild traumatic injury, allergy, and emotional stress.

    _____ Aphthous stomatitis is characterized by painful, small, whitish ulcerations that heal without complication in 4 to 12 days.

    _____ Herpetic gingivostomatitis is caused by herpes simplex virus, usually type 1.

    _____ Herpetic gingivostomatitis is commonly called "cold sores" or "fever blisters."

    _____ Treatment for stomatitis is aimed at relief of complications.

    _____ When examining herpetic lesions, the nurse uses her uncovered index finger to check for cracks in the skin surface.

    _____ Herpetic gingivostomatitis is associated with sexual transmission.

    _____ Treatment for children with severe cases of herpetic gingivostomatitis includes oral acyclovir.

    _____ Topical anesthetics like lidocaine (Xylocaine Viscous) can be prescribed for children who are old enough to keep the drug in the mouth for 2 to 3 minutes and then swallow the drug.

41. Anne, an 8-year-old, has been diagnosed with giardiasis. The nurse would expect Anne to have most likely been seen initially with which of the following signs and symptoms?
    a. Diarrhea with blood in the stools
    b. Nausea and vomiting with a mild fever
    c. Abdominal cramps with intermittent loose stools
    d. Weight loss of 5 lb in the past month

42. A drug used to treat children diagnosed with giardiasis is:
    a. metronidazole (Flagyl).
    b. amoxicillin
    c. erythromycin.
    d. tetracycline.

43. The nurse is instructing parents on the test-tape diagnostic procedure for enterobiasis. Which one of the following is included in the explanation?
    a. Use a flashlight to inspect the anal area while the child sleeps.
    b. Perform the test 2 days after the child receives the first dose of antiparasitic medication.
    c. Test all members of the family at the same time using frosted tape.
    d. Collect the tape in the morning before the child has a bowel movement or bath.

44. Children with pinworm infections are seen with the principal symptom of:
    a. perianal itching.
    b. diarrhea with blood.
    c. evidence of small, ricelike worms in their stool and urine.
    d. abdominal pain.

45. Care of bacterial skin infections in children may include all of the following *except*:
    a. good hand washing.
    b. keeping the fingernails short.
    c. puncturing the surface of the pustule.
    d. application of topical antibiotics.

46. Which one of the following is a fungal infection that lives on the skin?
    a. Tinea corporis
    b. Herpes simplex type 1
    c. Scabies
    d. Warts

47. Steve, age 8, has been diagnosed with tinea capitis. Which one of the following does the nurse include in the teaching plan for Steve and his parents?
    a. No animal-to-person transmission is associated with this infection.
    b. Steve can continue to share hair-grooming articles with his younger brother.
    c. Griseofulvin should be administered with high-fat foods.
    d. Cleanliness is the best way to prevent this disease.

48. Which one of the following statements about scabies is incorrect?
    a. Clinical manifestations include intense pruritus, especially at night, and papules, burrows, or vesicles on inter-digital surfaces.
    b. Treatment is the application of 5% Elimite for all family members.
    c. After treatment, all previously worn clothing is washed in very hot water and dried at the high setting in the dryer.
    d. The rash and itching will be eliminated immediately after treatment.

49. a. What would the nurse look for in assessing whether a child has pediculosis?

    b. When can the student with pediculosis return to school?

    c. Because of its efficacy and lack of toxicity, what is the drug of choice for infants and children with pediculosis?

50. In helping parents cope with pediculosis, the nurse should emphasize that:
    a. anyone can get pediculosis.
    b. lice will fly and jump from one person to another.
    c. cutting the child's hair short will prevent reinfestation.
    d. the condition can be transmitted by pets.

51. Bedbugs, although once considered to be practically nonexistent, have remerged within the past decade as troublesome. Which of the following does the nurse recognize as incorrect information about bedbugs?
    a. They tend to inhabit warm, dark areas such as furniture and emerge at night to feed.
    b. They act as vectors for disease transmission.
    c. The treatment of bedbugs should focus on proper identification, treatment of symptoms, and eradication.
    d. Their bites are often misdiagnosed as scabies, spider bites, or mosquito bites.

52. Match each term with its description.

    a. Histoplasmosis
    b. Coccidioidomycosis
    c. Rocky Mountain spotted fever

    d. Epidemic typhus
    e. Endemic typhus
    f. Rickettsialpox

    _____ Transmitted by flea bite or by inhaling or ingesting flea excreta

    _____ Transmitted from human to human by the body louse; requires that patient be isolated until deloused

    _____ Marked by maculopapular rash following primary lesion and eschar at site of bite; transmitted from mouse mite to humans

    _____ Infection caused by organism cultured from soil, especially where contaminated with fowl droppings

    _____ Transmitted by tick; maculopapular or petechial rash on palms and soles

    _____ Primary lung disease; endemic in the southwestern United States

53. Children with Lyme disease in the first stage are seen with clinical manifestations of:
    a. a small, erythematous papule that enlarges and has a circumferential ring with a raised, edematous, doughnut-like border resulting in a bull's-eye appearance.
    b. multiple, small secondary annular lesions without indurated centers that occur anywhere except on the palms and soles.
    c. flulike symptoms of headache, malaise, fever, fatigue, and generalized lymphadenopathy.
    d. musculoskeletal pains, swelling, and effusion characterized by intermittent painful swollen joints and spontaneous remissions and exacerbations.

54. Susan, age 10 years, has been diagnosed with Lyme disease. She has no allergies to medications. The nurse can expect the treatment to be:
    a. erythromycin.
    b. cefuroxime.
    c. ciprofloxin.
    d. doxycycline.

55. Children with cat scratch disease usually are seen with:
    a. headache, diarrhea, and fever.
    b. regional lymphadenopathy.
    c. maculopapular rash over the entire body.
    d. painful, pruritic papules at the site of inoculation.

56. Which of the following statements about cat scratch disease is true?
    a. It is caused by the scratch or bite of an animal, usually a cat or kitten.
    b. The animal will have a history of illness before transmission of the disease.
    c. Antibiotics shorten the duration of the illness.
    d. Analgesics are avoided during the disease process.

57. Harry, age 16, has been diagnosed, by culture, as having recurrent methicillin-resistant *Staphylococcus aureus* (MRSA) sores on his face, neck, and arm. He is in for a follow-up visit and asks the nurse the following question. "Why do I keep getting these sores, and how can I keep them from coming back?" What should be included in the answer to each part of this question?

Jimmy is a 4-year-old preschool student who is brought to the school nurse's office by his teacher. She is concerned because Jimmy has purulent discharge in the corner of both eyes, with inflamed conjunctiva. The nurse observes Jimmy wiping his eyes frequently with his hands.

58. Based on the information provided, the nurse suspects that Jimmy has:
    a. bacterial conjunctivitis.
    b. viral conjunctivitis.
    c. allergic conjunctivitis.
    d. conjunctivitis caused by a foreign body.

59. Based on knowledge of communicable diseases, the nurse identifies which one of the following as the priority goal for Jimmy's plan of care?
    a. Patient will not become infected.
    b. Patient will not spread disease.
    c. Patient will experience minimal discomfort.
    d. Patient will maintain skin integrity.

60. The nurse calls Jimmy's parents to request that they come and pick Jimmy up from school. What is the best rationale for this action?
    a. Jimmy is tired and needs additional rest because of the infection.
    b. Jimmy is at high risk for spreading the disease because of his age and his inability to wash his hands after touching his eyes.
    c. Jimmy needs immediate medical attention to prevent complications.
    d. The nurse needs to discuss causes of this disease with Jimmy's mother so that its recurrence can be prevented.

61. It is important to include what information in the teaching plan for Jimmy's parents?
    a. Jimmy needs to have his own face cloth and towel.
    b. Eye medication will need to be administered before the eyes are cleaned.
    c. Jimmy cannot return to school until all symptoms have stopped.
    d. Jimmy will need his own eating utensils.

62. The nurse can expect treatment for Jimmy's condition to include:
    a. use of continuous warm compresses held in place on each infected eye.
    b. application of fluoroquinolone ophthalmic agents.
    c. oral broad-spectrum antibiotics.
    d. all of the above.

63. The effectiveness of nursing interventions for Jimmy's condition is best demonstrated by which one of the following evaluations?
    a. There is no spread of the disease within the school and family.
    b. Parents are able to demonstrate appropriate eye care.
    c. Jimmy reports no eye discomfort.
    d. Child engages in normal activities.

7 Health Promotion of the Newborn and Family

1. The three chemical factors in the blood that stimulate the initiation of the first respiration in the neonate are:

2. The primary thermal stimulus that helps initiate the first respiration is:

3. The nurse recognizes that tactile stimulation probably has some effect on initiation of respiration in the neonate. Which one of the following is of *no* beneficial effect?
   a. Normal handling of the neonate
   b. Drying the skin of the neonate
   c. Slapping the neonate's heel or buttocks
   d. Placing the infant skin-to-skin with the mother

4. Which one of these neonates will most likely need additional respiratory support at birth?
   a. The infant born by normal vaginal delivery
   b. The infant born by cesarean birth
   c. The infant born vaginally after 12 hours of labor
   d. The infant born with high levels of surfactant

5. During the transition from fetal to neonatal circulation, the newborn's cardiovascular system accomplishes which of the following anatomic and physiologic alterations?
   i. Closure of the ductus venosus
   ii. Closure of the foramen ovale
   iii. Closure of the ductus arteriosis
   iv. Increased systemic pressure and decreased pulmonary artery pressure

   a. i, ii, iii, and iv
   b. i, ii, and iii
   c. ii, iii, and iv
   d. i, iii, and iv

6. Identify the following statements about infant adjustments to extrauterine life as true or false.

   _____ Factors that predispose the neonate to excessive heat loss are large surface area, thin layer of subcutaneous fat, and the lack of shivering to produce heat.

   _____ Nonshivering thermogenesis is an effective method of heat production in the neonate, because it is able to produce heat with little use of oxygen.

   _____ Brown fat, or brown adipose tissue, has a greater capacity to produce heat than does ordinary adipose tissue.

   _____ The longer the infant is attached to the placenta, the less blood volume will be received by the neonate.

   _____ Deficient production of pancreatic amylase impairs utilization of complex carbohydrates.

   _____ Deficiency of pancreatic lipase assists the neonate in the digestion of cow's milk.

_____ Most salivary glands are functioning at birth even though most infants do not start drooling until teeth erupt.

_____ The stomach capacity varies in the first few days of life, from about 5 ml on day one to about 60 ml on day three.

_____ The newborn is expected to have the first void within the first 48 hours.

_____ The liver is the most mature of the gastrointestinal organs at birth.

_____ At birth the skeletal system contains larger amounts of ossified bone than cartilage.

_____ After birth, development of the nervous system proceeds in a cephalocaudal-proximodistal pattern.

7. What three factors make the infant more prone to problems of dehydration, acidosis, and overhydration?

8. Match each term with its description.

   a. Meconium
   b. Breast-fed infant stools
   c. Formula-fed infant stools

   _____ Pale yellow to golden; pasty consistency

   _____ First stool; dark green with pasty, sticky consistency

   _____ Pale yellow to light brown; firmer in consistency with more offensive odor

9. Newborns receive passive immunity in the form of immunoglobulin G from the _____
   _____ and _____ _____.

10. The nurse recognizes that all of the following effects of maternal sex hormones are normal *except*:
    a. hypertrophied labia.
    b. secretion of milk from the newborn breasts during the first 2 months of life.
    c. pseudomenstruation.
    d. bleeding from the breast nipples.

11. Fill in the blanks in the following statements pertaining to sensory functions in the normal newborn.

    a. The newborn can fixate on a bright object that is within _____ _____ and in the midline of the visual field.

    b. Infants have visual preferences for the colors _____, _____, and _____ and for
       designs such as _____ _____ and _____.

    c. The newborn's response to _____-frequency sounds is one of decreased motor activity and crying. The
       newborn's exposure to _____-frequency sound elicits an alerting reaction.

    d. Newborn visual acuity is reported to be between _____ and _____.

12. The nurse is performing the 5-minute Apgar on a newborn. Which one of the following observations is included in the Apgar score?
    a. Blood pressure
    b. Temperature
    c. Muscle tone
    d. Weight

13. Match each period of reactivity with the observations the nurse is likely to make during that period.

    a. First period of reactivity
    b. Second stage of first period of reactivity
    c. Second period of reactivity

    _____ This is an excellent bonding period and the best time to start breast-feeding.

    _____ During this period, infant sleep lasts 2 to 4 hours; heart rate and respiratory rate decrease.

    _____ Gastric and respiratory secretions are increased; passage of meconium commonly occurs.

14. The nurse is using the Brazelton Neonatal Behavioral Assessment Scale to assess the newborn's behavioral responses. How should the nurse define habituation?
    a. Responsiveness of the newborn to auditory and visual stimuli
    b. Process whereby the newborn becomes accustomed to stimuli
    c. The ability of the infant to be easily aroused from sleep state
    d. A reactive Moro reflex by the infant, with good muscle tone and coordination

15. Which of the following is *not* correct about the relationship of newborn weight to gestational age?
    a. All infants below the weight of 2500 g (5 lb, 8 oz) are preterm by gestational age.
    b. Gestational age is more closely related to fetal maturity than is birth weight.
    c. Classification of infants by both weight and gestational age can be beneficial for predicting mortality risks.
    d. Hereditary influences are a normal part of assessment.

16. On assessment of a 24-hour-old newborn, the nurse makes the following observations. Which is normal?
    a. Cyanotic color centrally and peripherally
    b. Axillary temperature of 35.5° C (96° F)
    c. Flexion of the infant's head and extremities, which rest on the chest and abdomen
    d. Respirations of 68 breaths/min

17. Which of the following statements regarding measuring temperature in pediatric patients is correct?
    a. Rectal temperature is taken in newborn infants because it is the most accurate.
    b. Axillary temperatures are taken in the newborn because insertion of a thermometer into the rectum can cause perforation of the mucosa.
    c. Skin temperature is slightly higher than core body temperature; therefore, rectal temperature is less than axillary temperature.
    d. Infrared ear thermometry is the most accurate method of taking temperature in newborn infants and children under 2 years of age.

18. Match each term with its description.

    a. Milia
    b. Erythema toxicum
    c. Harlequin color change
    d. Nevus flammeus
    e. Acrocyanosis

    f. Cutis marmorata
    g. Mongolian spots
    h. Nevus simplex
    i. Caput succedaneum
    j. Cephalhematoma

    k. Vernix caseosa
    l. Lanugo
    m. Capillary hemangiomas

    _____ Bright red, raised, soft, lobulated tumor occurring on the head, neck, trunk, or extremities; does not blanch with pressure

    _____ Irregular areas of deep blue pigmentation, usually in sacral and gluteal regions, seen in the newborn

    _____ Distended sebaceous glands that appear as tiny white papules on the cheeks, chin, and nose in the newborn

    _____ Condition in which the lower half of the body becomes pink and upper half is pale when the newborn lies on side

    _____ Edema of the soft scalp tissue

    _____ Pink papular rash with vesicles superimposed on thorax, back, buttocks, and abdomen in the newborn

_____ Port-wine stain

_____ Hematoma between periosteum and skull bone

_____ Cyanosis of hands and feet

_____ "Stork bites"; flat, deep pink, localized areas usually seen at back of neck

_____ Transient mottling when infant is exposed to decreased temperature, stress, or overstimulation

_____ Fine downy hair present on the newborn's skin

_____ Cheeselike substance; mixture of sebum and desquamating cells covering the skin at birth

19. Newborns lose up to 10% of their birth weight by 3 or 4 days of age. The factor that does *not* contribute to this process is:
    a. limited fluid intake in breast-fed infants.
    b. incomplete digestion of complex carbohydrates.
    c. loss of excessive extracellular fluid.
    d. passage of meconium.

20. When assessing blood pressure (BP) in the newborn, the nurse knows which of the following is true?
    a. BP is affected by gestational age and birth weight.
    b. Routine BP measurements of full-term neonates are an excellent predictor of hypertension.
    c. A normal BP reading for a 3-day-old infant is approximately 90/60.
    d. BP should be measured routinely on all healthy newborns as recommended by the American Academy of Pediatrics.

21. Which of the following is an abnormal finding when assessing the head of a newborn?
    a. Molding found in an infant after vaginal birth
    b. Inability to palpate the sphenoidal and mastoid fontanels
    c. Head lag and hyperextension when the infant is pulled into a semi-Fowler position
    d. Posterior fontanel palpated at about 2 to 3 cm

22. Assessment of the newborn includes which of the following?
    i. Clinical gestational age assessment
    ii. General measurements
    iii. General appearance
    iv. Head-to-toe assessment
    v. Parent-infant attachment

    a. i, ii, iii, iv, and v
    b. i, ii, iii, and iv
    c. ii, iii, iv, and v
    d. ii, iii, and iv

23. Which of the following observations from the eye assessment of a newborn is recognized as normal?
    a. Purulent discharge at age 48 hours
    b. Absence of the red reflex at age 24 hours
    c. No pupillary reflex at age 3 weeks
    d. Presence of strabismus at age 48 hours

24. a. How should the nurse assess auditory ability in the newborn?

    b. How can the nurse assess for hearing loss in the newborn?

25. It is important to assess for nasal patency in the newborn, because newborns are usually _____
_____ .

26. The nurse correctly identifies the need to notify the physician for which of the following neonates?
    a. The 24-hour-old neonate found to have Epstein pearls on the side of the hard palate
    b. The 2-day-old neonate with periodic breathing
    c. The 24-hour-old neonate who has nasal flaring
    d. The 2-hour-old neonate who has a bluish, white, moist umbilical cord with one vein and two arteries visible

27. Match each term with its description.

    a. Anal patency   e. Moro reflex
    b. Periodic breathing   f. Apnea
    c. Rooting reflex   g. Grasp reflex
    d. Babinski reflex   h. Lingual frenulum

    _____ Restriction can interfere with adequate sucking

    _____ Response in which touching cheek along the side of the mouth causes infant to turn head toward that side
              and begin to suck

    _____ Fanning of the toes and dorsiflexion of the great toe; disappears after 1 year of age

    _____ Symmetric abduction and extension of the arms; fingers fan out; thumb and index finger form a C

    _____ Passage of meconium from rectum during first 48 hours of life

    _____ Flexion caused by touching soles of feet near bases of digits or palms of hands

    _____ Rapid nonlabored respirations followed by pauses of less than 20 seconds

    _____ Period of no respiration for 20 seconds

28. Which of the following means of identification for the newborn is recommended by the National Center for Missing
    and Exploited Children (NCMEC)?
    a. Color photographs kept in the medical record
    b. Storage of blood for DNA genotyping
    c. Use of footprints and a cord blood sample that is kept until after the newborn is discharged
    d. Use of password system between the staff and parent when the newborn is taken from the room

29. Fill in the blanks in the following statements.
    a. The loss of heat to cooler solid objects in the environment that are not in direct contact with an infant is called

    _____ .

    b. Heat loss from the body through direct contact of the skin with a cooler solid object is termed _____ .

    c. Placing an infant in the direct flow of air from a fan causes rapid heat loss through _____ .

    d. Loss of heat through skin moisture is termed _____ .

30. The nurse implements all of the following actions to maintain a patent airway in a newborn. Which one will be *least*
    effective?
    a. Maintaining the infant in a supine position during sleep
    b. Performing oropharyngeal suctioning for 5 seconds with sufficient time between attempts to allow infant to
       reoxygenate
    c. In the delivery room, suctioning the infant's pharynx first, then the nasal passages
    d. Continuing oral feedings for the infant with nasal flaring and intercostal retractions

31. Identify the following medications to be given as preventive care.

a. _____ Prophylactic eye treatment against ophthalmia neonatorum

b. _____ Administered by injection to prevent hemorrhagic disease of the newborn

c. _____ First dose given between birth and 2 days of age to decrease incidence of hepatitis B

32. In screening for phenylketonuria, the nurse knows:
a. that blood samples should be taken after 24 hours of age and again at 2 weeks of age.
b. that blood should be drawn using a venous blood sample.
c. that preparation includes instructing parents to keep the infant NPO for 2 hours before the test.
d. to completely saturate the filter paper by applying blood to both sides of the paper.

33. The nurse should involve the parents in the care of their newborn. Teaching is *least* likely to include:
a. the use of Ivory soap, oils, powder, and lotions with each bath.
b. bathing the infant, using plain warm water, no more than two or three times per week during the first 2 to 4 weeks of age.
c. care of the umbilical stump, including placing the diaper below the cord to avoid irritation and wetness of the site.
d. care of the circumcision site, explaining that on the second day a yellowish white exudate forms normally as part of the granulation process.

34. Describe the current policy of the American Academy of Pediatrics on circumcision of newborn male infants.

35. Human milk is preferable to cow's milk because:
a. human milk has a nonlaxative effect.
b. human milk has more calories per ounce.
c. human milk has greater mineral content.
d. human milk offers greater immunologic benefits.

36. Cultural beliefs and practices are significant influences on infant feeding. Identify which one of the following statements is true.
a. Many cultures do not give colostrum to newborns but wait until the milk has "come in" to start breastfeeding.
b. U.S.-born Hispanic women are more likely to initiate breast-feeding than those recently immigrated.
c. Muslim women typically continue exclusive breastfeeding until late in infancy.
d. Jewish cultures place little value on breastfeeding their infants.

37. Contraindications to breastfeeding include which of the following?
a. Mothers who have received chemotherapy in the past
b. Mothers with active tuberculosis and who are undergoing treatment
c. Mothers living in the industrialized world who have HIV
d. Mothers with herpes simplex lesion on the mouth

38. The nurse is instructing new parents about proper feeding techniques for their newborn. Indicate whether the following statements are true or false.

_____ Infants need at least 2 hours of sucking daily.

_____ Galactosemia in the infant is a contraindication for breastfeeding.

_____ Breast-fed infants tend to be hungry every 2 to 3 hours.

_____ Using a microwave oven to defrost frozen human milk destroys the antiinfective factors and vitamin C content in the milk.

_____ Supplemental water is not needed in breast-fed infants, even in hot climates.

_____ Propping the bottle is discouraged because it facilitates the development of middle ear infections in the infant.

51

39. Mrs. Gonzalez is a first-time mother. She comes to the clinic because of painful nipples and is afraid she will have to terminate breastfeeding. The breast physical examination is normal. Which of the following actions does the nurse recognize as most likely causing the painful nipples?

    i. Using an electric pump to express milk for the infant to drink when Mrs. Gonzalez is away from home
    ii. Washing the nipples before and after each feeding with soap and applying aloe vera gel
    iii. Using plastic-backed nipple pads
    iv. Letting warm water flow directly over the breast in the shower
    v. Leaving breast milk on the areola after feedings and letting it dry
    vi. Letting the infant breast-feed every 2 hours

    a. i and v
    b. iv and v
    c. iii and vi
    d. ii and iii

40. Which one of the following actions by the nurse will *least* likely promote the attachment process between the infant and parent?
    a. Recognizing individual differences present in the infant and explaining these normal characteristics to the parent
    b. Helping the mother assume the en face position when she is presented with her infant
    c. Explaining to the parents how to respond to their infant with the use of reciprocal interacting
    d. Explaining to the parents the need for infants to have an organized schedule of daily activities that allows them to remain in their crib during awake periods

41. List the five behavioral stages that occur during successful feeding, and give an example of each.

CRITICAL THINKING—CASE STUDY

Michael was born by normal vaginal delivery to Marilyn and Doug Madison. Assessment at birth reflects the following: heart rate of 120 beats/min; respiratory effort good with a strong cry; well-flexed muscle tone with active movement and reflex irritability; turns head away when nose is suctioned; and color assessment of body pink with feet and hands blue. Michael's weight is 2700 g (6 lb), and his length is 53 cm (21 inches). Mrs. Madison is allowed to hold Michael and put him to breast in the delivery room. The Madisons do not plan to have Michael circumcised.

42. What is the Apgar score for Michael?
    a. 8
    b. 10
    c. 9
    d. 7

43. The nurse is conducting a gestational age assessment of Michael based on the six neuromuscular signs. What are these signs, and what results would indicate a higher maturity rating?

44. Listed below are nursing actions that the nurse would perform during the transitional period. Arrange these actions in order of highest to lowest priority.
    i. Taking head and chest circumference measurements
    ii. Assessing for neonatal distress
    iii. Administering prophylactic medications
    iv. Scoring for gestational age
    v. Assessing vital signs

    a. ii, v, i, iii, iv
    b. i, ii, v, iii, iv
    c. ii, iii, i, v, iv
    d. ii, v, iv, i, iii

45. Identify, in order of highest to lowest priority, four nursing goals that are considered the basics for safe and effective care of the newborn.

46. Mrs. Madison and Michael are being discharged tomorrow. You are preparing to provide Mrs. Madison with the newborn discharge teaching plan. Michael is Mrs. Madison's first infant, and on assessment you find that she has several questions about her techniques of breastfeeding. You show her how to hold Michael for feeding, how to position him properly to facilitate sucking, and how to care for her breasts. You also provide her with a video to reinforce your instruction. When you return later, Mrs. Madison asks you about the use of supplemental feedings. Which of the following is your best response?
    a. "It is okay to give Michael supplements but only after he is put to the breast."
    b. "Why would you think about that now? We'll discuss it tomorrow when you are ready to go home."
    c. "There is no need to give Michael supplemental feedings. Supplemental feeding may decrease your milk production."
    d. "You will need to give Michael supplemental feedings sometimes because you may not have enough milk."

47. You correctly evaluate the teaching plan you provided in question 46 as effective when:
    a. Mrs. Madison is discharged to take Michael home.
    b. Mrs. Madison explains to the nurse how to successfully breast-feed Michael.
    c. Mrs. Madison is seen by the nurse successfully breastfeeding Michael. Additionally, Mrs. Madison discusses with the nurse the information that the nurse had previously shared with her on breastfeeding.
    d. Mrs. Madison verbalizes that she has no further questions about breastfeeding and is able to describe to the nurse the teaching that had been provided.

48. Mrs. Madison and Michael are being discharged just 24 hours after birth. What should the nurse include in the early discharge newborn home care instructions for each of the following areas?
    a. Wet diapers:

    b. Stools:

    c. Activity:

    d. Cord:

    e. Position for sleep:

    f. Safe transport of the newborn home from the hospital:

49. Mrs. Madison is concerned because she thinks Michael is getting a cold. She tells you that he is "sneezing a lot." Your best response would be:
    a. "It is because the nose has been flattened while going through the birth canal. It will go away in another day or two."
    b. "Michael cannot get a cold; he is breastfeeding and this gives him a natural immunity."
    c. "Sneezing is abnormal, and you will need to watch Michael for fever development and decreased sucking."
    d. "Most newborns are obligatory nose breathers, and sneezing is very common."

50. You are a nurse assigned to the newborn nursery. While assessing a newborn, you see white patches on the inside of the mouth. How would you correctly determine whether this is a normal or abnormal finding?

51. A nursing assistant has been assigned to work with you in the newborn nursery. Summarize what you would tell him or her about each of the following issues.
    a. The most important way to prevent cross-infection:

    b. Handling newborn infants before the first bath:

54

Chapter **7 Health Promotion of the Newborn and Family**

8 Health Problems of Newborns

1. Match each term with its description or associated term.

   a. Cephalopelvic disproportion
   b. Crepitus
   c. Congenital hemangioma
   d. *Staphylococcus aureus*
   e. Icterus
   f. Hemolytic

   g. Phototherapy
   h. Bronze-baby syndrome
   i. Erythema toxicum neonatorum
   j. Vulnerable child syndrome
   k. Infantile hemangioma
   l. Port-wine stain

   m. Ecchymoses
   n. Craniosynostosis
   o. Teratogen
   p. Pierre Robin sequence

   _____ Causes impetigo

   _____ Small hemorrhagic areas that may occur on the infant after traumatic birth

   _____ Exposing the infant's skin to an appropriate light source

   _____ Agent that produces congenital malformations

   _____ Results in fetal head not being able to pass through the maternal pelvis

   _____ Rare reaction to phototherapy in which the serum, urine, and skin turn grayish brown

   _____ Associated with glaucoma

   _____ Fully formed at birth and may or may not involute over time

   _____ Defect characterized by retroposition of the tongue and mandible

   _____ Also known as flea bite dermatitis or newborn rash; benign, self-limiting eruption that usually appears within the first 2 days of life

   _____ Coarse, crackling sensation that can be produced by rubbing together fractured bone fragments

   _____ Vascular tumor that usually grows after birth

   _____ The parents' belief that their child has suffered a "close call" and is at risk for serious injury

   _____ Related to destruction of red blood cells

   _____ Premature closure at birth of one or more cranial sutures

   _____ Jaundice

2. Birth injuries may occur during the delivery of the infant. Birth injuries are not usually the result of:
   a. forceful extraction.
   b. dystocia.
   c. excess amniotic fluid.
   d. breech presentations.

3. Which one of the following birth injuries is most likely to need further evaluation?
   a. Subcutaneous fat necrosis
   b. Ecchymoses
   c. Petechiae
   d. Scleral hemorrhage

4. Nursing care for soft tissue injury is typically *not* directed toward:
   a. assessing the injury.
   b. preventing breakdown and infection.
   c. providing explanations and reassurance to the parents.
   d. explaining the need for careful follow-up of injury after the infant's discharge.

5. Match each type of extracranial hemorrhagic injury with its description.

   a. Caput succedaneum
   b. Subgaleal hemorrhage
   c. Cephalhematoma

   _____ Bleeding into the area between the periosteum and bone; does not cross the suture line

   _____ Bleeding into the potential space that contains loosely arranged connective tissue

   _____ Edematous tissue above the bone; extends across sutures

6. An infant suffers a fracture of the clavicle during birth. Which one of the following would the nurse expect to observe on the physical examination of this infant?
   a. Crepitus felt over the affected area
   b. Symmetric Moro reflex
   c. Complete fracture with overriding fragments
   d. Positive scarf sign

7. Match each type of paralysis with its correct description. (Types may be used more than once.)

   a. Facial paralysis
   b. Brachial palsy
   c. Phrenic nerve paralysis

   _____ Arm hangs limp, the shoulder and arm are adducted and internally rotated.

   _____ The eye cannot close completely on the affected side; the corner of the mouth droops, and an absence of forehead wrinkling occurs. This type of paralysis is caused by injury to cranial nerve VII.

   _____ This usually disappears spontaneously in a few days but may take several months.

   _____ This causes diaphragmatic paralysis, with respiratory distress as the most common sign of injury; injury is usually unilateral, with affected side of lung not expanding.

   _____ Nursing care includes maintaining proper positioning and preventing contractures.

   _____ Nursing care is aimed at aiding the infant in sucking and the mother with feeding techniques.

   _____ Nursing care is aimed at assisting the infant with respiratory complications.

   _____ Artificial tears are instilled to prevent drying.

8. Posterior fontanel is closed by age _____. Anterior fontanel is closed by age _____.

   Sutures are unable to be separated by intracranial pressure by age _____.

9. Identify the following statements about microcephaly as true or false.

   _____ Fetal alcohol exposure has not been shown to increase the risk for microcephaly.

   _____ Primary microcephaly can be caused by autosomal recessive disorder or a chromosome abnormality.

   _____ Secondary microcephaly can be caused by maternal infection or chemical agents.

   _____ All children with microcephaly have cognitive delays.

   _____ There is no treatment for microcephaly.

   _____ Nursing care is supportive and directed toward helping parents adjust to the infant.

10. Therapeutic management for craniosynostosis is:
    a. placement of ventriculoperitoneal shunt.
    b. removal of neoplasm.
    c. release of fused sutures.
    d. supportive assistance for parents.

11. Nursing care after surgery for the infant with craniosynostosis includes:
    a. careful monitoring of hematocrit and hemoglobin because of expected large blood loss during surgery.
    b. applying ice compresses for 5 minutes every hour because eyelids are often swollen shut.
    c. avoiding sedation and pain medications because neurologic status may be altered.
    d. avoiding supine positioning.

12. In preparing the nursing care plan for the infant born with craniofacial abnormalities, the nurse recognizes which of the following as true?
    a. Children with this deformity always have some cognitive impairment.
    b. Abnormalities include deformities involving the skull, facial bones, and neck.
    c. A helmet is often required after surgery to protect the operative site and bone grafts for 5 years.
    d. Surgical correction involves peeling the patient's face away from the skull and remolding the understructures.

13. An important assessment for the nurse to perform in identifying cleft palate is to:
    a. assess sucking ability of infant.
    b. assess color of lips.
    c. palpate the palate with a gloved finger.
    d. do all of the above.

14. Describe long-term problems often experienced by children with cleft lip or cleft palate.

15. Which feeding practices should be used for the infant with a cleft lip or palate?
    a. Use a large, hard nipple with a large hole.
    b. Use a normal nipple and position it sideways in the mouth.
    c. Use a special nipple, positioned so it is compressed by the infant's tongue and existing palate.
    d. Withhold breastfeeding until after surgical correction of the defect.

16. Which of the following is acceptable in providing postoperative care for the infant with a cleft lip or palate?
    a. Use of tongue depressor in the mouth to assess surgical site
    b. Continuous elbow restraints to prevent injury
    c. Placement of infant in the prone position after cleft lip repair
    d. Position the infant in a side-lying position after cleft palate repair

17. In preparing the parents of a child with cleft palate, the nurse includes which of the following in the long-term family teaching plan?
    a. Explanation that tooth development will be delayed
    b. Guidelines to use for speech development
    c. Use of decongestants and acetaminophen to care for frequent upper respiratory tract symptoms
    d. All of the above

18. The priority nursing goal in the immediate care of a postoperative infant after repair of a cleft lip is to:
    a. keep the infant well hydrated.
    b. prevent vomiting.
    c. prevent trauma to operative site.
    d. administer medications to prevent drooling.

19. Which of the following is *not* correct in describing erythema toxicum neonatorum?
    a. It is a benign, self-limiting rash that appears within the first 2 days of life.
    b. The rash is most obvious during crying episodes.
    c. The rash may be located on all areas of the body, including the soles of the feet and the palms of the hands.
    d. Lesions appear as 1- to 3-mm, white or pale yellow pustules with an erythematous base. Smears of the pustules show increased numbers of eosinophils and lowered numbers of neutrophils.

20. You are preparing to teach a class to new parents about candidiasis. Identify whether each of the following statements is true or false.

_____ Candidiasis is a yeastlike fungus that can be transmitted by maternal vaginal infection during delivery, through person-to-person contact, and from contaminated articles.

_____ In the neonate, candidiasis is usually found in the oral and diaper areas.

_____ It is difficult to distinguish between oral candidiasis and coagulated milk in the infant's mouth because both are easily removed by simple wiping.

_____ Thrush appears when the oral flora are altered as a result of antibiotic therapy or poor hand washing by the infant's caregiver.

_____ Oral candidiasis can be treated with the administration of oral nystatin four times a day, after feedings and at night.

_____ Candidiasis appears most often in the newborn's first week of life.

_____ It is not necessary to boil bottles or nipples for infants with oral candidiasis, since the fungus is heat resistant.

_____ Oral nystatin should be placed in the far back of the throat to allow the infant to swallow it easily.

_____ Oral nystatin should be administered before feedings to help the medication provide better coverage of the gastrointestinal lesions.

21. Which of the following statements regarding herpes simplex virus (HSV) is correct?
    a. Lesions take several weeks to ulcerate and crust over.
    b. The mother always has a history of symptoms of infection at the time of vaginal transmission.
    c. Approximately 86% to 90% of transmission occurs during delivery.
    d. It always manifests with some type of rash.

22. Which one of the following statements concerning impetigo is *not* correct and should be omitted by the nurse from the teaching plan?
    a. Impetigo is treated with oral antibiotics and topical application of mupirocin (Bactroban).
    b. Impetigo is an eruption of vesicular lesions that occurs on skin that has not been traumatized.
    c. Distribution of impetigo lesions usually occurs on the perineum, trunk, face, and buttocks.
    d. The infected child or infant must be isolated from others until all lesions have healed.

23. Identify the type of birthmark described by each of the following statements.

    a. _____ These lesions are pink, red, or purple and often thicken, darken, and proportionately enlarge as the child grows.

    b. _____ These are red, rubbery nodules with a rough surface that are recognized as tumors that involve only capillaries.

    c. _____ These are flat, light brown marks that are often associated with the autosomal dominant hereditary disorder neurofibromatosis.

    d. _____ These involve deeper vessels in the dermis and have a bluish-red color and poorly defined margins.

24. Treatment for port-wine stain includes laser therapy. The teaching plan for treatment expectations includes which of the following?
    a. The lesion will have a bright pink appearance for 10 days after treatment.
    b. Expose the infant to sunlight for 15 minutes daily after treatments.
    c. Administer salicylates before each treatment for pain.
    d. After treatment, gently wash the area with water and dab it dry.

25. _____ is an excessive accumulation of bilirubin in the blood and is characterized by

    _____, a yellow discoloration of the skin.

26. In discussing the pathophysiology of bilirubin, the nurse knows that red blood cell destruction results in

_____ and _____. _____ _____ is an

insoluble substance bound to albumin. In the liver this is changed to a soluble substance, _____

_____.

27. The term used to describe the yellow staining of the brain cells that can result in bilirubin encephalopathy is:
    a. jaundice.
    b. physiologic jaundice.
    c. kernicterus.
    d. icterus neonatorum.

28. Which one of the following statements about bilirubin encephalopathy is true?
    a. Development may be enhanced by metabolic acidosis, lowered albumin levels, intracranial infections, and increases in the metabolic demands for oxygen or glucose.
    b. It produces no permanent neurologic damage.
    c. Serum bilirubin levels alone can predict the risk for brain injury.
    d. It produces permanent liver damage by deposits of conjugated bilirubin within the cell.

29. A newborn develops hyperbilirubinemia at 48 hours of age. The condition peaks at 72 hours and declines at about age 7 days. The most likely cause of this hyperbilirubinemia is:
    a. physiologic jaundice.
    b. pathologic jaundice.
    c. hemolytic disease of the newborn.
    d. breast milk jaundice.

30. Of the four infants described below, which one should the nurse recognize as being least likely to develop jaundice?
    a. An infant with subgaleal hemorrhage that is now resolving
    b. An infant with cephalhematoma that is now resolving
    c. An infant who has feedings started early, which will stimulate peristalsis and rapid passage of meconium
    d. An infant who is of Native American descent

31. Which one of the following therapies should the nurse expect to implement for jaundice associated with breastfeeding?
    a. Increased frequency of breastfeedings
    b. Permanent discontinuation of breastfeedings
    c. Discontinuation of breastfeedings for 24 hours with the use of home phototherapy
    d. Increased frequency of breastfeedings and addition of caloric supplements

32. Newborns are more prone to produce higher levels of bilirubin because they:
    i. have higher concentrations of circulating erythrocytes.
    ii. have red blood cells with a shorter life span.
    iii. have reduced albumin concentrations.
    iv. have anatomically underdeveloped livers.

    a. i, ii, iii, and iv
    b. i, ii, and iii
    c. ii, iii, and iv
    d. iii and iv

33. Which one of the following is true regarding diagnostic evaluations for bilirubin?
    a. Newborn levels of unconjugated bilirubin must exceed 5 mg/dl before jaundice is observable.
    b. Hyperbilirubinemia is defined as a serum bilirubin value above 8 mg/dl in full-term infants.
    c. When jaundice occurs before 24 hours of age, bilirubin level assessment is unnecessary.
    d. Transcutaneous bilirubinometry is an effective cutaneous measurement of bilirubin in full-term infants being treated with phototherapy.

34. List the risk factors that place the term and late-term infant at high risk for pathologic hyperbilirubinemia.

35. Which of the following statements about phototherapy is *false*?
    a. For phototherapy to be effective, the infant's skin must be fully exposed to an adequate amount of light or irradiance.
    b. The initiation of phototherapy should always be based on clinical judgment rather than serum bilirubin levels alone.
    c. For best results, the goal of phototherapy is to increase irradiance to the 460-490 nm band.
    d. The color of the infant's skin influences the efficacy of phototherapy, with darker-skinned infants needing double or intensive therapy.

36. Implementation of phototherapy for an infant with jaundice does *not* include:
    a. shielding the infant's eyes with an opaque mask.
    b. recognizing that once phototherapy has been started, visual assessment of jaundice increases in validity; therefore fewer serum bilirubin levels will be necessary.
    c. repositioning the infant frequently to expose all body surfaces to the light.
    d. assessing the infant for side effects, including loose, greenish stools; skin rashes; hyperthermia; dehydration; and increased metabolic rates.

37. Intravenous immunoglobulin (IVIG) is effective in reducing bilirubin levels in infants:
    a. with Rh isoimmunization and ABO incompatibility.
    b. with breast-feed jaundice.
    c. who are late-term and term infants.
    d. when administered to the mother immediately before delivery.

38. Complete the following:
    a. Erythroblastosis fetalis is caused by _____ _____.
    b. Problems of Rh incompatibility may arise when the mother is _____ _____ and the infant is _____ _____. The most common blood group incompatibility in the neonate occurs when the mother has type _____ blood and the infant has either type _____ or type _____ blood.
    c. The nurse is reviewing maternal laboratory results. The nurse knows that the _____ _____ test monitors anti-Rh antibody titers. The test performed postnatally to detect antibodies attached to the circulating erythrocytes of affected infants is called the _____ _____ test.
    d. To be effective in preventing maternal sensitization to the Rh factor, the nurse must administer Rh immune globulin (RhoGam) to the Rh-negative mother within _____ _____ after the first delivery or abortion and with each subsequent pregnancy. To further decrease the risk for Rh alloimmunization, RhoGam is administered at _____ to _____ weeks of gestation. RhoGam is administered only to the mother by the _____ route.
    e. Exposure to Rh antigen with significant antibody formation occurring and causing a sensitivity response is known as _____.

39. Explain how the nurse is expected to assist the practitioner with a blood exchange transfusion in the newborn.

40. Which of the following statements about hypoglycemia in the newborn is true?
    a. Hypoglycemia is present when the newborn's blood glucose is lower than the baby's requirement for cellular energy and metabolism.
    b. In the healthy term infant who is born without complications, blood glucose is routinely monitored within 24 hours of birth to detect hypoglycemia.
    c. A plasma glucose level less than 60 mg/dl requires intervention in the term newborn.
    d. Pregnancy-induced hypertension and terbutaline administration have not been found to alter infant metabolism or increase the hypoglycemia risk in the newborn.

41. What assessment finding is the nurse most likely to see in the infant as a result of hypoglycemia?
    a. Forceful, low-pitched cry
    b. Tachypnea
    c. Jitteriness, tremors, twitching
    d. Vomiting, refusal to eat

42. Which of the following nursing interventions are recognized as appropriate for the infant with hypoglycemia?
    i. Institute early bottle-feeding or breastfeeding.
    ii. Increase environmental stimulants.
    iii. Protect from cold stress and respiratory difficulty that predispose the infant to decreased blood glucose levels.
    iv. Force early oral glucose feedings, avoiding formula and breast milk until the newborn is stable.

    a. i, ii, iii, and iv
    b. i and iii
    c. iii and iv
    d. i, ii, and iii

43. Full-term infants at risk for hypoglycemia shortly after birth include which of the following?
    i. Those born to diabetic mothers
    ii. Those who are small for gestational age
    iii. Those with perinatal hypoxia

    a. i, ii, and iii
    b. i and ii
    c. ii and iii
    d. i and iii

44. Bruce, a full-term newborn, has symptomatic hypoglycemia and inability to tolerate oral feedings. An intravenous glucose infusion has been ordered. Which of the following does the nurse recognize as correct?
    a. Too rapid infusion of the hypertonic solution can cause intracellular overload.
    b. An initial bolus infusion of 10% dextrose will be given over a 10-minute interval, followed by continuous dextrose infusion for 24 hours.
    c. The infusion is maintained at the ordered flow rate via an intravenous pump with hourly intake charting to decrease the risk of circulatory overload.
    d. Termination of the glucose solution should be rapid to prevent hyperinsulinism.

45. Hyperglycemia in the newborn is defined as a blood glucose concentration greater than _____ in the full-term infant and greater than _____ in the preterm infant.

46. Infants at risk for early-onset hypocalcemia include:
    a. postterm infants.
    b. infants who develop jaundice.
    c. infants born to hypertensive mothers.
    d. small-for-gestational-age infants who experience perinatal hypoxia.

47. The nurse caring for the infant who has hypocalcemia and is receiving intravenous calcium gluconate recognizes that which one of the following is included in the care plan?
    a. The scalp veins are the preferred site for intravenous administration of calcium gluconate.
    b. Signs of acute hypercalcemia include vomiting and bradycardia.
    c. Rapid infusion administration is best tolerated by the infant.
    d. Calcium gluconate is compatible with sodium bicarbonate.

48. The nurse is assessing Sarah, a neonate born at home, and observes slight blood oozing from the umbilicus. What is the most likely cause of Sarah's hemorrhagic disease?
    a. The neonate was born with an anatomically immature liver.
    b. Coagulation factors (II, VII, IX, X) are deactivated in the neonate.
    c. Vitamin K was administered to the neonate shortly after birth.
    d. The newborn was born with a sterile intestine and was unable to synthesize vitamin K until feedings began.

49. The goal is to prevent hemorrhagic disease in the newborn by prophylactic administration of vitamin K (AquaMEPHYTON). How does the nurse correctly administer this drug?

50. Which of the following has a teratogenic effect on the fetus?
    a. Folic acid
    b. X-rays taken of the pelvis and abdomen 1 week after menstruation
    c. Amoxicillin
    d. Valproic acid

CRITICAL THINKING—CASE STUDY

Mrs. Becker had a normal pregnancy and delivery without complications at 39 weeks of gestation.
She is breastfeeding her 2-day-old neonate, Ben, when she notices that Ben's skin looks yellow.
Tests reveal that Ben's total serum bilirubin level is 13 mg/dl.

51. Mrs. Becker asks the nurse about Ben's condition and the seriousness of his illness. Which one of the following is the best response?
    a. "Ben has pathologic jaundice, a serious condition."
    b. "Ben has breast milk jaundice, and you will need to stop breastfeeding."
    c. "Ben probably has physiologic jaundice, a normal finding at his age."
    d. "Infants with serum bilirubin levels of 13 mg/dl will develop bilirubin encephalopathy and severe brain damage."

52. The physician tells Mrs. Becker to increase her frequency of breastfeeding to every 2 hours and to avoid supplementation. The nurse is discussing the rationale for this management with Mrs. Becker. Which one of the following is the basis for the ordered treatment?
    a. The jaundice is related to the process of breastfeeding, probably from decreased caloric and fluid intake by breast-fed infants.
    b. The jaundice is caused by a factor in the breast milk that breaks down bilirubin to a lipid-soluble form, which is reabsorbed in the gut.
    c. The jaundice is caused by the mother's hemolytic disease.
    d. The jaundice is increased because the infant was put to breast early, which increases the amount of time meconium is kept in the gut before excretion.

53. Ben's serum bilirubin level has not decreased as the physician hoped, and phototherapy has been ordered. Which of the following is the priority goal at this time?
    a. The family will be prepared for home phototherapy.
    b. The infant will receive adequate intravenous hydration.
    c. The infant will experience no complications from phototherapy.
    d. The infant will have hourly bilirubin level testing completed.

54. When caring for Ben, the nurse should take all the following actions to prevent complications *except*:
    a. making certain that eyelids are closed before applying eye shields; checking eyes at least every 4 to 6 hours for discharge or irritation.
    b. monitoring axillary temperature closely to detect hyperthermia and/or hypothermia.
    c. maintaining an 18-inch distance between infant and light.
    d. applying oil daily to skin to avoid breakdown.

55. Which of the following is the best expected patient outcome for Ben while he is on phototherapy?
    a. Newborn begins feeding soon after birth.
    b. Family demonstrates an understanding of therapy and prognosis.
    c. Newborn displays no evidence of infection.
    d. Newborn displays no evidence of eye irritation, dehydration, temperature instability, or skin breakdown.

56. Accurate charting is an important nursing responsibility when caring for the newborn receiving phototherapy. What is included in the charting?

57. Once phototherapy is considered permanently completed, the nurse should expect what to occur in relation to the bilirubin level?

58. Ben's condition has improved, and the physician has ordered him off phototherapy and released him for discharge. What home care instructions should the nurse provide?

9 The High-Risk Newborn and Family

1. Provide the correct term for each of the following descriptions.
   a. An infant whose birth weight is less than 2500 g (5.5 lb), regardless of gestational age: _____-_____- _____ _____

   b. An infant whose birth weight is less than 1000 g (2.2 lb): _____ _____-_____ _____ _____

   c. An infant whose birth weight falls below the 10th percentile on intrauterine growth curves: _____- _____-_____-_____ _____

   d. An infant whose birth weight falls above the 90th percentile on intrauterine growth curves: _____- _____-_____-_____ _____

   e. An infant born before completion of 37 weeks of gestation: _____ _____

   f. An infant born between the 38th week and completion of the 42nd week of gestation: _____- _____ _____

   g. An infant born after 42 weeks of gestation: _____ _____

   h. Death of a fetus after 20 weeks of gestation: _____ _____

   i. Death that occurs in the first 27 days of life: _____ _____

   j. Describes the total number of fetal and early neonatal deaths per 1000 live births: _____ _____

   k. An infant born between 34⅟ and 36⅟ weeks of gestation, regardless of birth weight: _____- _____ _____

2. Which one of the following is *not* used as a category in the classification of high-risk newborns?
   a. Birth size
   b. Gestational age
   c. Mortality
   d. Birth age

3. Which of the following is a neonatal intensive care facility that provides care for extremely low-birth-weight infants plus offers extracorporeal membrane oxygenation and surgical repair of serious congenital cardiac malformations?
   a. Level I facility
   b. Level IIB facility
   c. Level IIIC facility
   d. Level IV facility

4. When a high-risk neonate needs transportation to a facility that can provide intensive care, the nurse recognizes that priority care for this neonate must include:
   a. transfer of both the mother and infant.
   b. immediate transport, often before stabilization of the neonate.
   c. complete life support system available during transport.
   d. prevention of transport delay by carrying the infant in the nurse's arms to the waiting transport vehicle.

5. A thorough, systematic physical assessment is a must in the care of the high-risk neonate. Subtle changes in

_____ _____, _____, _____,

_____ _____, or _____ _____ often indicate an under-lying problem.

6. At birth the newborn is immediately assessed to determine any apparent problems and to identify those that demand immediate attention. The assessment *not* usually conducted at birth or immediately after birth is:
   a. assignment of a gestational age score.
   b. assignment of an Apgar score.
   c. evaluation for obvious congenital anomalies.
   d. evaluation for neonatal distress.

7. Identify whether the following statements about care of the high-risk neonate are true or false.

   _____ Neonates under intensive observation are placed in a controlled environment and monitored for heart rate, respiratory activity, and temperature.

   _____ Sophisticated monitoring and life-support systems can replace the observations of the infant by nursing personnel.

   _____ When hydrogel electrodes are used on the neonate's skin, they are easily removed by lifting the edge and wiping with alcohol.

   _____ Infants who are mechanically ventilated and have low Apgar scores can have lower blood pressures.

   _____ An accurate output measurement can be obtained in the neonate by using a urine collecting bag or by weighing the infant's diaper (40-g weight of urine would be recorded as 40 ml of urine).

   _____ Studies have shown that infants receiving a heel puncture for blood collection demonstrated less pain response than those receiving a venipuncture.

   _____ Nurses are allowed to turn off alarm systems for electronic monitoring devices when their sounds disturb the infant's parents.

8. Identify the two most critical goals in caring for the high-risk infant.

9. The major source of increased production of heat during cold stress in the high-risk neonate is _____

_____.

10. Low-birth-weight infants are at a disadvantage for heat production when compared with full-term infants because they have:
    i. small muscle mass.
    ii. fewer deposits of brown fat.
    iii. less insulating subcutaneous fat.
    iv. poor reflex control of skin capillaries.

    a. i, ii, iii, and iv
    b. ii, iii, and iv
    c. i, ii, and iii
    d. i, iii, and iv

11. Identify three major consequences produced by cold stress that create additional hazards for the neonate.

12. Match each term with its description.

a. Thermal stability
b. Neutral thermal environment
c. Convective heat loss
d. Radiant heat loss
e. Conductive heat loss
f. Evaporative heat loss

_____ Capacity to balance heat production, heat conservation, and heat dissipation

_____ Allows one to maintain normal core temperature with minimal oxygen consumption and caloric use

_____ Occurs by transfer of body heat to a cooler solid object not in direct contact

_____ Occurs when infants are exposed to drafts or when surrounding air is cool

_____ Can be decreased by drying the neonate thoroughly with warm towels

_____ Loss of heat through direct contact with a cooler surface

13. Which of the following interventions is *least* likely to be effective for high-risk neonates?
   a. Keeping the infant on servocontrol in an incubator or radiant warmer
   b. Placing the heat-sensing probe on the infant's abdomen when the infant is in the prone position
   c. Ensuring that the oxygen supplied to the infant via a hood around the head is warmed and humidified
   d. Warming all items that come in direct contact with the infant, including the hands of caregivers

14. A primary objective in the care of high-risk infants is to maintain respiration. Describe how the nurse should complete the respiratory assessment.

15. The best way to prevent infection in the high-risk neonate begins with:
   a. meticulous and frequent hand washing of all persons coming in contact with the infant.
   b. observing continually for signs of infection.
   c. requiring everyone working in the neonatal intensive care unit (NICU) to put on fresh scrub clothes before entering the unit.
   d. performing epidemiologic studies at least monthly.

16. Baby girl Miller has been admitted to the NICU with low birth weight and possible infection. Parenteral fluids have been ordered for hydration and antibiotic administration.
   a. What are the preferred sites for peripheral intravenous (IV) infusions for this infant?

   b. The nurse starts a peripheral line and places the neonate on an infusion pump to regulate the rate of IV administration. Ten minutes later the nurse observes for signs of infiltration. What signs should the nurse be looking for?

17. A complication that develops with the use of the umbilical catheter is thrombi. This complication is best recognized by the appearance of:
   a. blanching of the buttocks and genitalia.
   b. bluish discoloration seen in the toes, called "cath toes."
   c. bounding pedal pulses.
   d. hemorrhage from the umbilical catheter area.

18. Introduction of minimal enteral feedings in the metabolically stable preterm infant:
   a. increases incidence of necrotizing enterocolitis.
   b. increases mucosal atrophy incidence.
   c. stimulates the infant's gastrointestinal tract.
   d. maintains serum glucose homeostasis.

19. Identify whether the following statements are true or false.

_____ Although infants demonstrate some sucking and swallowing activities before birth, coordination of these mechanisms does not occur until approximately 32 to 34 weeks of gestation, and they are not fully synchronized until 36 to 37 weeks.

_____ Research has shown that infants receiving trophic feedings versus no feedings have an overall higher number of days to full feedings and a longer hospital stay.

_____ Preterm infants receiving continuous feedings show better weight gain than those receiving intermittent bolus feedings.

_____ Milk produced by mothers of preterm infants changes in content over the first 30 days postnatally, until its content is similar to that of full-term human milk.

_____ Milk produced by mothers whose infants are born at term contains higher concentrations of protein, sodium chloride, and immunoglobulin A (IgA).

_____ Low-birth-weight infants (<1500 g) who are fed only human milk demonstrate decreased growth rates and nutritional deficiencies.

_____ Preterm infants who are fed fortified human milk have shorter hospital stays and less infection than infants given preterm formulas.

_____ Fortified human milk is mixed as close to feeding time as possible and stored in the refrigerator.

_____ IgA concentration is higher in the milk of mothers of term infants as compared with mothers of preterm infants.

_____ Pasteurization of donor human milk serves little purpose, since all donors are carefully screened.

_____ Preterm infants have the same capacity to digest and absorb protein, carbohydrates, and fats as full-term infants.

_____ The number of calories required for optimal growth in sick and very low-birth-weight infants is higher than for healthy infants.

_____ Studies have shown that preterm infants who received human milk during their hospitalization demonstrated better intellectual performance scores at 7½ to 8 years of age compared with children who received formula.

20. The amount to be fed to the infant by nipple is:
    a. determined by the infant's tolerance to previous feedings.
    b. increased when the infant requires 25 minutes or more for feeding completion.
    c. increased when the infant reaches the postnatal age of 34 weeks.
    d. increased when prodding techniques are used to increase sucking and decrease aspiration.

21. Feeding facilitation techniques for preterm infants include:
    a. using a pliable nipple with faster flow.
    b. using a slightly firm nipple with slow flow.
    c. manipulating the nipple frequently by twisting and turning when the infant stops sucking.
    d. positioning the infant on the back with the head supported.

22. What is the best measurement of feeding success in the infant?
    a. Soft abdomen
    b. No aspirated gastric residual
    c. Ability to suck on pacifier
    d. Coordinated sucking and swallowing ability

23. An infant who weighs 1400 g appears to be ready for enteral feedings. Which one of the following should the nurse include in the implementation of gavage feedings?
    a. Insert the tube into the unobstructed nares.
    b. Perform the procedure with the infant in a supine position with the head elevated 45 degrees.
    c. Aspirate the contents of the stomach, measure these contents, and replace the residual as part of the feeding.
    d. Allow the feeding to flow by gravity; then push a small amount of the feeding into the stomach; then allow the remainder of the feeding to flow by gravity.

24. _____ _____ decreases hospital stay, enhances transition from tube to bottle-feeding, and results in better bottle-feeding performance in preterm infants.

25. In caring for a preterm infant's skin, the nurse knows to:
    a. use scissors to remove dressings or tape from the infant's extremities.
    b. use solvents to remove tape from the neonate's skin.
    c. use alkaline-based soaps in removal of stool.
    d. use zinc oxide–based tape to secure monitoring equipment or intravenous infusions.

26. Which of the following is a correct nursing intervention to prevent skin damage in the neonate?
    a. Instruct parents before discharge on regular use of sunscreen for all infants under 6 months of age.
    b. Apply adhesive tape to protect arms, elbow, and knees from friction rubs.
    c. Use powders on diaper dermatitis areas as a moisture barrier.
    d. Use gel mattresses to decrease skin breakdown.

27. a. _____ _____, a common preservative in bacteriostatic water and saline, has been shown to be toxic to newborns and is not used to flush intravenous catheters or reconstitute medications.

    b. Oral or parenteral medications should be sufficiently diluted if they are _____ solutions to prevent necrotizing enterocolitis.

28. Identify the following as true or false.

    _____ Each infant is different; therefore supportive developmental care requires ongoing data collection by the nurse.

    _____ Developmentally supportive care uses both physiologic and behavioral information to evaluate the needs of the infant in an NICU setting.

    _____ Developmental maturation for the young preterm infant is seen by a decrease in quiet sleep.

    _____ Nursing care for the neonate should include modification of care to provide longer episodes of undisturbed sleep.

    _____ Prolonged "clustering" of care for the ill infant promotes physiologic stability.

    _____ The best time for care of an infant is when the infant is awake.

    _____ Containment or facilitated tucking positioning of the infant during procedures has been shown to increase physiologic and behavioral stressors.

    _____ Stroking a preterm infant who is not physiologically stable can result in distress, including oxygen desaturation.

    _____ Preterm infants are less responsive to visual stimulation and have less acuity and accommodation than full-term infants.

    _____ Therapeutic positioning for preterm and high-risk infants should provide support to maintain flexed and midline postures.

    _____ Using earmuffs in the NICU is an important intervention to prevent later speech and language difficulties.

    _____ Strong visual stimulation such as high-contrast black-and-white patterns can evoke an obligatory staring response by the immature infant, who is unable to break away from it.

29. The _____ sleeping position is recommended by the American Academy of Pediatrics for healthy infants in the first year of life as a preventive measure for sudden infant death syndrome.

30. Which of the following is the best way for the nurse to promote a healthy parent-infant relationship for the family with a high-risk neonate?
    a. Reinforce parents during their caregiving activities and interactions with their infant.
    b. Help parents understand that the preterm infant offers no behavioral rewards.
    c. Reassure parents that the infant is doing well.
    d. Encourage the mother to stay by the infant's bedside to promote bonding.

31. a. The term _____ _____ _____ is applied to physically healthy children who are perceived by parents to be at high risk for medical or developmental problems.

    b. The term _____ _____ is used when parents show hesitancy to embark on a relationship with their infant, unconsciously preparing themselves for the infant's death.

32. Discharge instructions for the parents of the preterm infant should *not* include:
    a. warning parents that their infant may still be in danger and will need constant attention.
    b. providing information to the parents on how to contact personnel for later questions.
    c. instructions about car safety seats, including how these seats can be adapted for smaller infants with the placement of blanket rolls on each side of the infant to support the head and trunk.
    d. providing adequate information about immunization needs.

33. To help parents deal with neonatal death, the nurse should:
    a. discourage the parents from staying with the infant before death to prevent overattachment.
    b. explain to the parents that the infant would have had many developmental problems and it is better that the infant did not suffer.
    c. give the parents the opportunity to hold and talk with the infant before and after death.
    d. force the parents to see the infant after death because closure is necessary.

34. A physical characteristic usually observed in the preterm infant and not observed in the full-term infant is:
    a. proportionately equal head in relation to the body.
    b. skin that is translucent, smooth, and shiny with small blood vessels clearly visible underneath the epidermis.
    c. distinct creases extending across the entire palms of the hands and down the soles of the feet.
    d. absence of lanugo and little vernix caseosa.

35. A cause of fetal and neonatal mortality in postterm infants as compared with term infants is:
    a. absence of lanugo.
    b. skin cracking, parchmentlike, and peeling.
    c. depletion of subcutaneous fat.
    d. macrosomia and meconium aspiration syndrome.

36. Apnea in the preterm infant is defined as a lapse of spontaneous breathing lasting for how many seconds?
    a. 5
    b. 10
    c. 15
    d. 20

37. Bryan, a 2-day-old preterm infant being cared for in the NICU, had some periods of apnea yesterday. Today when you arrive to work, you learn in report that the infant has had no further apneic episodes since yesterday. However, shortly after you begin your shift, Bryan's apnea monitor alarm sounds. What should you do first?
    a. Use tactile stimulation, rubbing on the infant's back to stop the apneic spell.
    b. Suction his nose and oropharynx.
    c. Assess the infant for color and for presence of respiration.
    d. Place the infant on his abdomen.

38. The preterm infant is having respirations with absence of diaphragmatic muscle function. This is causing a lack of respiratory effort because the central nervous system is not transmitting signals to the respiratory muscles. What is this type of apnea called?
   a. Obstructive apnea
   b. Central apnea
   c. Periodic apnea
   d. Mixed apnea

39. A late and serious sign of respiratory distress in the neonate is:
   a. central cyanosis.
   b. respiratory rate of 90 breaths/min.
   c. substernal retractions.
   d. nasal flaring.

40. Discuss the importance of surfactant to the preterm infant's lungs.

41. Match each term with its description.

   a. Pulmonary interstitial emphysema
   b. Lung compliance of distensibility
   c. Continuous positive airway pressure (CPAP)
   d. Intermittent mandatory ventilation (IMV)
   e. Positive end-expiratory pressure (PEEP)
   f. Nasal flaring

   g. Grunting
   h. Synchronized intermittent mandatory ventilation (SIMV)
   i. High-frequency ventilation (HFV) modalities
   j. Lecithin/sphingomyelin ratio

   _____ Method that infuses air or oxygen under a preset pressure by means of nasal prongs, a face mask, or an endotracheal tube

   _____ Perinatal diagnostic test for lung maturity

   _____ Method that allows infant to breathe spontaneously at his or her own rate but provides mechanical cycled respirations and pressure at regular preset intervals by means of an endotracheal tube and ventilator

   _____ Condition that develops in the preterm infant with respiratory distress syndrome and immature lungs as a result of overdistention of distal airways

   _____ Method that provides increased end-expiratory pressure during expiration and between mandatory breaths, preventing alveolar collapse

   _____ Lung distensibility

   _____ Abnormal sounds made on respiration as a result of increased effort required to fill the lungs; associated with atelectasis

   _____ Widening of the nostrils during inspiration; signals respiratory distress

   _____ Infant-triggered ventilator with signal detector and assist/control mode

   _____ Method that delivers gas at very rapid rates to provide adequate minute volumes using lower proximal airway pressures

42. The administration of exogenous surfactant to preterm neonates with respiratory distress syndrome:
   a. shows no difference in improvement when synthetic surfactant is used versus natural surfactant.
   b. is done by intravenous infusion.
   c. requires adjustment of ventilator settings.
   d. requires suctioning the infant during administration.

43. Suctioning of the infant with respiratory distress syndrome:
    a. is performed by applying intermittent suction as the catheter is withdrawn.
    b. is performed routinely every 30 minutes to keep the airway open.
    c. is performed by slowly and gently inserting the catheter.
    d. is performed by advancing the catheter until resistance is met and then withdrawing.

44. Susie, a neonate born 20 minutes ago, was observed at birth to have meconium staining. If Susie has meconium in the lungs, this most likely will:
    a. prevent air from entering the lungs.
    b. trap inspired air in the lungs.
    c. cause no problems with breathing.
    d. lead to respiratory alkalosis.

45. An important nursing function is close observation of neonates at risk for developing air leaks. These infants include:
    a. those with respiratory distress syndrome.
    b. those with meconium-stained amniotic fluid.
    c. those receiving continuous positive airway pressure (CPAP) or positive-pressure ventilation.
    d. all of the above.

46. Which of the following is a correct statement about persistent pulmonary hypertension of the newborn (PPHN)?
    a. PPHN is primarily a condition of preterm infants.
    b. PPHN is rarely associated with meconium aspiration.
    c. A loud pulmonary component of the second heart sound and often a systolic ejection murmur are present with PPHN.
    d. Vasodilators, such as tolazoline, are used to decrease cardiac output.

47. Infants diagnosed with bronchopulmonary dysplasia have special care needs. These needs include:
    a. adequate rest.
    b. avoiding diuretics.
    c. decreasing caloric intake.
    d. rapid weaning from ventilator.

48. Why are diagnosis and treatment of sepsis sometimes delayed in the neonate?

49. The laboratory evaluation for the diagnosis of sepsis is *least* likely to include:
    a. blood cultures.
    b. spinal fluid culture.
    c. urine culture.
    d. gastric secretions culture.

50. Clinical signs seen in necrotizing enterocolitis are:
    i. increased abdominal girth.
    ii. increased gastric residual.
    iii. positive stool hematest.
    iv. hypertension.

    a. i, ii, and iv
    b. i and iii
    c. ii, iii, and iv
    d. i, ii, and iii

51. Clinical manifestations of patent ductus arteriosus (PDA) include which of the following?
    a. Increased $Paco_2$, decreased Pao_2, and decreased Fio_2
    b. Narrow pulse pressure with increased diastolic blood pressure
    c. Systolic or continuous murmur heard as a "machinery-type" sound
    d. Bradycardia

71

Chapter **9** **The High-Risk Newborn and Family**

52. Therapy for preterm infants who develop PDA often includes the administration of:
    a. theophyllin.
    b. indomethacin.
    c. digoxin.
    d. heparin.

53. Why does the nurse carefully monitor and record amounts of all blood drawn for tests in the preterm infant?
    a. Early prevention of anemia
    b. Prevention of infection
    c. Prevention of polycythemia
    d. Detection of factors that contribute to hypothermia

54. Define polycythemia and identify the infants who are most at risk for this condition.

55. Retinopathy of prematurity nursing care management includes:
    a. decreasing or avoiding events known to cause fluctuations in systemic blood pressure and oxygenation.
    b. using cool compresses to decrease the edema of the eyelids after the infant undergoes laser surgery.
    c. delaying all eye medication administration until the eye edema has subsided and the infant can open his/her eyes.
    d. delay breastfeeding or bottle-feeding for 24 hours after laser eye surgery.

56. Brenda is a 1-hour-old newborn who suffered asphyxia before birth, resulting in hypoxic-ischemic brain injury. What signs can the nurse expect to see indicating encephalopathy?

57. Which of the following interventions is contraindicated in the preterm infant with increased intracranial pressure?
    a. Avoiding interventions that produce crying
    b. Avoiding rapid volume expansion following hypotension
    c. Administering analgesics to reduce discomfort
    d. Turning the head to the right without body alignment

58. _____, the most common type of intracranial hemorrhage, occurs in both term and preterm infants. Small hemorrhages of venous origin with underlying contusion may occur.
    a. Subdural hemorrhage
    b. Intracerebellar hemorrhage
    c. Subarachnoid hemorrhage
    d. Hematoma

59. Which one of the following statements about neonatal stroke is true?
    a. It is the number one leading cause of seizures in term neonates.
    b. It is more common in females, where there is a tendency toward left-sided involvement.
    c. Known risk factors include maternal and/or fetal factor V Leiden, antiphospholipid, and prothrombin factors.
    d. Diagnosis is most accurate with head ultrasonography.

60. The nurse must be able to distinguish between seizures and jitteriness in the neonate. Which of the following is true about seizures?
    a. Seizures are not accompanied by ocular movement.
    b. Seizures have their dominant movement as tremor.
    c. In seizures the dominant movement cannot be stopped by flexion of the affected limb.
    d. Seizures are highly sensitive to light manual stimulation.

61. John is a newborn just delivered of a diabetic mother. The nurse will watch John for signs that he is rapidly developing:
    a. hyperglycemia.
    b. hypoglycemia.
    c. failure of the pancreas.
    d. dehydration.

62. Infants born to drug-dependent mothers may exhibit all of the following clinical manifestations *except*:
    a. tremors and restlessness.
    b. frequent sneezing.
    c. coordinated suck and swallow reflex.
    d. high-pitched, shrill cry.

63. The nurse recognizes which of the following as true about the infant diagnosed with neonatal abstinence syndrome (NAS)?
    a. Methadone treatment by the mother will prevent withdrawal reaction in neonates.
    b. Meconium sampling for fetal drug exposure is less accurate than neonatal urine sampling because it does not take into account recent drug use by the mother.
    c. Mothers of NAS infants usually do not want the pregnancy or the infant.
    d. The most severe symptoms are observed in the infants of mothers who have taken large amounts of drugs over a long period.

64. Identify the following as true or false.

    _____ Methadone withdrawal in the fetus is less severe than heroin withdrawal.

    _____ The methadone-exposed fetus shows no signs of congenital anomalies.

    _____ The mother using methadone is not allowed to breastfeed her infant.

    _____ Infants exposed to methadone have a higher than normal incidence of sudden infant death syndrome.

    _____ Cocaine can affect fetal cardiac function and suppress fetal immune system.

    _____ Infants exposed to cocaine in utero demonstrate immediate untoward effects at birth.

    _____ A higher incidence of preterm delivery and placental abruption are associated with methamphetamine use during pregnancy.

    _____ Infants exposed to methamphetamine in utero have significantly smaller head circumferences and birth weights than those not exposed.

    _____ Marijuana is the most common illicit drug used by women of childbearing age in the United States.

    _____ Marijuana use during pregnancy can result in infants with larger head circumference and developmental delays.

    _____ Fetal alcohol syndrome is the leading cause of preventable cognitive impairment.

    _____ Fetal abnormalities are not related to the amount of the mother's alcohol intake but to the amount of alcohol consumed in excess of the liver's ability to detoxify it.

    _____ It is necessary for the woman wanting to become pregnant to understand that she should stop drinking 3 months before she plans to conceive.

65. The nurse can expect the infant with fetal alcohol syndrome to exhibit which of the following on assessment?
    a. Normal prenatal growth patterns
    b. Normal feeding patterns
    c. Thicker upper lip and longer palpebral fissures
    d. Irritability

66. When mothers smoke:
    a. their infants will have normal birth weights as long as the number of cigarettes smoked does not exceed one pack per day.
    b. their level of nicotine is higher than that of their newborn.
    c. their breast milk will not be affected.
    d. their rate of preterm births is increased.

67. TORCHS complex is a group of microbial agents that cause similar manifestations in the neonate. Identify what each letter stands for.

    T:

    O:

    R:

    C:

    H:

    S:

68. How can human immunodeficiency virus (HIV) be transmitted from the mother to the infant?

CRITICAL THINKING—CASE STUDIES

Baby Mark was born at 36 weeks of gestation and weighed 2300 g (5 lb) at birth. At 1 minute of age, his Apgar score was 5. Mark was suctioned, and oxygen administration was started. He responded with spontaneous respirations. You are the nurse who has been assigned to care for Mark in the special care nursery. His admission vital signs are heart rate 150 beats/min, respirations 56 breaths/min, and axillary temperature of 35.8° C (96.4° F). Mark is placed in a radiant warmer, and oxygen administration is continued by oxygen hood.

69. You would classify Baby Mark as a:
    i. full-term infant.
    ii. preterm infant.
    iii. low-birth-weight infant.
    iv. small-for-gestational-age infant.

    a. i and iv
    b. ii and iv
    c. ii and iii
    d. i and iii

70. You identify Mark as being at risk for developing respiratory distress syndrome based on his:
    i. gestational age.
    ii. low Apgar score.
    iii. hypothermia.
    iv. respiratory rate of 56 breaths/min.

    a. i, ii, iii, and iv
    b. i, ii, and iii
    c. ii, iii, and iv
    d. ii and iii

74

Chapter **9**   **The High-Risk Newborn and Family**

71. The nurse's plan for oxygen administration includes:
    a. frequent suctioning.
    b. frequent assessment to include unobstructed nares.
    c. nipple feeding with respiratory rates of 70 breaths/min and below.
    d. turning off monitor alarms to allow the neonate to rest.

72. Baby Mark's parents are visiting him for the first time. How can the nurse assist the parents in feeling more comfortable in the NICU atmosphere?
    a. Discourage questions of a technical nature.
    b. Tell the parents that Mark is going to be fine.
    c. Explain what is happening with Mark and why he is receiving this type of care.
    d. Leave the parents alone with the infant.

73. The nurse will develop a care plan for Mark that recognizes which of the following as the best expected outcome?
    a. Oxygen is administered correctly, and arterial blood gases are within normal limits.
    b. Monitor for changes in thermal environment.
    c. Record oxygen delivery rates every 2 hours.
    d. Assess respiratory status every hour.

74. Mark has had an apneic episode. What should the nurse include in the documentation of this episode?

    As a nurse in the NICU, you are assigned to care for an 1815-g (4-lb) preterm infant named Maria. In report you learn that Maria is still on gavage feedings and that tomorrow she is scheduled to begin bottle-feeding. If Maria tolerates her bottle-feedings well, she is scheduled to go home in a few days. You observe Maria closely for behaviors that indicate readiness for bottle-feedings.

75. Name the behaviors indicating readiness for bottle-feedings.

76. Describe how you as the nurse in the special care nursery should position Maria, the preterm infant.

10 Health Promotion of the Infant and Family

1. Match each psychosocial development term with its description.

a. Acquiring a sense of trust, overcoming a sense of mistrust
b. Primary narcissism
c. Grasping
d. Biting
e. Cognition
f. Sensorimotor phase

g. Separation
h. Object permanence
i. Symbols
j. Use of reflexes
k. Primary circular reactions
l. Secondary circular reactions
m. Imitation

n. Play
o. Affect
p. Secondary schemas
q. Reactive attachment disorder (RAD)
r. Solitary play
s. Weaning

_____ A stage of the sensorimotor period; lasts until 8 months of age; primary circular reactions are repeated and prolonged for the response that results; phase in which grasping and holding become shaking, banging, and pulling

_____ The phase with which the infant is concerned, according to Erikson

_____ Process of giving up one method of feeding for another; usually refers to relinquishing the breast or bottle for a cup

_____ Reaching out to others; initially reflexive; has powerful social meaning for the parents

_____ Total concern for oneself; at its height in the newborn

_____ The ability to know; most commonly explained by Piaget's theory of development

_____ Mental representations; a major intellectual achievement of the sensorimotor period

_____ Occurs in the second stage of infancy; infants learn they can hold onto what is their own and more fully control their environment; also brings internal relief from teething discomfort and a sense of power or control

_____ A crucial event in the sensorimotor phase, in which infants learn to detach themselves from other objects in the environment

_____ The term used by Piaget to describe the period from birth to 24 months

_____ Marks the beginning of the replacement of reflexive behavior with voluntary acts in the sensorimotor period; occurs from 1 to 4 months; sucking and grasping become deliberate acts to elicit certain responses

_____ The realization that objects that exit the visual field still exist; a major accomplishment for the infant in the sensorimotor phase

_____ Identifies the first stage of the sensorimotor period; the experience of perceiving patterns or ordering; provides a foundation of the subsequent stages

_____ Occurs during the fourth sensorimotor stage of Piaget; characterized by infants using previous behavior achievements as the foundation for adding new skills

_____ Human behavior that requires the differentiation of selected acts from several events; developed by infants in the second half of the first year

_____ The type of play that infants engage in; denotes one-sided play

_____ Activity in which infants take pleasure in performing acts after they have mastered them; consumes most of the infant's waking hours

_____ Outward manifestation of emotion and feeling; seen as infants begin to develop a sense of permanency

_____ A psychologic and developmental problem that stems from maladaptive or absent attachment between the infant and parent (or caregiver)

2. If the infant weighs 8 kg at age 5 months, about how many kilograms was his or her probable birth weight?
   a. 7.0
   b. 6.0
   c. 4.0
   d. 15.0

3. The nurse can expect an infant whose birth weight was 7 pounds to weigh _____ pounds by 12 months of age.
   a. 14 pounds
   b. 21 pounds
   c. 28 pounds
   d. 32 pounds

4. The infant's posterior fontanel usually closes by:
   a. 6 to 8 weeks.
   b. 3 to 6 months.
   c. 12 to 18 months.
   d. 9 to 12 months.

5. A 4-month-old infant who does not express vocalization such as cooing, gurgling, or laughing should be evaluated for:
   a. tongue-tie (ankyloglossia).
   b. hearing impairment.
   c. cleft palate.
   d. vocal cord paralysis.

6. Of the following characteristics of vision, the one that is developed at the earliest age is:
   a. binocularity.
   b. stereopsis.
   c. corneal reflex.
   d. convergence.

7. The characteristic of the respiratory system that predisposes the infant to middle ear infection is the:
   a. short, angled eustachian tube.
   b. short, straight eustachian tube.
   c. close proximity of the trachea to the bronchi.
   d. size of the lumen of the eustachian tube.

8. The nurse can expect that an infant will begin to respond discriminately to others, particularly the mother, and respond by crying, smiling, and vocalizing at about _____ months of age:
   a. 2
   b. 4
   c. 6
   d. 8

9. Of the following hematopoietic changes that occur in infancy, the one that is considered abnormal in the first 5 months of life is:
   a. low iron levels.
   b. physiologic anemia.
   c. presence of fetal hemoglobin.
   d. low hemoglobin level.

10. All of the following digestive processes are deficient in an infant until about 3 months *except*:
    a. amylase.
    b. lipase.
    c. saliva.
    d. trypsin.

11. The _____ is the most immature of all the gastrointestinal organs throughout infancy.
    a. large intestine
    b. pylorus
    c. liver
    d. lower esophageal sphincter

12. The purpose of nonnutritive sucking is to:
    a. satisfy the basic sucking urge.
    b. take in food.
    c. collect food and propel it into the esophagus.
    d. provide an efficient way to process fluids.

13. Which of the following is a characteristic of the somatic swallow reflex?
    a. The mandible does not thrust forward.
    b. The tongue remains in front of the central incisors.
    c. The tongue is concave and inclined against the palate.
    d. It is efficient for fluids but not for solids.

14. After birth, maximum levels of immunoglobulin A, D, and E in humans are:
    a. reached during infancy.
    b. attained in early childhood.
    c. transferred from the mother.
    d. reached before 9 months of age.

15. The infant is predisposed to a more rapid loss of total body fluid and dehydration because:
    a. of a high proportion of extracellular fluid.
    b. of a high proportion of intracellular fluid.
    c. total body water is at about 40%.
    d. extracellular fluid is 20% of the total.

16. Complete maturity of the kidneys occurs:
    a. at birth.
    b. by 6 months.
    c. by 1 year.
    d. by 24 months.

17. Separation anxiety begins between ages _____ and _____ months, when the infant progresses through the first stage of separation-individuation and begins to have some awareness of self and mother as separate beings.

18. The expected immaturity of the infant's functioning endocrine system will be demonstrated in the infant's:
    a. growth patterns.
    b. thyroid levels.
    c. homeostatic control.
    d. immunoglobulin levels.

19. Fine motor development is evaluated in the 10-month-old infant by observing the:
    a. ability to stack blocks.
    b. pincer grasp.
    c. righting reflexes.
    d. tonic neck reflex.

20. If parents are concerned about the fact that their 14-month-old infant is not walking, the nurse should evaluate the cephalocaudal gross motor skill patterns and particularly evaluate whether the infant:
    a. pulls up to furniture.
    b. uses a pincer grasp.
    c. transfers objects.
    d. has developed object permanence.

21. The factor that best determines the quality of the infant's formulation of trust is the:
    a. quality of the interpersonal relationship.
    b. degree of mothering skill.
    c. quantity of the mother's breast milk.
    d. length of suckling time.

22. According to Piaget's theory of cognitive development, the three crucial events of the sensorimotor phase are:
    a. trust, readjustment, and the regulation of frustration.
    b. separation, object permanence, and mental representation.
    c. imitation, personality development, and temperament.
    d. ordering, comfort, and satisfaction with his or her body.

23. The development of gender identity is reported to begin:
    a. after the first year.
    b. during the phallic stage.
    c. in utero.
    d. at puberty.

24. Separation anxiety and stranger fear normally begin to appear by:
    a. 4 weeks.
    b. 6 months.
    c. 8 months.
    d. 12 months.

25. A formerly maltreated child who manifests behaviors such as limited eye contact and poor impulse control may be suffering from:
    a. separation anxiety.
    b. stranger fear.
    c. reactive attachment disorder.
    d. spoiled child syndrome.

26. Which of the following play activities would be *least* appropriate to suggest to parents for their 3-month-old infant?
    a. Provide bright objects.
    b. Use rattles.
    c. Place in an infant walker.
    d. Place infant on floor to crawl and roll.

27. Limit-setting and discipline should begin in:
    a. middle childhood or adolescence.
    b. infancy, with voice tone and eye contact.
    c. early infancy, with voice tone and eye contact.
    d. infancy, with time-out in a chair for misbehavior.

28. In guiding parents who are choosing a daycare center, the nurse should stress that state licensure represents a program that maintains:
    a. optimal care.
    b. health features.
    c. minimum requirements.
    d. safety features.

29. A 12-month-old infant would be likely to have:
    a. 2 teeth.
    b. 4 teeth.
    c. 6 teeth.
    d. 12 teeth.

30. Which one of the following techniques is recommended to assist in weaning an infant?
    a. Gradually replace one bottle-feeding or breastfeeding at a time.
    b. Always wean to a bottle first.
    c. Always wean directly to a cup.
    d. Eliminate the nighttime feeding first.

31. In order to prevent rickets, the mother who is exclusively breastfeeding should consider the administration of:
    a. iron.
    b. calcium.
    c. vitamin E.
    d. vitamin D.

32. A recent survey of breastfeeding mothers identified causes for the mother stopping breastfeeding before 6 months. Which of the following was *not* a cause for stopping breastfeeding?
    a. Concern about infant weight gain
    b. Difficulties with lactation
    c. Effort to pump and maintain milk supply
    d. Infant refusing to nurse

33. The primary reason for introducing solid food to infants is to:
    a. increase their overall caloric intake.
    b. provide a substitute for the milk source.
    c. introduce a taste and chewing experience.
    d. increase their weight.

34. Studies have shown that excessive fruit juice consumption in infants and small children increases the risk for:
    a. hypervitaminosis.
    b. fluorosis.
    c. rickets.
    d. growth problems.

35. When introducing new food, the parents should *not*:
    a. decrease the quantity of the infant's milk.
    b. mix food with formula to feed through a nipple.
    c. introduce new foods in small amounts.
    d. offer the new food by itself at first.

36. According to recent studies, the best place for the infant car restraint is in the:
    a. back seat of the car, facing the rear.
    b. back seat of the car, facing front.
    c. front passenger seat of the car with an air bag, facing front.
    d. front passenger seat of the car without an air bag, facing back.

37. Which of the following infant traits is most likely to contribute to shaken baby syndrome (traumatic brain injury)?
    a. laughing out loud
    b. crying
    c. soiling the diaper
    d. pulling up to furniture

38. Identify the three leading causes of accidental injury in infants.

39. List three infant care practices that contribute to the development of early childhood caries.

40. Indicate whether each of the following statements is true or false.

   a. _____ Iron-fortified rice cereal is recommended as the infant's first solid food.

   b. _____ Pasteurized whole cow's milk is an acceptable alternative to breastfeeding in a 6-month-old infant.

   c. _____ The American Academy of Pediatric Dentistry recommends fluoride supplementation in infants beginning at 6 months of age.

   d. _____ The American Academy of Pediatrics recommends that infants be started on solid foods beginning between 4 and 6 months of age.

CRITICAL THINKING—CASE STUDY

Jennifer, a 4-month-old infant, is admitted to the pediatric unit with bronchiolitis. Both of the parents work, and Jennifer attends daycare. Jennifer is the first child, and the parents seem quite anxious about the admission, as well as about her care at home and her normal development. Jennifer's mother tells the nurse caring for her that they feel inadequate as parents and need information about general health promotion for their infant.

41. Place a check next to each of the following areas that should be assessed to determine the status of the parents' current health promotion practices. (Check all that apply.)

   _____ Respiratory status (lung sounds)

   _____ Nutrition

   _____ Fever patterns

   _____ Sleep and activity

   _____ Number and condition of teeth

   _____ Fluid and hydration status

   _____ Condition of the mucous membranes of the mouth

   _____ Immunization status

   _____ Safety precautions used in the home

42. Which of the following nursing diagnoses would be used most often for health promotion related to development in an infant Jennifer's age?
   a. Activity Intolerance
   b. Ineffective Thermoregulation
   c. High Risk for Injury
   d. Altered Parenting

43. Of the following strategies, the one used most often to help new parents like Jennifer's adjust to the parenting role is:
   a. parenting classes.
   b. anticipatory guidance.
   c. first aid courses.
   d. cardiopulmonary resuscitation courses.

11 Health Problems of the Infant

1. The following terms are related to nutritional disturbances and feeding difficulties. Match each term with its description.

   a. Atopy
   b. Lactase
   c. Congenital lactase deficiency
   d. Sensitization
   e. Primary lactase deficiency
   f. Diarrhea

   g. Food intolerance
   h. Late-onset lactase deficiency
   i. Food allergy
   j. Oral allergy syndrome
   k. Allergens

   _____ Allergy with a hereditary tendency

   _____ Condition in which a food or food component elicits a reproducible adverse reaction but does not have an established or likely immunologic mechanism

   _____ A major factor in malnutrition in many developing and underdeveloped nations

   _____ Hypersensitivity; refers to those reactions to food that involve immunologic mechanisms, usually immunoglobulin E (IgE)

   _____ Lactose intolerance that occurs when the intestinal lumen is damaged, causing a decrease in or destruction of the enzyme lactase

   _____ Occurs when a food allergen (commonly fruits and vegetables) is ingested and subsequent edema and pruritus develop, involving the lips, tongue, palate, and throat; recovery from symptoms usually is rapid

   _____ An enzyme needed for the digestion of lactose in the small intestine

   _____ Usually involve proteins capable of inducing IgE antibody formation

   _____ The initial exposure of an individual to an allergen, resulting in an immune response, after which subsequent exposure induces a much stronger response that is clinically apparent

   _____ A rare disorder that appears soon after the infant has consumed lactose-containing milk; an inborn error of metabolism that involves the complete absence or severely reduced presence of lactase

   _____ The most common type of lactose intolerance; manifested at around 3 to 7 years of age; more common in Asians, southern Europeans, Arabs, Israelis, and African-Americans; characterized by abdominal pain, bloating, flatulence, and diarrhea that occur 30 minutes to several hours after lactose consumption

2. Identify 4 populations at risk for vitamin D deficiency or rickets.

   a.

   b.

   c.

   d.

3. Which of the following vitamins when taken in excess would be most likely to cause problems for the infant or child?
   a. Folate
   b. Vitamin A
   c. Biotin
   d. Vitamin C

4. Vitamin A deficiency has been reported with increased morbidity and mortality in children:
   a. with sickle cell disease.
   b. exposed to environmental tobacco smoke.
   c. with measles.
   d. who are breast-fed.

5. The greatest concern with minerals is:
   a. deficiency.
   b. excess, causing toxicity.
   c. nervous system disturbances from excess.
   d. hemochromatosis.

6. An imbalance in the intake of calcium and phosphorus may occur in infants who are fed _____ instead of infant formula.

7. Which of the following vitamin supplements is recommended for all women of childbearing age to prevent neural tube defects?
   a. Vitamin D
   b. Vitamin B_{12}
   c. Folic acid
   d. Vitamin K

8. The Whole Cows Milk _____ standardized growth reference charts are now recommended for all children from birth to 24 months; they are based on the growth of healthy breast-fed infants throughout the first year of life.

9. A 6-month-old infant who is being exclusively breast-fed (no solid foods are being given) should optimally receive a daily supplement of:
   a. iron
   b. folic acid
   c. vitamin A
   d. vitamin B_{12}

10. In the United States, severe acute malnutrition (SAM) may occur where:
    a. the food supply is inadequate.
    b. the food supply may be adequate.
    c. the adults eat first, leaving insufficient food for children.
    d. the diet consists mainly of starch grains.

11. Kwashiorkor occurs in populations where:
    a. the food supply is inadequate.
    b. the food supply is adequate for protein.
    c. the adults eat first, leaving insufficient food for children.
    d. the diet consists mainly of starch grains.

12. Childhood nutritional marasmus usually results in populations where:
    a. the food supply is inadequate.
    b. the food supply is adequate for protein.
    c. the adults eat first, leaving insufficient food for children.
    d. the diet consists mainly of starch grains.

13. Kwashiorkor, SAM, and marasmus would be *least* likely to be managed by:
    a. providing a high-protein, high-carbohydrate diet.
    b. replacing fluids and electrolytes.
    c. providing a high-fiber, high-fat diet.
    d. providing for essential physiologic needs.

14. Which of the following would be considered the *least* allergenic?
    a. Orange juice
    b. Eggs
    c. Bread
    d. Rice

15. Sensitivity to cow's milk in an infant may be manifested clinically by:
    a. irritability.
    b. excessive crying.
    c. vomiting and diarrhea.
    d. all of the above.

16. Which one of the following diagnostic strategies is the most definitive for identifying a milk allergy?
    a. Stool analysis for blood
    b. Serum IgE levels
    c. Challenge testing with milk
    d. Skin testing

17. The American Academy of Pediatrics recommends treating cow's milk allergy in infants by changing the formula to:
    a. soy formula.
    b. goat's milk.
    c. hydrolysate formula.
    d. milk pretreated with microbial-derived lactase.

18. Which of the following is a less expensive alternative to hydrolyzed formulas and may be recommended by health care providers for cow's milk allergy?
    a. Yogurt
    b. Soy formula
    c. Amino acid formula
    d. Goat's milk

19. Congenital lactase deficiency is:
    a. a rare form of lactose intolerance.
    b. the form of lactose intolerance associated with giardiasis.
    c. an intolerance that is manifested later in life.
    d. a form of lactose intolerance caused by intestinal damage.

20. Late-onset lactase deficiency is also known as:
    a. congenital lactase deficiency.
    b. secondary lactase deficiency.
    c. primary lactase deficiency.
    d. congenital lactose intolerance.

21. One strategy for parents of infants with lactase deficiency would be to:
    a. substitute human milk for cow's milk.
    b. substitute a low-lactose or lactose-free formula for human milk.
    c. drink milk alone without other food or drink.
    d. substitute frozen yogurt for fresh yogurt.

22. If cow's milk intolerance is suspected as the cause of an infant's colic, the parents should:
    a. try substituting hydrolysate formula.
    b. try substituting soy formula.
    c. be reassured that the symptoms will disappear spontaneously at about 3 months of age.
    d. be assessed for areas of improper feeding techniques.

23. Which one of the following factors is *not* considered to be a possible etiology for colic?
    a. Lactase deficiency
    b. Excessive air swallowing
    c. Gastroesophageal reflux
    d. Infant temperament
    e. Maternal depression

24. Other terms for failure to thrive include:
    a. growth failure and pediatric undernutrition.
    b. growth failure and organic failure to thrive.
    c. pediatric undernutrition and nonorganic failure to thrive.
    d. organic failure to thrive and nonorganic failure to thrive.

25. List five etiologic factors associated with growth failure.

26. Which of the following categories of failure to thrive is based on pathophysiology rather than etiology?
    a. Growth failure related to inadequate caloric intake
    b. Growth failure related to inadequate absorption
    c. Growth failure related to increased metabolism
    d. All of the above.

27. If failure to thrive has been a longstanding problem, the infant will show evidence of:
    a. both weight and height being decreased.
    b. weight restriction only.
    c. height restriction only.
    d. increased head circumference.

28. One important strategy for feeding a child with failure to thrive would be to:
    a. avoid having the same nurse feed the child.
    b. distract the child during meals with television and toys.
    c. maintain a calm, even temperament during feedings.
    d. vary the feeding routines to make the feeding time more interesting.

29. To increase the caloric intake of an infant with failure to thrive, the nurse might recommend:
    a. using developmental stimulation by a specialist during feedings.
    b. avoiding solids until after the bottle is well accepted.
    c. restricting juice intake.
    d. varying the schedule for routine activities on a daily basis.

30. The three factors that are known to cause diaper dermatitis are:

31. Parents of an infant with diaper dermatitis are encouraged to:
    a. wash the skin frequently.
    b. mix zinc oxide thoroughly with antifungal cream.
    c. use a hand-held dryer on the open lesions.
    d. allow the excoriated area to air dry as much as possible.

32. Seborrheic dermatitis is usually manifested primarily in:
    a. infants.
    b. toddlers.
    c. adults.
    d. children with atopy.

33. List the 4 major goals in the management of atopic dermatitis.

34. Identify the following statements as true or false.

_____ The incidence of sudden infant death syndrome (SIDS) is associated with diphtheria, tetanus, and pertussis vaccines.

_____ Maternal smoking during and after pregnancy has been implicated as a contributor to SIDS.

_____ Parents should be advised to place infants on their side to sleep prevent SIDS.

_____ The nurse should encourage the parents to sleep in the same bed as the infant who is being monitored for apnea of infancy in order to detect subtle clinical changes.

_____ Parents should avoid using soft, moldable mattresses and pillows in the bed to prevent SIDS.

35. The condition that often occurs when an infant is placed supine which results in an oblique or asymmetric head is:
   a. microcephaly
   b. cranisosynostosis
   c. hydrocephaly
   d. positional plagiocephaly

36. List 4 modifiable risk factors that are associated with an increase in the incidence of SIDS.

37. List 4 factors that place infants at an increased risk for SIDS.

38. Which of the following is *not* considered a characteristic associated with ALTE?
   a. Apnea
   b. Cyanosis
   c. Coughing
   d. Hypotonia
   e. Acrocyanosis

39. Which of the following may be used to treat positional plagiocephaly in the first few months of life?
   a. Serial casting
   b. Molded helmet
   c. Pavlik harness
   d. Ventricular shunting

40. Identify 2 important nursing interventions to help parents of an infant with colic.

41. Which of the following strategies are effective in helping an infant sleep well at night?
   i. Place infant to sleep in its own bed.
   ii. Give the infant a bottle if it awakes during the night.
   iii. Establish and enforce a bedtime routine.
   iv. Allow the infant to watch a movie before bedtime.
   v. Allow the crying infant to sleep with parents or sibling.
   vi. Avoid picking up and rocking the infant who awakens during the night.

   a. i, iii, and vi
   b. ii, iii, and v
   c. ii, iii, and vi
   d. i, ii, and vi

CRITICAL THINKING—CASE STUDY

Six-month-old Jason has come to the office today for his routine immunizations. His mother says she thinks everything is just fine, except that Jason seems to have a lot of food intolerances. The nurse continues the assessment and finds that Jason is eating many of the food items the rest of the family eats, including milk products in very small amounts. There is no particular pattern to the way the new foods are being introduced. Jason exhibits a variety of symptoms related to skin irritations. He is developing rashes around his mouth and rectum and elsewhere on his body when he eats certain foods.

42. Based on the prevalence of the common health problems of infancy, what areas should the nurse include in an initial assessment of a 6-month-old?
   a. Nutrition
   b. Temperament
   c. Sleep patterns
   d. All of the above

43. Based on the data from the assessment interview, which one of the following goals is best for the nurse to establish?
   a. To prevent outbreaks of food allergy
   b. To prevent death from anaphylaxis
   c. To prevent genetic transmission
   d. All of the above

44. Which one of the following recommendations would be most appropriate for Jason's mother?
   a. Reconsider breastfeeding.
   b. Eliminate cow's milk.
   c. Avoid adding new foods at same time.
   d. Eliminate solids until 9 months of age.

45. At an earlier visit with Jason's family, the nurse had determined that there was Altered Parenting related to lack of knowledge. Which one of the following outcome criteria would help the nurse evaluate the mother's ability to provide a constructive environment for Jason?
   a. Jason's mother is able to identify eating patterns that contribute to symptoms.
   b. Jason's mother is able to share her feelings regarding her parenting skills.
   c. Jason's mother is able to practice appropriate precautions to prevent infection.
   d. Jason's mother is able to identify the rationale for prevention of the skin rashes.

12 Health Promotion of the Toddler and Family

1. Match each term with its description.

   a. Regression
   b. Tertiary circular reactions
   c. Sibling rivalry
   d. Ritualism
   e. Parallel play
   f. Autonomy versus doubt and shame
   g. Negativism
   h. Separation
   i. Egocentrism

   j. Domestic mimicry
   k. Individuation
   l. Preoperational phase
   m. Inventions of new means through mental combinations
   n. Egocentric speech
   o. Preoperational thinking
   p. Socialized speech

   _____ Imitation of household activity

   _____ The persistent negative response to requests; characteristic of the toddler's behavior

   _____ The developmental task of the toddler years

   _____ The toddler's need to maintain sameness and reliability; provides a sense of comfort

   _____ The fifth stage of the sensorimotor phase of development, when the child uses active experimentation to achieve previously unattainable goals

   _____ The final sensorimotor stage that occurs during ages 19 to 24 months

   _____ The inability to envision situations from perspectives other than one's own

   _____ Consists of repeating words and sounds for the pleasure of hearing oneself and is not intended to communicate

   _____ Spans ages 2 to 7 years; characterized by egocentrism, transductive reasoning, magical thinking, and inability to conserve

   _____ Those achievements that mark children's assumption of their individual characteristics in the environment

   _____ The child's emergence from a symbiotic fusion with the mother

   _____ Playing alongside, not with, other children

   _____ The natural jealousy and resentment of children to a new child in the family

   _____ Implies that children think primarily based on their own perception of an event; phase in which problem solving is based on what children see or hear directly, rather than on what they recall about objects and events

   _____ A retreat from a present pattern of functioning to past levels of behavior; usually occurs in instances of stress, when the child attempts to cope by reverting to patterns of behavior that were successful in earlier stages of development; common in toddlers

   _____ One of the two types of speech used by children in the toddler years; used for communication; egocentric in that children communicate about themselves to others

2. The toddler years cover the period from _____ to _____ months of age.

3. By the age of two years, most toddlers demonstrate increased gross motor skills by:
   a. jumping using both feet.
   b. walking up and down stairs.
   c. running and skipping on alternate feet.
   d. jumping from a height of 3 feet without falling.

4. Which of the following characteristics most likely predisposes toddlers to frequent infections?
   a. Short straight internal ear canal and enlarged lymph tissue
   b. Slower pulse and respiratory rate and higher blood pressure
   c. Abdominal respirations
   d. Less efficient defense mechanisms

5. One of the most important digestive system changes completed during the toddler period is the:
   a. increased acidity of the gastric contents.
   b. voluntary control of the sphincters.
   c. protective function of the gastric contents.
   d. increased capacity of the stomach.

6. Which one of the following statements is most characteristic of a 24-month-old child in regard to motor development?
   a. Motor skills are fully developed but occur in isolation from the environment.
   b. The toddler walks alone, but falls easily.
   c. The toddler's activities begin to produce purposeful results.
   d. The toddler is able to grasp small objects, but cannot release them at will.

7. Using Erikson's theory as a foundation, the primary developmental task of the toddler period is to:
   a. satisfy the need for basic trust.
   b. achieve a sense of accomplishment.
   c. learn to give up dependence for independence.
   d. acquire language or mental symbolism.

8. Piaget's theory of cognitive development depicts the toddler as a child who:
   a. repeatedly explores the same object each time it appears in a new place.
   b. is able to transfer information from one situation to another.
   c. has a persistent negative response to any request.
   d. has the rudimentary beginning of a superego.

9. The principal characteristics of Piaget's preoperational phase are:
       i. dependence on perception in problem solving.
      ii. egocentric use of language.
     iii. the ability to manipulate objects in relation to one another in a logical manner.
      iv. the ability to problem solve based on what is recalled about objects and events.

   a. i, ii, and iii
   b. i and ii
   c. ii and iii
   d. ii, iii, and iv

10. According to Kohlberg, the best way to discipline children is to:
    a. use a punishment and obedience orientation.
    b. withhold privileges.
    c. use power to control behavior.
    d. give explanations and help the child to change.

11. By the age of 3, the toddler generally:
    a. has clear body boundaries.
    b. participates willingly in most procedures.
    c. has a sense of maleness or femaleness.
    d. is unable to learn correct terms for body parts.

12. Which of the following skills is *not* necessary for the toddler to acquire before separation and individuation can be achieved?
    a. Object permanence
    b. Lack of anxiety during separations from parents
    c. Delayed gratification
    d. Ability to tolerate a moderate amount of frustration

13. The typical number of words acquired by the age of 2 years is:
    a. 50.
    b. 100.
    c. 300.
    d. 500.

14. One recommended method to foster language development in the toddler is to:
    a. read books together.
    b. watch an educational program on the television.
    c. increase the toddler's exposure to a large number of adults and older children.
    d. Encourage the toddler to watch at least 2 hours of children's television shows per day.

15. As the child moves through the toddler period, there is a decrease in the frequency of:
    a. solitary play.
    b. imitative play.
    c. tactile play.
    d. parallel play.

16. List at least five characteristics in a toddler that would indicate readiness for toilet training.

17. Of the following techniques, which is the best to use when toilet training a toddler?
    a. Limit sessions to 5 to 8 minutes of practice.
    b. Remove child from the bathroom to flush the toilet.
    c. Ensure the toddler's privacy during the sessions.
    d. Place potty chair near a television to help distract the child during the sessions.

18. Which one of the following statements is *false* in regard to toilet training?
    a. Bowel training is usually accomplished after bladder training.
    b. Nighttime bladder training is usually accomplished after bowel training.
    c. The toddler who is impatient with soiled diapers is demonstrating readiness for toilet training.
    d. Fewer wet diapers signal that the toddler is physically ready for toilet training.

19. Of the following strategies, which is most appropriate for parents to use to prepare a toddler for the birth of a sibling?
    a. Explain the upcoming birth as early in the pregnancy as possible.
    b. Move the toddler to his or her own new room.
    c. Provide a doll for the toddler to imitate parenting.
    d. Tell the toddler that a new playmate will come home soon.

20. The best approach toward tapering temper tantrums requires _____ and developmentally appropriate expectations and rewards.

21. The best approach to stop a toddler's attention-seeking behavior of a temper tantrum with head banging is to:
    a. ignore the behavior.
    b. provide time-out.
    c. offer a toy to calm the child.
    d. protect the child from injury.

22. Of the following techniques, which is the best one to deal with the negativism of the toddler?
    a. Quietly and calmly ask the child to comply.
    b. Provide few or no choices for the child.
    c. Provide acceptable choices.
    d. Remain serious and intent.

23. Which of the following statements about stress in toddlers is true?
    a. Toddlers are rarely exposed to stress or the results of stress.
    b. Any stress is destructive because toddlers have a limited ability to cope.
    c. Most children are exposed to a stress-free environment.
    d. Small amounts of stress help toddlers develop effective coping skills.

24. Regression in toddlers occurs when there is:
    a. stress.
    b. a threat to their autonomy.
    c. a need to revert to dependency.
    d. all the above.

25. Which of the following statements is true in regard to nutritional changes from the infant to the toddler years?
    a. Growth rate increases.
    b. Caloric requirements decrease.
    c. Protein requirements are minimal.
    d. Fluid requirements increase.

26. Which nutritional requirement may be difficult to meet in the toddler years?
    a. Calories
    b. Proteins
    c. Minerals
    d. Fluids

27. Physiologic anorexia in toddlers is characterized by:
    a. strong taste preferences.
    b. extreme changes in appetite from day to day.
    c. heightened awareness of social aspects of meals.
    d. all of the above.

28. Healthy ways of serving food to toddlers include:
    a. establishing a pattern of sitting at a table for meals.
    b. permitting nutritious nibbling in lieu of meals.
    c. discouraging between-meal snacking.
    d. allowing the toddler to choose preferred foods at every meal.

29. Developmentally by 12 months of age most children:
    a. use a spoon adeptly.
    b. relinquish the bottle voluntarily.
    c. eat the same food as the rest of the family.
    d. reject all solid food in preference for the bottle.

30. Adequate intakes (AIs), a category of the Dietary Reference Intakes, are based on nutrient intake of:
    a. preterm breast-fed infants.
    b. preterm bottle-fed infants.
    c. full-term breast-fed infants.
    d. full-term bottle-fed infants.

31. The toddler's decreased nutritional requirements are manifested in a phenomenon known as _____ _____.

32. Briefly describe the role of ritualism in relation to feeding behaviors in toddlers.

33. Serving size may affect toddler feeding habits. What would be an appropriate feeding serving size of a vegetable for a 3-year-old?

    _____

34. The main source of calcium and phosphorus in a toddler is _____, which should optimally average _____ to _____ oz per day.

35. Studies in adults, which presumably may apply to children as well, indicate that benefits of an adequate intake of dietary fiber:
    i. decrease constipation
    ii. increase body weight
    iii. decrease body weight
    iv. prevent type 2 diabetes mellitus
    v. prevent type 1 diabetes mellitus

    a. i, iii, and iv
    b. i, iii, and v
    c. ii and iv
    d. iii, iv, and v

36. Children on strict vegetarian and macrobiotic diets should be evaluated for:
    a. constipation and heart disease
    b. rickets and iron-deficiency anemia
    c. scurvy
    d. severe acute malnutrition

37. Which of the following is *not* considered a complementary and alternative medicine therapy?
    a. Multivitamin
    b. St. John's wort (herb)
    c. Massage therapy
    d. Probiotic

38. Which of the following would be an *inappropriate* method to help a toddler adjust to the initial dental checkup?
    a. Explain to the child that a checkup will not hurt.
    b. Have the child observe his or her sibling's examination.
    c. Have the child perform a checkup on a doll.
    d. Ask the dentist to reserve a thorough examination for another visit.

39. Flossing is necessary:
    a. to remove plaque from below the gum margin.
    b. to remove debris from between the teeth.
    c. to reach areas where brushing is ineffective.
    d. All of the above

40. Adequate fluoride ingestion in children:
    a. prevents gingivitis.
    b. prevents fluorosis.
    c. helps retain enamel protein.
    d. reduces the amount of plaque.

41. To prevent fluorosis, parents of toddlers should use all of the following strategies *except*:
    a. supervise the use of toothpaste.
    b. use fluoride mouthrinses.
    c. store fluoride products out of reach.
    d. administer fluoride supplements on an empty stomach.

42. Early childhood caries may result from:
    a. using a pacifier coated with honey.
    b. feeding the last bottle just before bedtime.
    c. long, frequent nocturnal breastfeeding.
    d. all of the above.

43. _____ _____ injuries cause more accidental deaths in all pediatric age-groups than any other type of injury.

44. Studies indicate that toddlers up to 24 months of age are safest when they are:
    a. placed in a car restraint seat in the front seat of the car.
    b. placed in a car restraint seat facing the rear in the back seat.
    c. placed in a front passenger seat with a deactivated airbag.
    d. allowed to stand in the back seat holding on to a shoulder belt.

45. In 2014, NHTSA made a recommendation to use the lap-shoulder seat restraint instead of the LATCH system if the child's and restraint seat's combined weight is more than _____ pounds.

46. One of the best ways to prevent drowning in the toddler group is for parents to:
    a. learn cardiopulmonary resuscitation (CPR).
    b. supervise children within arm's reach whenever they are near any source of water.
    c. enroll the toddler in a swimming program.
    d. not allow the child to swim.

47. Burn injuries in the toddler age-group are most often the result of:
    a. flame burns from playing with matches.
    b. scald burn from hot liquids.
    c. hot object burns from cigarettes or irons.
    d. electric burns from electrical outlets.

48. Accidental poisonings in toddlers can be best prevented by:
    a. consistently using safety caps.
    b. storing poisonous substances in a locked cabinet.
    c. keeping ipecac syrup in the home.
    d. storing poisonous substances out of reach.

49. For each of the following potentially hazardous categories, give an example of an item that could cause aspiration or suffocation in the toddler (e.g., foods: hard candy).

    Foods:

    Play objects:

    Common household objects:

    Electrical items:

Tasha Jackson is a 14-month-old infant who is visiting the clinic for her well-baby checkup. Tasha's mother, Dora, is expecting her second child in 3 months. Dora works full time and will be home for 6 weeks with the new baby. Tasha has been in daycare since she was a baby. Dora's husband also works full time during the day.

50. List four areas that the nurse should assess to obtain the information necessary to adequately provide anticipatory guidance for a toddler Tasha's age.

51. The most appropriate initial nursing intervention would be to:
    a. allow Mrs. Jackson to express her feelings.
    b. provide Mrs. Jackson advice about daycare.
    c. provide Mrs. Jackson advice about sibling rivalry.
    d. evaluate Mrs. Jackson's knowledge about growth, development, and behavior in toddlers

52. Dora Jackson shares with the nurse that she is concerned about toilet training Tasha before bringing the new baby home. List major points to discuss with Dora about toilet training Tasha and the birth of a new sibling.

53. Ms. Jackson also tells the nurse in a side comment that Tasha has become a very picky eater and Dora is concerned that she has lost some weight. How should the nurse address these concerns?

13 Health Promotion of the Preschooler and Family

1. The approximate age range for the preschool period begins at age _____ years and ends at age _____ years.

2. The average annual weight gain during the preschool years is _____ to _____ kg, or _____ to _____ lb.

3. Which one the following statements about the preschooler's physical proportions is true?
   a. Preschoolers have a squat and potbellied frame.
   b. Preschoolers have a slender but sturdy frame.
   c. The muscle and bones of the preschooler have matured.
   d. Sexual characteristics can be differentiated in the preschooler.

4. By _____ years of age, the child skips on alternate feet, jumps rope, and begins to skate and swim.

5. According to Erikson, the chief psychosocial task of the preschool period is acquiring a sense of _____

   and overcoming a sense of _____.

6. Uninhibited scribbling and drawing can help the child to develop:
   a. symbolic language.
   b. fine muscle skills.
   c. eye-hand coordination.
   d. all of the above.

7. The resolution of the Oedipus/Electra complex occurs when the child:
   a. identifies with the same-sex parent.
   b. realizes that the same-sex parent is more powerful.
   c. wishes that the same-sex parent were dead.
   d. notices physical sexual differences.

8. Because of the preschooler's egocentric thought, the best approach for effective communication is through:
   a. speech.
   b. play.
   c. drawing.
   d. actions.

9. Magical thinking, according to Piaget, is the belief that:
   a. events have cause and effect.
   b. God is an imaginary friend.
   c. thoughts are all-powerful.
   d. if the skin is broken, the child's insides will come out.

10. The moral and spiritual development of the preschooler is characterized by:
    a. concern for why something is wrong.
    b. actions that are directed toward satisfying the needs of others.
    c. thoughts of loyalty and gratitude.
    d. a very concrete sense of justice.

11. The preschooler's body image has developed to include:
    a. a well-defined body boundary.
    b. knowledge about his or her internal anatomy.
    c. fear of intrusive experiences.
    d. anxiety and fear of separation.

12. Sex typing involves the process by which the preschooler develops:
    a. a strong attachment to the same-sex parent.
    b. an identification with the opposite-sex parent.
    c. behavior and beliefs for his or her culture and sex.
    d. all of the above.

13. The average child can be expected to have a vocabulary of more than _____ words by the age of 6 years.

14. Language during the preschool years:
    a. includes telegraphic speech.
    b. is simple and concrete.
    c. uses phrases, not sentences.
    d. includes the ability to follow complex commands.

15. Research has shown that when two languages are presented to children simultaneously in early childhood, bilingual children are most likely to experience:
    a. adverse effects in their receptive language development.
    b. adverse effects in performance in the majority language.
    c. language milestones at similar stages to monolinguals.
    d. adverse effects to areas in addition to language.

16. Which one of the following statements about social development of the preschooler is *false*?
    a. Imaginary playmates are a normal part of the preschooler's play.
    b. Preschoolers have overcome much of their anxiety regarding strangers.
    c. Preschoolers use telegraphic speech between the ages of 3 and 4 years.
    d. Preschoolers particularly enjoy parallel play.

17. In regard to the development of temperament in the preschool years:
    a. temperamental characteristics change considerably during the preschool years.
    b. the effect of temperament on adjustment in a group becomes important during the preschool years.
    c. children need to be treated the same regardless of differences in temperament.
    d. there really is no tool that will adequately identify temperamental characteristics during the preschool years.

18. List at least two strategies parents may use to help their child prepare for the preschool or kindergarten experience.

19. Identify three functions served by imaginary playmates.

20. To guide parents in their quest to find a school with comprehensive services, the nurse should advise the parent to:
    a. find a school that focuses primarily on skill acquisition.
    b. visit the schools to observe their services personally.
    c. select a licensed program to ensure the highest standard.
    d. do all of the above.

21. The best way for parents to respond to a child's questions about sexuality is to give the child:
    a. an honest answer and find out what the child thinks.
    b. one or two sentences that answer specific questions only.
    c. an honest, short, and to-the-point answer.
    d. an honest answer but a little less information than the child expects.

22. Which of the following characteristics is *not* typically seen in a gifted or talented child?
    a. Asynchrony across developmental domains
    b. Insatiable curiosity
    c. Less need for attention than other children
    d. Intensity of feelings and emotions

23. Which one of the following factors influences aggressive behavior?
    a. Frustration
    b. Modeling
    c. Gender
    d. All of the above

24. Which one of the following dysfunctional speech patterns is a normal characteristic of the language development of a preschooler?
    a. Lisp
    b. Stuttering
    c. Nystagmus
    d. Echolalia

25. Which one of the following sources of stress is typical of a 3-year-old?
    a. Insecurity
    b. Masturbation
    c. Jealousy
    d. Sexuality

26. Briefly define the concept of animism.

27. What are some of the most common fears of preschoolers? (list 6)

28. Which one of the following examples would best help a preschooler dispel his or her fear of the water when learning to swim?
    a. Fear of the water is a healthy fear. It should not be dispelled.
    b. Allow the child to sit by the water with other children, play with water toys, and get splashed lightly with the water.
    c. Reassure the child as he or she is brought slowly into the water with an adult who knows how to swim.
    d. Throw the child in the water and have an adult keep the child's head above water.

29. When educating the preschool child about injury prevention, the parents' emphasis should be on:
    a. setting a good example.
    b. helping children establish basic safety habits.
    c. protection and education for injury prevention.
    d. all of the above.

30. In comparison to the nutritional requirements for toddlers, preschoolers' caloric requirements:
    a. increase slightly.
    b. decrease slightly.
    c. remain the same.

31. One way to decrease total fat intake in the preschooler is to:
   a. drink less milk.
   b. eat fewer quantities of dairy products.
   c. substitute for low-fat food sources.
   d. consume more fruit juice.

CRITICAL THINKING—CASE STUDY

Sheila Roth arrives at the office for a routine preschool physical. Her son Jacob, who is almost 3 years old, will attend the 3-year-old preschool program at a local private school this year. Since he was a baby, Jacob has attended a home daycare program, while his mother managed her own interior decorating business. The daycare where Jacob will attend is run by an older woman who treats the 12 children in her program as if they were family. The helper at the daycare also seems very loving. The program is highly structured in regard to schedule and usual routines. Ms. Roth tells the nurse that she is looking forward to Jacob's new environment. His teacher is very creative and approaches the classroom from the perspective of the child's development. There will be a lot of choices for activities during the day.

32. Based on the information provided, which of the following is the best analysis?
   a. Jacob needs some preparation for this new preschool experience.
   b. Jacob will have less trouble adjusting than a child who has never attended daycare.
   c. Jacob is too young for such a drastic change.
   d. Jacob needs the individual attention he is getting at the daycare.

33. Which one of the following expected outcomes would be most reasonable to establish?
   a. The nurse will help Ms. Roth assess Jacob's readiness for preschool.
   b. Jacob will attend preschool without any behavioral indications of stress.
   c. Ms. Roth will verbalize at least five strategies that can be used to help prepare Jacob for his preschool experience.
   d. Jacob will demonstrate behavior that indicates that he is adjusting to his preschool experience.

34. Which one of the following interventions would be inappropriate for the nurse to suggest?
   a. Introduce Jacob to the teacher.
   b. Leave quickly the first day.
   c. Talk about the new school as exciting.
   d. Be confident the first day.

35. Which of the following characteristics would indicate that Jacob is ready for preschool?
   a. Social maturity
   b. Good attention span
   c. Academic readiness
   d. All of the above

14 Health Problems of Early Childhood

1. Which one of the following does *not* contribute to sleep disturbances during preschool years?
   a. Evening media use
   b. Inconsistent bedtime routines
   c. Limit setting
   d. Nighttime fears

2. Janie, age 3 years, has inadequate sleep patterns. The nurse, in preparing the care plan, recognizes seven consequences associated with inadequate sleep. List them.
   - daytime tiredness
   - hyperactivity
   - behavior changes
   - difficulty concentrating
   - impaired learning ability
   - poor control of emotions/impulses
   - strain on fam. relationships

3. The nurse has conducted an assessment of the sleep patterns of Janie and found that Janie delays going to bed each night. Which of the following interventions does the nurse recognize as *least* helpful?
   a. Consistent bedtime ritual, like reading a book before bedtime
   b. Not allowing the child to stay up past a reasonable hour
   c. Keeping a light on in the room
   d. Taking the child into the parents' bed

4. Match each term with its description. Terms are used more than once.

   a. Nightmares
   b. Sleep terrors

   ___A___ A scary dream taking place during REM (rapid-eye-movement) sleep

   ___B___ A partial arousal from very deep REM sleep

   _B_ _B_ Usually occurs after 1 to 4 hours after falling asleep

   ___A___ Crying in younger children and fright in all children; behaviors persistent when child is awake

   ___A___ Return to sleep may be considerably delayed because of persistent fear

   ___B___ Return to sleep usually rapid, often difficult to keep child awake

   ___B___ Initially may sit up, thrash, or run in bizarre manner, scream, talk, show anger or obvious confusion, which disappears when child is fully awake

5. Reduction of poisonings in children and infants can be accomplished by:
   a. use of child-resistant containers.
   b. educating parents and grandparents to place products out of reach of small children.
   c. educating parents to relocate plants out of reach of infants, toddlers, and small children.
   d. all of the above.

6. Ingestion of injurious agents by children:
   a. occurs most frequently at grandparents' or friend's home.
   b. occurs because infants and toddlers explore their environment through oral experimentation.
   c. has increased despite the use of child-resistant containers.
   d. can be avoided by teaching preschoolers which substances are dangerous.

7. The first action parents should be taught to initiate in a poisoning is to:
   a. induce vomiting.
   b. take the child to the family physician's office or emergency center.
   c. call the poison control center.
   d. follow the instructions on the label of the product.

8. Gastric lavage for pediatric poison ingestions:
   a. can be associated with serious complications of gastrointestinal perforation, hypoxia, and aspiration.
   b. is recommended in the emergency department for all cases of ingestion.
   c. has been proven to decrease morbidity.
   d. is most useful when the child comes to the emergency department within 3 hours of ingestion of the toxin.

9. Identify the general guidelines for emergency treatment of poisoning.
   - assess victim
   - stop exposure to poison
   - identify poison
   - call poison control
   - call doctor / seek ER treatment

10. Which of the following statements about ipecac use for poisonous substance ingestion is true?
    a. Ipecac helps to absorb the toxin.
    b. Ipecac is no longer recommended for routine home treatment of poisoning.
    c. Ipecac is useful when a corrosive substance has been ingested.
    d. Ipecac is useful when an overdose of a calcium channel blocker has been ingested.

11. Which one of the following actions taken by the nurse is *least* likely to prevent recurrence of poisonings?
    a. In the emergency department, begin a discussion of ways to injury-proof the home.
    b. Do a home visit to assess safety before the child is discharged.
    c. Administer questionnaire for poison prevention to the parents when the child is discharged.
    d. Advise parents to kneel down to the child's level when determining what products need to be placed out of reach.

12. The nurse expects to assist with administration of a specific antidote for poisoning in which one of the following pediatric patients?
    a. The 8-month-old child admitted to the emergency department after eating 8 or 10 holly berries
    b. The 13-year-old girl who ingested an overdose of diazepam (Valium)
    c. The 8-year-old child who ingested three of his mother's birth control pills
    d. The 6-year-old child who ingested an overdose of an unidentified corrosive substance

13. Activated charcoal:
    a. is odorless, tasteless, and delivered with fewer complications via gastric lavage.
    b. stimulates the gastric mucosa.
    c. is often mixed with diet soda and served through a straw from an opaque container.
    d. has a bitter taste.

14. Potential causes of heavy metal poisoning in children include lead , mercury , and iron .

15. The nurse, while conducting a home visit, finds that the mother of 4-year-old Nathan is using a mercury thermometer to take his axillary temperature. Which one of the following is the best intervention for the nurse at this time?
    a. Tell the mother to stop using mercury thermometers because if the mercury is ingested, it can cause mercury toxicity.
    b. Explain to the mother that mercury poisoning can cause acrodynia.
    c. Explain to the mother that mercury thermometers are no longer recommended and that if broken, the inhaled vapors can cause toxicity.
    d. Reassure the mother that as long as the mercury thermometer is not broken, it is okay to continue to use it.

16. On routine physical examination, 2-year-old Zach is found to have an elevated blood lead level. The most likely cause for this finding is:
    a. Zach is allowed to play in the local sandbox at the park.
    b. Zach lives in a house built after 1980.
    c. Zach is fed from pottery that the family brought in Mexico.
    d. Zach's father is an artist and works at home.

17. Identify the following statements as true or false.

    ___T___ The neurologic system is of most concern when young children are exposed to lead, since the developing brain is very vulnerable.

    ___T___ Mild to moderate lead poisoning can cause a number of cognitive and behavioral problems in young children, including aggression, hyperactivity, impulsivity, disinterest, and withdrawal.

    ___T___ Lead-based nonintact paint in structures built before 1978 remains a frequent source of lead poisoning in children.

    ___F___ Lead-containing pottery or leaded dishes do not contribute to lead poisoning, because food does not absorb lead.

    ___T___ If the venous blood value is below 5 mcg/dl of lead, the child is considered to have a safe blood lead value.

    ___F___ At the cellular level, lead assists the regulating action of calcium.

    ___T___ The primary nursing goal in lead exposure is to prevent the child's initial contact.

    ___T___ Universal screening guidelines for blood lead level testing include all children between 1 and 2 years of age and between the ages of 3 and 6 years who have not been previously screened.

    ___T___ Mercury thermometers can cause toxicity if they are broken and vapors are inhaled.

    ___T___ Chelation treatment works by the use of a chemical compound that combines with the metal for excretion.

    ___F___ A level of lead not harmful to the pregnant woman is also not harmful to the fetus.

    ___F___ High lead levels are of most concern when they occur in children who are ages 12 and under.

    ___T___ Children who are iron deficient absorb lead more readily than those with sufficient iron stores.

18. The nurse is to give an injection of the chelation drug calcium disodium edentate. Which of the following does the nurse recognize as most appropriate?
    a. Keeping the child NPO for 24 hours after administration of the drug
    b. Mixing the drug with procaine to lessen the pain associated with the injection
    c. Maintaining seizure precautions at the bedside
    d. Making certain the patient has no peanut allergy before injection

19. Diagnostic evaluations for lead poisoning include:
    a. blood levels for lead concentration, including screening by finger and heel sticks, with blood collected by venipuncture to confirm diagnosis.
    b. recommended universal screening for all children, with those ages 6 years or older given priority.
    c. identifying children at high risk for anemia, since these children will most likely have higher lead levels.
    d. understanding that a blood level for lead in the 3 to 5 mcg/dl range is normal and the child should be rescreened in 1 year unless exposure status changes.

20. Therapeutic interventions for lead poisoning do *not* include:
    a. removal of the source of lead.
    b. improving nutrition.
    c. using chelation therapy.
    d. intravenous administration of dimercaprol.

21. Discharge planning for children with lead poisoning includes:
    a. confirmation that the child will be discharged to a home without lead hazards.
    b. immediate referral for development and speech therapy.
    c. visiting nurse care for continuation of intravenous treatment at home.
    d. explanation that there is little need for follow-up, because lead levels have returned to normal.

22. Match each term with its description.

    a. Child neglect
    b. Physical neglect
    c. Emotional neglect
    d. Emotional abuse
    e. Physical abuse

    f. Munchausen syndrome by proxy
    g. Abusive head trauma (shaken baby syndrome)
    h. Child maltreatment
    i. Child abuse

    ___D___ Deliberate attempt to destroy a child's self-esteem

    ___G___ Violent shaking of infant that can cause fatal intracranial trauma

    I ___A___ Any recent act or failure to act on the part of a parent or caretaker that results in death, serious physical or emotional harm, sexual abuse, or exploitation of a child

    ___C___ Failure to meet the child's needs for affection

    ___B___ Deprivation of necessities such as food and clothing

    H ___I___ Intentional physical abuse or neglect, emotional abuse or neglect, and sexual abuse of children

    A ___h___ Failure to provide for the child's basic needs and adequate level of care

    ___E___ Deliberate infliction of physical injury on a child

    ___F___ An illness that one person fabricates or induces in another person

23. Identified characteristics of parents who are at higher risk for abusing their children do *not* include:
    a. older parents who waited until their mid-30s before having their first child.
    b. isolated parents with few supportive relationships.
    c. parents who grew up with poor role models.
    d. single-parent family.

24. A child who unintentionally contributes to an abusive situation most likely:
    a. fits into the "easy-child pattern."
    b. has demands, both physical and emotional, that are incompatible with the parents' ability to meet these needs.
    c. has low self-esteem.
    d. comes from a low socioeconomic background.

25. Which one of the following statements is *false*?
    a. Most reporting of abuse has been from the middle socioeconomic population.
    b. One child is usually the victim in an abusive family; removal of this child often places the other sibling(s) at risk.
    c. The abusive family environment is one of chronic stress, including problems of divorce, poverty, unemployment, and poor housing.
    d. Child abuse is a problem of all socioeconomic groups.

26. Match each term with its description.

   a. Incest
   b. Molestation
   c. Exhibitionism

   d. Pedophilia
   e. Sexual abuse

   ___E___ The use, persuasion, or coercion of any child to engage in sexually explicit conduct

   ___D___ Preference for a prepubertal child by an adult as a means of achieving sexual excitement

   ___A___ Any physical sexual activity between family members

   ___B___ "Indecent liberties," such as touching or fondling

   ___C___ Indecent exposure

27. Identify each of the following statements related to sexual abusers as true or false.

   ___F___ The typical abuser is a male who is unknown to the victim.

   ___T___ Boys are less likely to report both intrafamilial and extrafamilial abuse than are girls.

   ___T___ Many sexual offenders are active in the community and hold full-time jobs.

   ___F___ The incestuous relationship between stepfather and daughter is generally shorter and more often reported than the incestuous relationship between biologic father and daughter.

   ___F___ Sexual abuse by relatives who have a strong emotional bond with the victim is the least devastating to the child.

   ___F___ The youngest daughter is typically the child in the incestuous relationship.

   ___T___ Children may not reveal the truth about the abuse because they fear their parents would not believe them.

28. Sexual abusers:
     i. can be anyone but most often a male who is known by the victim.
     ii. can hold full-time jobs and are active in community affairs.
     iii. are most often not family members.
     iv. often spend time with the victims to gain their trust before initiating any sexual contact.
     v. rarely abuse the younger child if the older child is not present.

   a. ii, iii, iv, and v
   b. i, iii, and iv
   c. i, ii, iv, and v
   d. iii, iv, and v

29. In identification of the abused child, the nurse knows:
   a. physical abuse can be readily identified during the physical examination.
   b. specific behavioral problems can be seen in the abused child.
   c. maltreated children easily admit to the abuse they received from their parents.
   d. incompatibility between the history and the injury is probably the most important criterion on which to base the decision to report suspected abuse.

30. In obtaining a history pertaining to an incident of abuse, the nurse should:
   a. expect the child to betray the parents by admitting to the abuse received.
   b. expect the child to defend the parents out of a sense of loyalty.
   c. recognize that the child will have a sense of relief after telling someone about the abuse.
   d. avoid biasing the child's retelling of the events.

31. Which of the following parental behavioral responses should alert the nurse to the possibility of maltreatment of the child?
    a. Parent displays extreme care for the child, not wanting to leave the child's side.
    b. Parent displays signs of guilt, not being able to eat or sleep.
    c. Parent displays abnormal interest in the incident, going over each detail repeatedly.
    d. Parent displays anger at the child for being injured.

32. Physical assessment for child physical abuse:
    a. should identify all injuries.
    b. should always begin with rapid assessment of airway, breathing, circulation, and neurologic systems.
    c. should recognize that all forms of physical abuse have obvious signs.
    d. should occur only after legal authorities have been notified.

33. Physical assessment for child sexual abuse:
    a. includes documentation of only abnormal genital findings.
    b. includes collecting forensic evidence obtained directly from a prepubertal victim's body as much as 3 days after the incident.
    c. includes examination of the anal area.
    d. includes documentation of the size of the hymenal opening, since it is predictive of sexual abuse.

34. The nurse working with the abused child and family:
    i. should view the parent and child as victims.
    ii. should teach the parents through demonstration and example rather than lecture.
    iii. recognizes that parents need to correct abnormal behavior in the child—for example, "We told you not to go with strangers."
    iv. recognizes that the goal of the nurse-child relationship is to provide a role model for the parents in helping them to relate positively to their child.

    a. i, ii, iii, and iv
    b. ii, iii, and iv
    c. i and iii
    d. ii and iv

CRITICAL THINKING—CASE STUDY

Malcolm is a 4-year-old brought to the emergency room by his mother. Malcolm's mother tells the nurse that Malcolm was being swung around by his old brother, who accidently hurt Malcolm's arm. During the interview process, the mother says that Malcolm has not stopped complaining and crying about his arm and will not use it. The mother tells Malcolm that he needs to "stop crying. It's all your fault." When the mother leaves to fill out admission paperwork, Malcolm tells the nurse, "My mom hurt my arm." On physical exam, the nurse views that Malcolm's left arm is deformed and painful when moved. The nurse notes that Malcolm's legs are covered with bruises and there appears to be an old healing burn on Malcolm's back.

35. Based on the information provided, the nurse suspects that Malcolm is being physically abused. Which one of the following best supports this theory?
    a. Malcolm's mother is distant and angry with Malcolm about his injuries.
    b. Malcolm's mother blames his older brother for Malcolm's injuries.
    c. Malcolm tells the nurse, "My mom hurt my arm."
    d. Malcolm has physical evdence of previous injuries that are in various stages of healing.

36. Based on the above physical findings, documentation should include:
    i. location and detailed description of arm injury, including asymmetry of injury and pain degree.
    ii. color, size, and location of all bruising, including distinguishing characteristics such as shape.
    iii. location, pattern, demarcation lines, and presence of escar, blisters, or scarring for burns.
    iv. photographs of the injuries using a measurement tool.

    a. i, ii, iii, and iv
    b. ii and iii
    c. i, ii, and iv
    d. ii, iii, and iv

37. The best nursing goal for Malcolm at this time is:
    a. identification of all injuries.
    b. identification of abuse pattern.
    c. reassuring Malcolm that everything is going to be fine.
    d. protecting Malcom from further abuse.

38. Malcolm has been admitted to the hospital for closed reduction of his fracture. The suspected child abuse has been reported to the state welfare department and a caseworker has been assigned. Which one of the following is the most appropriate nursing intervention for Malcolm at this time?
    a. Provide consistent caregiver during hospitalization.
    b. Educate Malcolm's mother on the physical and emotional needs of Malcolm.
    c. Treat Malcolm as a child who is a victim of specific physical abuse.
    d. Promise Malcom that what he tells you is a secret and you will not tell anyone.

15 Health Promotion of the School-Age Child and Family

1. Middle childhood is also referred to as the middle years, the school years, or the school-age years. What ages does this period represent?
   a. Ages 5 to 13 years
   b. Ages 4 to 14 years
   c. Ages 6 to 12 years
   d. Ages 6 to 16 years

2. Identify when the middle childhood years physiologically begin and end.

3. Which finding should the nurse expect when assessing physical growth in the school-age child?
   a. Weight increase of 2 to 3 kg per year
   b. Height increase of 3 cm per year
   c. Little change in refined coordination
   d. Decrease in body fat and muscle tissue

4. Identify the following statements about the school-age child as true or false.

   _____ In middle childhood there are fewer stomach upsets, better maintenance of blood glucose levels, and an increased stomach capacity.

   _____ Caloric needs are higher in relation to stomach size when compared with the needs of preschool years.

   _____ The heart is smaller in relation to the rest of the body during the middle years.

   _____ During the middle years, the immune system develops little immunity to pathogenic microorganisms.

   _____ Backpacks, when worn correctly, are preferred to other book totes during middle years.

   _____ Physical maturity correlates well with emotional and social maturity during the middle years.

   _____ School-age children's muscles are still functionally immature compared with those of the adolescent and are more easily damaged by muscular injury and overuse.

   _____ Wider physical differences between children are seen at the beginning of middle childhood than at the end.

   _____ There is no universal age at which the child assumes the characteristics of preadolescence.

   _____ Early appearance of physical sexual characteristics in girls and late appearance in boys have been linked to participation in risk-taking behaviors.

5. What period begins toward the end of middle childhood and ends at age 13?
   a. Puberty
   b. Preadolescence
   c. Early maturation
   d. All of the above

6. According to Freud, middle childhood is described as which one of the following periods?
   a. Anal
   b. Latency
   c. Oral
   d. Oedipal

7. According to Erikson, what is the developmental goal of middle childhood?
   a. Autonomy
   b. Trust
   c. Initiative
   d. Industry

8. Which of the following descriptions of school-age children is most closely linked to Erikson's theory?
   a. During this time, children experience relationships with same-sex peers.
   b. During this time, there is an overlapping of developmental characteristics between childhood and adolescence.
   c. During this time, temperamental traits from infancy continue to influence behavior.
   d. During this time, interests expand and children, with a growing sense of independence, engage in tasks that can be carried through to completion.

9. According to Piaget, what is the stage of development for middle childhood?
   a. Concrete operational
   b. Preoperational
   c. Formal operational
   d. Sensorimotor

10. Early appearance of secondary sex characteristics of girls during preadolescence may be associated with which of the following feelings?
    a. Satisfaction with physical appearance and higher self-esteem
    b. Increase in self-confidence and a more outgoing personality
    c. Dissatisfaction with physical appearance and lower self-esteem
    d. Increased substance use and reckless vehicle use

11. Toward the end of middle childhood, the discrepancies in growth and maturation between boys and girls becomes apparent. Which of the following statements is true?
    a. There is usually a 4-year difference between the onset of pubescence in girls and boys.
    b. The universal age at which the first physiologic signs appear in girls is 9 years of age.
    c. The onset of puberty at age 7 years is considered normal.
    d. The average age of puberty is 12 years in girls and 14 years in boys.

12. Middle childhood is the time when children:
    i. learn the value of doing things with others.
    ii. learn the benefits derived from division of labor in accomplishing goals.
    iii. achieve a sense of industry and accomplishment.
    iv. expand interests and engage in tasks that can be carried to completion.

    a. i, ii, iii, and iv
    b. i, iii, and iv
    c. i and iv
    d. ii and iii

13. Dillon is a 6-year-old starting in a new neighborhood school. On the first day of school, he complains of a headache and tearfully tells his mother he does not want to go to school. Dillon's mother takes him to school, and the nurse is consulted. The nurse recognizes that Dillon is slow to warm up to others and suggests which one of the following?
    a. Put Dillon in the classroom with the other children and leave him alone.
    b. Insist that Dillon join and lead the class song.
    c. Include Dillon in activities without assigning him tasks until he willingly participates in activities.
    d. Send Dillon home with his mom because he has a headache.

14. Which of the following accurately describes the expected cognitive development during the concrete-operational period of middle childhood?
    a. Children are able to follow directions but unable to verbalize the actions involved in the process.
    b. Children are able to use their thought processes to experience events and actions and make judgments based on what they reason.
    c. Children are able to see things from an egocentric outlook that is rigidly developed around the action to be completed.
    d. Children progress from conceptual thinking to perceptual thinking when making judgments.

15. Children who are identified as having a difficult or easily distracted temperament:
    a. rarely pose a problem.
    b. usually exhibit discomfort when introduced to new situations.
    c. benefit from practice sessions before an event.
    d. should not be told when to stop activities, since this can trigger a reaction event.

16. The following terms relate to the accomplishment of cognitive tasks of middle childhood. Match each term with its description.

    a. Conservation   f. Serialize
    b. Identity   g. Combinational skills
    c. Reversibility   h. Metalinguistic awareness
    d. Reciprocity   i. Perceptual thinking
    e. Classification skills   j. Conceptual thinking

    _____ Arrange objects according to some ordinal scale

    _____ Ability to manipulate numbers and to learn the skills of addition, subtraction, multiplication, and division

    _____ Ability to group objects according to the attributes they share in common

    _____ Ability to think through an action sequence, anticipate the consequences, and return and rethink the action in a different direction

    _____ Ability to deal with two dimensions at one time and to comprehend that a change in one dimension compensates for a change in another

    _____ Ability to distinguish a shape change when nothing has been added or subtracted

    _____ Ability to comprehend that physical matter does not appear and disappear by magic

    _____ Ability to think about language and to comment on its properties

    _____ Ability to make decisions based on what one reasons

    _____ Ability to make decisions based on what one sees

17. A major difference in moral development between young school-age children and older school-age children is best described by which one of the following?
    a. Younger children believe that standards of behavior come from within themselves.
    b. Children 6 to 7 years of age know the rules and understand the reasons behind the rules.
    c. Older school-age children are able to judge an act by the intentions that prompted it and not only by the consequences.
    d. Rewards and punishments guide older school-age children's behavior.

18. Which one of the following best identifies the spiritual development of school-age children?
    a. They have little fear of "going to hell" for misbehavior.
    b. They begin to learn the difference between the natural and the supernatural.
    c. They petition to God for less tangible rewards.
    d. They view God as a deity with few human traits.

19. Which one of the following would the nurse *not* expect to observe as characteristic of peer group relationships of 8-year-old Mark?
    a. Mark demonstrates loyalty to the group by adhering to the secret code rules.
    b. Mark demonstrates a greater individual egocentric outlook when compared with other peer group members.
    c. Mark is willing to conform to the group's rule of "not talking to girls."
    d. Mark has a best friend within the peer group with whom he shares his secrets.

20. During the school-age years, children learn valuable lessons from age-mates. How is this accomplished?
    a. The child learns to appreciate the varied points of view within the peer group.
    b. The child becomes sensitive to the social norms and pressures of the group.
    c. The child's interactions among peers lead to the formation of intimate friendships between same-sex peers.
    d. All of the above

21. Which of the following is most characteristic of the relationship between school-age children and their families?
    a. Children desire to spend equal time with family and peers.
    b. Children are prepared to reject parental controls.
    c. The group replaces the family as the primary influence in setting standards of behavior and rules.
    d. Children need and want restrictions placed on their behavior by the family.

22. Ms. Jones is a single mother caring for her 10-year-old son, James. At an office appointment for James, his mother asks the nurse how to prevent her son from becoming involved in gang violence. The best response is which one of the following?
    a. "Try to be more of a pal to James so that he won't seek outside approval."
    b. "Relax restrictions on James. He needs to increase his independence, and this will show that you trust him."
    c. "Become aware of any gang-related activities in your community and become acquainted with your son's friends."
    d. "Don't allow James to join any 'boys only' groups."

23. Children's self-concepts are developed by:

24. Which of the following statements related to bullying is correct?
    a. Bullying usually occurs in school hallways and playgrounds where supervision is minimal but peers are present to witness the attack.
    b. Bullying or cyberbullying affects 50% of elementary school students either as the bully or the victim.
    c. The victim of bullying is usually male, depressed, has poor academic performance, and poor relationships and communication with parents.
    d. Victims of bullying are at higher risk for development of future problems of school dropout, unemployment, and participation in criminal behavior.

25. The nurse plans to conduct a sex education class for 10-year-olds. Which one of the following does the nurse recognize as most appropriate for this age-group?
    a. Present sex information as a normal part of growth and development.
    b. Discourage question-and-answer sessions.
    c. Because sexual information supplied by parents usually produces feelings of guilt and anxiety in children, avoid parental assistance in conducting the program.
    d. Segregate boys from girls and include information related only to same sex in the discussion.

26. In relation to body image, school-age children:
    a. are not aware of physical disabilities in others.
    b. pay little attention to their own body capabilities.
    c. seldom express concerns about their bodies to their families.
    d. do not model themselves after their parents or compare themselves with images observed in the media.

27. List team membership characteristics that promote child development during the middle years.

28. School-age children:
    a. have little interest in complex board, card, or computer games.
    b. rarely collect items.
    c. tire of having stories read aloud.
    d. participate in hero worship.

Chapter **15 Health Promotion of the School-Age Child and Family**

29. Identify the following statements as true or false.

_____ Successful adjustment to school entrance has little relationship to the child's physical and emotional maturity.

_____ Children's attitudes toward school are influenced by the attitudes of their parents.

_____ Television can increase the child's vocabulary, extend the child's horizon, and enrich the school experience.

_____ Television can encourage children to believe that violence is an effective solution to conflict.

_____ Children respond poorly to teachers who have attributes of caring parents.

_____ The teacher's primary goal is guiding the child's intellectual development.

_____ The reward and punishment administered by the teacher have little effect on the child's self-concept.

_____ Interaction between teacher and individual pupil affects the pupil's acceptance by the other children.

_____ Being responsible for school work helps children learn to keep promises, meet deadlines, and succeed at jobs as adults.

_____ Punitive interactions and corporal punishment are associated with decreasing disruptive behaviors in children.

30. A factor that most influences the amount and manner of discipline and limit-setting imposed on school-age children is:
    a. the parent's age.
    b. the parent's education.
    c. the child's response to rewards and punishments.
    d. the parent's ability to communicate with the school system.

31. List the purposes of discipline.

32. Seven-year-old Andy was caught taking a playmate's toy. Which of the following is an important understanding of this behavior?
    a. At this age, Andy's sense of property rights is limited, and he took the item simply because he was attracted to it.
    b. If Andy is caught and punished and promises "not to do it again," he will keep his promise.
    c. This stealing act is an indication that something is seriously lacking in Andy's life.
    d. Andy will learn the importance of respecting others' property if the parents unexpectedly give away an item of Andy's.

33. To assist school-age children in coping with stress in their lives, the nurse should:
    i. be able to recognize signs that indicate the child is undergoing stress.
    ii. teach the child how to recognize signs of stress in herself or himself.
    iii. help the child plan a means for dealing with any stress through problem solving.
    iv. reassure the child that the stress is only temporary.

    a. ii, iii, and iv
    b. i, ii, and iii
    c. ii and iv
    d. i and iii

34. Identify which one of the following statements describing fears in the school-age child is true.
    a. School-age children are increasingly fearful of body safety.
    b. Most of the new fears that trouble school-age children are related to school and family.
    c. School-age children should be encouraged to hide their fears to prevent ridicule by their peers.
    d. School-age children with numerous fears need continuous protective behavior by parents to eliminate these fears.

110

35. The term *latchkey children* refers to whom?

36. By the end of middle childhood, children should be able to assume personal responsibility for self-care in the areas
    of _____, _____, _____,
    _____, _____, and _____.

37. Jim, a 7-year old boy, has just been diagnosed with childhood obesity. Which one of the following does the nurse
    recognize as being most likely to contribute to Jim's obesity?
    a. Caloric needs are diminished in relation to body size during middle childhood.
    b. When Jim entered school, he developed an eating style that was increasingly independent from parental
       influence.
    c. The availability of inexpensive high-caloric foods and the tendency toward sedentary activities.
    d. Jim is a latchkey child and makes his own breakfast and lunch.

38. Sleep problems in the school-age child are often demonstrated by:
    a. delaying tactics because the child does not wish to go to bed.
    b. night terrors that awaken the child during the night.
    c. the development of somatic illness that awakens the child during the night.
    d. the increasing need for larger amounts of sleep compared with preschool and adolescent children.

39. The nurse knows that sleepwalking in childhood can best be described by which of the following statements?
    a. During sleepwalking, the movements are clumsy and repetitive.
    b. Sleepwalking occurs in the first 1 to 2 hours of sleep.
    c. During sleepwalking, speech is comprehensible.
    d. The child remembers the episode in the morning.

40. The nurse is planning to advise a school-age child's parents about appropriate physical activity for their child. Which
    fact does the nurse include?
    a. School-age children have the same stamina and control as 15-year-old teens.
    b. School-age children are prepared for participation in strenuous competitive athletics.
    c. Activities that promote coordination in the school-age child include running and skipping rope.
    d. Most children need continued encouragement to engage in physical activity.

41. Identify the following as true or false.

    _____ In children 6 and 7 years old, the task of going to bed can be facilitated by encouraging quiet activity
              before bedtime.

    _____ Twelve-year-old children usually offer the most difficulty in regard to bedtime.

    _____ The best approach to sleepwalking is to awaken the child and put him or her back to bed.

    _____ Nightmares are a part of the normal developmental process, and all children will experience nightmares
              during childhood.

    _____ Sleepwalking is usually self-limiting and requires no treatment.

    _____ Eruption of permanent teeth begins with the first, or 6-year, molar.

    _____ Children under 10 years of age often need parental assistance to brush the back teeth.

    _____ Toothbrushes for school-age children should be soft nylon brushes with an overall length of about
              8 inches.

    _____ During middle childhood, girls and boys have the same basic structure and can compete against one
              another in sports.

_____ Parents who pressure their children to perform beyond their capabilities risk injury and lowered self-esteem in their child.

_____ School-age children demonstrate little ability and interest in music.

_____ Children under the age of 13 years should ride in the front passenger seat of vehicles equipped with air bags.

_____ Children ages 5 to 9 years restrained in adult-type seatbelts are at increased risk for head injury from impact with interior vehicle parts.

_____ All-terrain vehicles (ATVs) have been approved by the American Academy of Pediatrics for children as young as 14 years of age.

_____ Skateboard, roller skate, or in-line skate injuries among children mostly involve the wrist and forearm.

_____ Warnings with new trampoline equipment recommend avoiding somersaults, restricting multiple jumpers, and limiting trampoline use to children 6 years or older.

_____ The normally shallow bony orbit of school-age children makes them vulnerable to eye trauma.

_____ School buses should be equipped with lap-shoulder restraint systems that can accommodate safety seats, booster seats, and harness systems.

42. Parent and teacher education relating to television, video games, and the Internet should include what recommendations?

43. List six components that should be included in the content of school health services.

44. The nurse is planning an educational session for a group of 9-year-olds and their parents aimed at decreasing injuries and accidents among this group. The nurse would best accomplish this goal by reviewing:
    a. safety rules to prevent burns when dealing with fire.
    b. safety rules to prevent poisonings when dealing with toxic substances.
    c. pedestrian safety rules and skills training programs to prevent motor vehicle accidents.
    d. safety rules for the use of all-terrain vehicles, encouraging their use only with supervision.

CRITICAL THINKING—CASE STUDY

Allen Thomas, age 9, is taken to the clinic by his mother for a school physical examination. Allen's mother is concerned because Allen wants to join the school soccer team this year. On physical examination, the nurse discovers that Allen has grown 5 cm (2 inches) in height and gained 5.4 kg (12 lb) since last year. His health history is unchanged from the previous year. Allen tells the nurse that he rides his bike more now than last year because he has a new best friend to go riding with.

45. Based on the information given, the nurse should expand assessment with Allen in which of the following areas at this visit?
    i. His diet
    ii. His knowledge and use of safety precautions when riding his bike
    iii. His hygiene habits
    iv. His reasons for wanting to play soccer

    a. i, ii, and iii
    b. ii and iv
    c. i and ii
    d. i and iv

46. Which of the following would be the nurse's best response to the mother's concern about Allen playing soccer?
    a. "Allen is healthy, and playing soccer will allow him to increase strength and develop motor skill performance."
    b. "Allen is overweight for his age and should be encouraged to ride his bike less. Soccer is a better activity for him since it will help decrease his weight."
    c. "Allen is still too young to participate in strenuous sports like soccer. He should be able to participate in another year."
    d. "Let Allen play what he wants to. You worry too much about his activities."

47. Based on the information provided, the nurse plans an educational session for Allen and his mother. Which knowledge deficit would the nurse most likely identify for this family?
    a. Modified nutrition because of improper dietary habits
    b. Improper nutrition related to less daily intake than the body needs
    c. Lack of proper physical activity related to bike riding
    d. Improper parenting skills related to overprotective mother

48. Mrs. Thomas asks the nurse how she can foster Allen's development. What would be the best response by the nurse?
    a. "Don't interfere with Allen as long as he is doing well in school."
    b. "Give Allen recognition and positive feedback for his accomplishments."
    c. "Always point out to Allen how he incorrectly performs tasks so he can improve his accomplishments."
    d. "Try not to set rules for Allen. He needs to set his own limits during this period of development."

49. The nurse realizes that Allen's weight gain:
    a. is normal during this growth period.
    b. is probably related to a high-fat diet, rich in junk food intake.
    c. will be corrected by the increase in exercise of soccer and bike riding.
    d. is not influenced by the mass media.

50. The nurse is discussing bicycle safety with Allen's mother. Mrs. Thomas says that Allen will soon need a new bike and helmet. Describe what should be included in the conversation about selecting the bike and safety helmet.

16 Health Problems of the School-Age Child

1. Skin in the infant and small child, as compared with skin in older children and adults:
   a. is tightly bound to the dermis.
   b. is less likely to have blister formation from an inflammatory process.
   c. is more likely to react to a sensitizing allergen than to a primary irritant.
   d. is more susceptible to superficial bacterial infection.

2. List three etiologic factors that can result in lesions of the skin in children.

3. Match each term related to assessment of the skin with its description.

   a. Pruritus   d. Paresthesia
   b. Anesthesia   e. Hypesthesia
   c. Hyperesthesia

   _____ Excessive sensitiveness

   _____ Absence of sensation

   _____ Diminished sensation

   _____ Itching

   _____ Abnormal sensation

4. Match each wound-related term with its description.

   a. Acute   g. Incision
   b. Chronic   h. Penetrating
   c. Pressure ulcer   i. Puncture
   d. Abrasion   j. Regeneration
   e. Avulsion   k. Allodynia
   f. Laceration

   _____ Rapid replacement by similar cells

   _____ Accidental cut, with either torn or jagged edges

   _____ Disruption of the skin that extends into the underlying tissue or into a body cavity

   _____ Heals uneventfully within the usual time frame

   _____ Does not heal in the expected time frame and can be associated with complications

   _____ Removal of the superficial layers of skin by scraping

   _____ Develops when soft tissue is compressed between a bony prominence and a firm surface and often becomes a chronic skin injury

   _____ Forcible pulling out or extraction of tissue

   _____ Wound with an opening that is small compared with its depth

   _____ Division of the skin made with a sharp object

   _____ Sensation of pain from normally nonpainful stimuli

114

5. Cindy, age 8 years, is brought to the clinic with a sore on her arm. She tells the nurse that she scratched it on a piece of metal at the playground about 1 week ago. Which one of the following signs would the nurse expect to find if the sore has become infected?
   a. Itching at the site of the sore
   b. Rough edges around the sore
   c. No pain at the site
   d. Increased erythema, especially around the sore

6. Epithelial wound healing:
   a. begins 72 hours after the wound is incurred.
   b. occurs by migration and proliferation of epithelial cells from the wound center toward the wound margins.
   c. occurs more rapidly when the wound is covered with a transparent or other occlusive-type dressing.
   d. occurs more rapidly when the skin is allowed to dry and to form an eschar, or scab.

7. Major aims of skin treatment include all of the following *except*:
   a. eliminate the cause.
   b. obtain an accurate account of child's symptoms.
   c. effective treatment and symptom relief.
   d. prevent complications.

8. During wound healing, immature connective tissue cells migrate to the healing site and begin to secrete collagen into the meshwork spaces. What is this phase called?
   a. Scar contracture
   b. Inflammation
   c. Fibroplasia
   d. Scar maturation

9. Mary, age 7 years, fell and sustained a deep laceration to her chin. She was taken to the emergency department, where the laceration was sutured with the edges well approximated. The nurse expects the repair healing to take place by:
   a. primary intention.
   b. secondary intention.
   c. tertiary intention.

10. The nurse recognizes that which of the following is not indicated for use in promoting wound healing?
    a. Nutrition with sufficient protein, calories, vitamins C and D, and zinc
    b. Irrigation of wounds with normal saline
    c. Application of povidone-iodine (Betadine) solution
    d. Application of an occlusive dressing

11. Jimmy, age 9 years, has fallen and scraped his knee at school. He is brought to the school nurse for treatment. Which one of the following does the nurse recognize as being *least* likely to promote healing?
    a. Changing the dressing when it becomes loose or soiled.
    b. Washing the injury with hydrogen peroxide and applying a dry gauze dressing.
    c. Applying an occlusive dressing.
    d. Washing the area with mild soap and water and applying a topical antibiotic with a nonadherent dressing.

12. Which one of the following statements about use of topical therapy in the pediatric population is true?
    a. Use of silver impregnated in dressing as foam decreases the bacterial burden and bioburden of the wound and has little absorption effect in the pediatric population.
    b. Application of heat provides a soothing effect to reduce inflammatory processes.
    c. The use of immunomodulators is suggested as first-line treatment in children younger than 2 years of age.
    d. Topical immunomodulators have been linked to possible skin cancer and lymphoma.

13. Which of the following does the nurse include in the educational plan when instructing parents about the use of topical corticosteroids?
    a. Do not use this cream on a fungal infection.
    b. Apply a thick layer of the cream and rub into the skin well.
    c. Do not use for longer than 3 days in chronic conditions.
    d. All of the above should be included.

14. Which of the following is true about topical therapy for acute treatment of dermatologic problems?
    a. Application of heat to the area will relieve itching.
    b. Apply the topical application in a systematic manner following the contour of the body surface.
    c. Chemicals that are nonirritating to intact skin will be nonirritating to inflamed skin.
    d. Emollient action of soaks, baths, or lotions increases skin irritation.

15. Skin disorder assessment includes the objective data collected by inspection and palpation. Which one of the following is *not* an example of objective data?
    a. The lesion has an increased erythematous margin edge.
    b. The rash appears as macules and papules.
    c. The lesion is painful and itches.
    d. The lesion is moist.

16. List the signs of wound infection.

17. Wound care instructions to parents should include which of the following?
    a. Use betadine, alcohol, and hydrogen peroxide to prevent infection.
    b. Use hydrocolloid dressing that just covers the wound with little overlap.
    c. Formation of yellow gel with a fruity odor under hydrocolloid dressings is a sign of infection.
    d. Remove the hydrocolloid dressings by raising one edge of the dressing and pulling parallel to the skin to loosen the adhesive.

18. During the physical exam of 8-year-old Kevin, the nurse sees a rash at the umbilicus and surrounding area. Kevin tells the nurse that the rash "comes and goes" but "does itch." The nurse recognizes the rash as contact dermatitis. Which one of the following is the most likely cause of this rash?
    a. Insect bite
    b. Nickel used in Kevin's belt
    c. Laundry detergent used to clean Kevin's clothes
    d. Kevin has developed a food allergy

19. Billy has come in contact with poison ivy on a school picnic. The best intervention for the nurse to implement at this time is to:
    a. wash the area with a strong soap and water solution.
    b. apply Calamine lotion to the area.
    c. prevent spread by instructing Billy not to scratch the lesions.
    d. flush the area immediately with cold water.

20. Which of the following foreign bodies is *least* likely to be successfully removed with tweezers?
    a. Small wooden splinter
    b. Large spines of cactus
    c. Embedded needle in the foot
    d. All of the above

21. When advising parents about the use of sunscreen for school-age children, the nurse should tell them that:
    a. a waterproof sunscreen with a minimum 15 SPF is recommended for children.
    b. the lower the number of SPF, the higher the protection.
    c. sunscreens are not as effective as sunblockers.
    d. the sunscreen should be applied 1 hour before the child is allowed in the sun.

22. Which of the following statements about sunscreen containing PABA is *false*?
    a. It may stain clothes.
    b. It can cause an allergic reaction.
    c. It provides little protection when the child is swimming or sweating.
    d. It is an effective sunscreen against ultraviolet B.

23. Match each term with its description.

    a. Chilblain
    b. Frostbite
    c. Sunscreen
    d. Sunblocker

    e. Ultraviolet A (UVA)
    f. Ultraviolet B (UVB)
    g. Hypothermia
    h. Contact dermatitis

    _____ Blocks out ultraviolet rays by reflecting sunlight

    _____ Partially absorbs ultraviolet light

    _____ An inflammatory reaction of the skin to a substance that evokes a hypersensitivity response or a direct irritation

    _____ Shorter light waves, responsible for tanning, burning, and most of the harmful effects attributed to sunlight

    _____ Longest light waves, causing only minimum burning but playing a significant role in photosensitive and photoallergic reactions

    _____ Condition in which ice crystals form in tissues

    _____ Redness and swelling of the skin from cold exposure

    _____ Cooling of the body's core temperature below 35° C (95° F)

24. In caring for the child with frostbite, the nurse remembers that:
    a. slow thawing is associated with less tissue necrosis.
    b. the frostbitten part appears white or blanched, feels solid, and is without sensation.
    c. rewarming produces a small return of sensation with a small amount of pain.
    d. rewarming is accomplished by rubbing the injured tissue.

25. Therapeutic management for mild hypothermia includes:
    a. having the child assume the fetal position.
    b. having the child in water move constantly.
    c. rapid rewarming of the extremities by applying heated blankets.
    d. external application of heat lamps or immersion in warm water.

26. Manifestations of drug reactions may be delayed or immediate. A period of _____ _____ is usually required for a child to develop sensitivity to a drug that has never been previously administered. With prior sensitivity, the

    reaction appears _____ _____. Frequent offenders in drug reactions are

    _____ and _____.

27. Erythema multiforme:
    a. can be caused by fungal infections.
    b. can be caused by flea bites.
    c. is characterized by lesions appearing primarily on the palms, soles and extensor surfaces.
    d. can be life threatening.

28. Erythema multiforme exudativum (Stevens-Johnson syndrome):
    a. is rare and occurs most often in females.
    b. is a hypersensitivity reaction to certain drugs.
    c. begins with generalized rash over the entire body except for palms, soles, and extensor surfaces.
    d. is caused by a bite from a flea.

29. Neurofibromatosis:
    i. is an autosomal dominant genetic disorder.
    ii. is suspected when the 5-year-old child is seen with six or more café-au-lait spots larger than 5 mm in diameter.
    iii. is suspected when the infant develops axillary or inguinal freckling.
    iv. is known to cause developmental delays and cognitive impairment.
    v. has the risk of being transmitted to 75% of the offspring.
    vi. therapy is limited to excision of tumors that produce pain or impair function and symptomatic management of symptoms.

    a. i, ii, iii, iv, and v
    b. i, ii, iii, iv, and vi
    c. i, iii, v, and vi
    d. ii, iii, iv, v, and vi

30. Hypersensitivity to which of the following drugs is most likely to cause toxic epidermal necrolysis?
    a. Aspirin
    b. Acetaminophen
    c. Phenytoin
    d. Erythromycin

31. Johnny's mother is calling the clinic because Johnny has developed a rash over his entire body. Two days ago he was prescribed amoxicillin for an ear infection, and now his mother tells the nurse she thinks Johnny may have gotten a small rash with this medication when he took it before. Which one of the following would be the best intervention by the nurse at this time?
    a. Question the mother about other symptoms that Johnny may have developed.
    b. Continue the medication and have Johnny come in tomorrow to see the practitioner.
    c. Stop the medication and inform the practitioner.
    d. Tell the mother to give only half the prescribed dose of the medication until Johnny can return to the clinic to see the practitioner.

32. Cindy is 12 years old and is brought to the clinic because of a bald spot developing on her head. Cindy wears her hair tightly braided with beads. Which one of the following should the nurse suspect?
    a. Alopecia from trauma
    b. Tinea capitis
    c. Psoriasis
    d. Urticaria

33. Billy has been stung by a bee. A small reaction has occurred at the site. What is the most appropriate action at this time?
    a. Wait until Billy is at home to completely remove the stinger with forceps.
    b. Remove the stinger as soon as possible by scraping it off the skin.
    c. Wash the area with hot water and soap.
    d. Arrange for Billy to undergo skin testing.

34. The most effective method for tick removal in a child is to:
    a. use curved forceps and grasp close to the point of attachment; then pull straight up with a steady, even pressure.
    b. apply mineral oil to the back of the tick and wait for it to back out.
    c. use the fingers to pull the tick out with a straight, steady, even pressure.
    d. place a hot match on the back of the tick and pick it up with gloved hands when the tick falls off.

35. The nurse is assisting Billy, aged 10 years, in applying an all-purpose insect repellent that contains the active ingredient DEET. Which one of the following should be included in the nurse's discussion with Billy?
    a. DEET is effective against most insects and arachnids, but not ticks.
    b. Protection will last for several hours but will need to be washed off with soap and water before he goes to bed tonight.
    c. DEET should be applied to the whole body including the face and hands for better protection.
    d. DEET must be reapplied after sweating, swimming, wiping, or exposure to rain.

36. The nurse is conducting a review of health records for incoming fifth grade students and discovers that Mary has a history of having had a severe life-threatening systemic response to a Hymenoptera sting. Which of the following is most important for the nurse to do at this time?
    a. Make sure that Mary has an identification bracelet to alert others of her allergy.
    b. Contact Mary's parents and physician and obtain an EpiPen for Mary to use if necessary at school.
    c. Contact Mary's parents about which hospital Mary should be taken to if a sting occurs at school.
    d. Talk to Mary and see if she has had skin testing to confirm her allergy.

37. Management of brown recluse spider bites includes:
    a. possible skin graft.
    b. administration of antivenin.
    c. applying lemon juice mixed with baking soda directly to the bite.
    d. administering epinephrine and corticosteroids for impending shock.

38. Dog bites in children occur most often:
    a. on the upper extremities in young children.
    b. from dogs owned by the family or by a neighbor.
    c. from stray dogs.
    d. in schoolyards and neighborhood parks.

39. Nora has been brought to the emergency department by her father after having been bitten by the family dog. Examination reveals three puncture wounds of the hand. Expected therapeutic management for these wounds includes:
    a. suturing the wounds.
    b. administering prophylactic antibiotics.
    c. irrigating with hydrogen peroxide.
    d. administering a tetanus toxoid booster, since Nora's last booster was given 13 months ago.

40. On a field trip to a remote area with his Boy Scout troop, Peter is bitten by a snake. Which one of the following actions would be contraindicated?
    a. Remove Peter from the area and have him rest in a reclined position.
    b. Feel for a pulse distal to the bite area.
    c. Place ice from the ice cooler on the bite area.
    d. Immobilize the limb.

41. Human bites:
    a. are treatable at home.
    b. do not require tetanus immunization.
    c. should not have ice applied to the area.
    d. should receive medical attention.

42. During middle childhood:
    a. children are less susceptible to development of dental caries.
    b. plasticized sealant, applied to deep fissures and grooves of healthy teeth, can prevent cavity formation.
    c. periodontal disease contributes to tooth loss.
    d. regular administration of fluoride dental varnish is no longer recommended.

43. The most common cause of malocclusion is:
    a. thumb sucking.
    b. tongue thrusting.
    c. hereditary factors.
    d. abnormal growth patterns.

44. Which of the following statements about children with orthodontic braces is true?
    a. There is pain when the child has the braces applied or adjusted, which lasts about 30 minutes.
    b. The bands and brackets offer protection and prevent plaque.
    c. If an arch wire breaks, cover the broken wire with dental wax and keep the regularly scheduled appointment with the orthodontist.
    d. Forbidden foods during orthodontic treatment include chewing gum, ice, nuts, uncut apples, corn on the cob, hard candy, hard taco shells, nachos, and popcorn.

45. Emergency care for tooth evulsion includes:
    a. replanting the tooth after bleeding has stopped.
    b. storing the tooth in tap water until it and the child can be transported to the dentist.
    c. holding the tooth by the root.
    d. rinsing the dirty tooth gently under running water before replanting.

46. The major nursing consideration in assisting the family of a child with nocturnal enuresis is to prevent the child from developing alterations in:
    a. body image.
    b. self-esteem.
    c. autonomy.
    d. peer acceptance.

47. The nurse is assisting the family of a child with a history of encopresis. Which one of the following should be included in the nurse's discussion with this family?
    a. Instructing the parents to sit the child on the toilet at two daily routine intervals
    b. Instructing the parents that the child will probably need to have daily enemas for the next year
    c. Suggesting the use of stimulant cathartics weekly
    d. Reassuring the family that most problems resolve successfully, with some relapses during periods of stress

48. Barbara has been diagnosed with attention deficit/hyperactivity disorder and placed on methylphenidate (Ritalin) by her physician. Which one of the following statements, made by the nurse to Barbara's parents, is correct?
    a. "This drug is usually administered twice daily, at breakfast and at noon with lunch."
    b. "Dosage is usually unchanged until adolescence."
    c. "This medication takes 2 to 3 weeks to achieve an effect."
    d. "Barbara's appetite will be increased with this drug."

49. Match each learning disability with its description.

    a. dyslexia
    b. dysgraphia
    c. dyscalculia

    _____ Reading letters in reverse

    _____ Difficulty with reading

    _____ Difficulty with calculation

50. Therapeutic management for a child with a tic disorder primarily consists of:
    a. behavioral modification to teach the child to suppress the tic disorder.
    b. administration of haloperidol to suppress the tic disorder.
    c. education and support for the child and family with reassurance about the prognosis.
    d. genetic counseling for the parents.

51. Which of the following statements about Tourette syndrome (TS) is true?
    a. Manifestations are stable in intensity and rarely change once developed.
    b. Children with TS have no associated obsessive-compulsive symptoms.
    c. Tics lead to physical deterioration and affect life expectancy.
    d. Behaviors are involuntary.

52. Which of the following statements about posttraumatic stress disorder (PTSD) is true?
    a. PTSD is the development of characteristic symptoms after exposure to a traumatic experience or event that is usually not life threatening.
    b. The second phase of PTSD lasts approximately 4 weeks and is one of coping.
    c. The third phase of PTSD extends over 6 months and is a period of direct inquiry. The victim wants to know what happened and appears to be getting better when actually getting worse.
    d. Any child exhibiting a sudden change in behavior needs to be assessed for exposure to a traumatic event.

53. Which of the following statements about school phobia is correct?
    a. School phobia is most common in boys over the age of 12.
    b. School phobia produces symptoms in children that are unrelieved when the student stays home from school.
    c. Students with school phobia that have separation anxiety are not afraid to go to school but rather afraid to leave home.
    d. School phobia fear is helped by a close intense relationship between the child and mother.

54. When caring for the child diagnosed with recurrent abdominal pain (RAP), the nurse recognizes which of the following as correct?
    a. Children with RAP have imagined pain usually located in the periumbilical and/or epigastric region of the abdomen.
    b. Children at high risk for RAP are those with high expectations and extensive personal goals or whose parents have unusually high expectations for them.
    c. Diagnosis is based on physical, laboratory, and radiographic findings.
    d. Initial efforts for therapeutic management include dietary modifications and cognitive-behavioral therapy and biofeedback.

55. Conversion reaction:
    a. is a psychophysiologic disorder associated with sudden onset.
    b. is more common in girls during childhood and adolescence.
    c. has an organic cause.
    d. is diagnosed on the basis of seizures and abnormal electroencephalogram.

56. Childhood depression:
    a. is easily detected because children tend to act out their problems and feelings.
    b. has characteristics that are determined by parallel developments in symbolism, language, and cognitive development.
    c. does not interrupt normal growth and development.
    d. treatment consists of antidepressants that must be at a therapeutic level for at least 6 to 8 weeks to achieve beneficial effect.

57. The cause of childhood schizophrenia is unknown. List three risk factors that have been identified with schizophrenia.

CRITICAL THINKING—CASE STUDY

Carol, age 9, went on a picnic yesterday with her family. Today she returns to school and is showing her classmates several leaves that she collected yesterday. The teacher notices that three of the leaves are from a poison ivy plant. The teacher takes Carol to the school nurse because of a rash that has developed on her arms and legs. Carol tells the nurse that the rash is "very itchy."

58. The nurse completes a diagnostic assessment of the skin rash to include a complete history and physical examination. The nurse knows that this history should include:
    a. inspection of the rash, including size and shape of lesions.
    b. symptoms, past and recent exposure to causative agents, medications taken, and history of previous similar rashes.
    c. palpation of the rash for increased heat, edema, and tenderness.
    d. skin scrapings from the site for microscopic examination.

59. The primary action the school nurse should take at this time is to:
    a. call Carol's parents to pick her up at school. Isolate Carol from other classmates until her parents arrive.
    b. give the poison ivy leaves to the school janitor to be destroyed in the school incinerator.
    c. instruct the teacher to make certain all classmates who had contact with the poison ivy plant flush these areas with cold running water.
    d. reassure Carol that everything is going to be fine, apply Calamine lotion to her rash, and instruct Carol not to scratch the rash.

60. What is the best nursing diagnosis for Carol at this time?
    a. Impaired Skin Integrity related to environmental factors
    b. High Risk for Infection related to presence of infectious organisms
    c. Pain related to skin lesions
    d. Body Image Disturbance related to presence of rash

61. Goals for Carol should include which of the following?
    a. Carol will not experience secondary damage, such as infection, from scratching.
    b. Carol will demonstrate acceptable levels of comfort from itching.
    c. Carol will be able to recognize and avoid the precipitating agent in the future.
    d. All of the above should be included.

62. In educating Carol and her parents about caring for the rash, the nurse should tell them to:
    i. bathe in tepid or cool water.
    ii. bathe in hot water.
    iii. apply hydrogen peroxide to the rash daily.
    iv. apply Calamine lotion to the rash.
    v. administer over-the-counter diphenhydramine orally to decrease itching.
    vi. keep Carol's fingernails short.
    vii. wear heavy clothing to prevent contamination.
    viii. understand that the rash is contagious and will weep.

    a. i, iii, iv, vi, and vii
    b. i, iv, v, and vi
    c. ii, v, vi, and vii
    d. iii, iv, v, and viii

17 Health Promotion of the Adolescent and Family

1. Growth and development during middle adolescence includes which one of the following?
   a. Characterized by a transition to a dominant peer orientation
   b. Characterized by the changes of puberty and the responses to those changes
   c. Characterized by the taking on of adult roles
   d. Characterized by excellent conflict resolution over parental control

2. In the female adolescent who has reached puberty, the luteinizing hormone initiates which of the following actions?
   a. Production of estrogen
   b. Growth of ovarian follicles
   c. Production of gonadotropin-releasing hormone
   d. Ovulation

3. The hormone in the female that causes growth and development of the vagina, uterus, fallopian tubes, and breasts is:
   a. estrogen.
   b. progesterone.
   c. follicle-stimulating hormone (FSH).
   d. luteinizing hormone (LH).

4. Match each term with its description.

   a. Thelarche
   b. Pubarche
   c. Physiologic leukorrhea
   d. Menarche
   e. Gynecomastia
   f. Puberty

   g. Ovulation
   h. Pubertal delay
   i. Precocious puberty
   j. Pubertal growth spurt
   k. Genetic endowment

   _____ Occurs when girls fail to develop breasts by age 13

   _____ Biologic changes of adolescence

   _____ Onset of menstrual periods

   _____ Development of breast tissue

   _____ When boys develop secondary sexual characteristics before the age of 9 years

   _____ Male breast enlargement and tenderness

   _____ General increase in in growth of the skeleton, muscles, and internal organs; reaches a peak of about 12 years of age in girls and 14 years of age in boys

   _____ Most important determinant of the onset, rate, and duration of pubertal growth

   _____ Development of pubic hair

   _____ Normal vaginal discharge

   _____ Release of an ovum by a follicle

5. Julie, 12 years old, is brought to the nurse practitioner's office by her mother. Julie has started to develop breast tissue and some pubic hair. Both the mother and daughter are concerned because Julie has been having increased vaginal discharge. Julie tells the nurse, "I wash my private area every day, but I still have fluid that comes out." What is the nurse's best response?
   a. "It sounds like you have an infection. We'll have the nurse practitioner check you to see what is causing this discharge."
   b. "Have you been using soap when you wash?"
   c. "This sounds like a normal discharge that happens to all girls as they start to mature. It is a sign that your body is preparing for your periods to begin."
   d. "This is probably not related to hygiene. Are you concerned that this discharge might be causing an odor?"

6. The first pubescent change in boys is:
   a. appearance of pubic hair.
   b. testicular enlargement with thinning, reddening, and increased looseness of the scrotum.
   c. penile enlargement.
   d. temporary breast enlargement and tenderness.

7. Tommy is brought in by his father for his yearly physical. On examination, the nurse notes that since last year Tommy has developed pubic hair, testicular enlargement, and related scrotal changes. In planning anticipatory guidance, the nurse recognizes that which one of the following subjects would best be discussed with Tommy as soon as possible?
   a. Nocturnal emission
   b. Sexually transmitted infection prevention
   c. Pregnancy prevention
   d. Hygiene needs

8. During assessment, the nurse observes that Gail has sparse growth of downy hair extending along the labia. Which of the following Tanner stages would be suspected?
   a. Stage 1
   b. Stage 2
   c. Stage 4
   d. Stage 5

9. Ben has just turned 16 years of age and is in for his routine physical. The nurse notes that Ben has pubescent changes and determines that Ben is in Tanner stage 3. What findings would best describe this Tanner stage?
   a. Testes, scrotum, and penis are adult in size and shape.
   b. No pubic hair is present.
   c. There is initial enlargement of scrotum and testes; reddening and texture changes of the scrotal skin; long, straight, downy hair at base of penis.
   d. There is initial enlargement of penis in length; testes and scrotum are enlarged; hair is darker, coarser, and curly over entire pubis.

10. Which one of the following statements about pattern of growth during adolescence is true?
    a. Knowing the correct sequence of the growth pattern is useful only when assessing abnormal growth patterns versus normal growth patterns.
    b. Girls usually begin puberty and reach maturity about 2 years earlier than boys do.
    c. Girls and boys experience an increase of muscle mass that begins during early puberty and lasts throughout adolescence.
    d. Girls and boys experience an increase in linear growth that begins for both during midpuberty.

11. Which one of the following best describes the formal operational thinking that occurs between the ages of 11 and 14 years?
    a. Thought process includes thinking in concrete terms.
    b. Thought process includes information obtained from the environment and peers.
    c. Thought process includes thinking in abstract terms, possibilities, and hypotheses.
    d. Thought process is limited to what is observed.

12. Jimmy, a 13-year-old, is sent to the school nurse because he and some of his peers were caught chewing tobacco while playing baseball. The nurse knows that the best way to influence Jimmy's behavior for health promotion would be which of the following?
    a. Tell Jimmy that he will be suspended from school if he continues to chew the tobacco.
    b. Show Jimmy pictures of oral cancer from chewing tobacco.
    c. Tell Jimmy about the dangers of chewing tobacco and stress the fact that girls do not like boys who chew tobacco.
    d. Arrange for a local baseball hero to talk with Jimmy and his friends, stressing that he does not use chewing tobacco, his friends do not chew tobacco, and chewing tobacco causes ugly teeth.

13. Adolescent egocentrism may lead to a pattern of personal fable. An example of a personal fable is:
    a. "Everyone is coming to the play just to see me."
    b. "Mary Sue got pregnant, but it won't happen to me."
    c. "I hate taking my clothes off for gym class because everyone stares at me."
    d. "Mary is very envious of how I dress."

14. Adolescents develop the social cognition change of mutual role-taking. Which one of the following is the best description of this ability?
    a. Heightened sense of self-consciousness
    b. Understanding the perspectives of others and that actions can influence others
    c. Beliefs that are more abstract and rooted in ideologic principles
    d. Realization that others have thoughts and feelings

15. The development of a personal value system or value autonomy during adolescence usually occurs by what age?
    a. 14 to 16 years
    b. 18 to 20 years
    c. 13 to 14 years
    d. 16 to 18 years

16. Elements of principled moral reasoning emerge during adolescence. Which of the following is the best description of this moral development?
    a. Moral guidelines are seen to emanate from authority figures.
    b. Moral standards are seen as objective and not to be questioned.
    c. Absolutes and rules are questioned and subject to disagreement.
    d. A personal value system is developed.

17. Spiritual development during adolescent years can best be described by which of the following?
    a. Places less emphasis on what a person believes
    b. Places more emphasis on whether a person attends religious services
    c. Becomes more focused on spiritual and ideologic matters and less on observing religious customs
    d. Becomes more focused on observing religious customs and less on ideologic matters

18. According to Erikson, a key to identity achievement in adolescence is:
    a. related to the adolescent's interactions with others and serves as a mirror reflecting information back to the adolescent.
    b. linked to the role the adolescent plays within the family.
    c. related to the adolescent's acceptance of parental guidelines.
    d. related to the adolescent's ability to complete his or her plans for future accomplishments.

19. Expected characteristics of emotional autonomy during early adolescence include:
    a. increased independence from friends.
    b. increased need for parental approval.
    c. belief that parents are all-knowing and all-powerful.
    d. less emotional dependence on parents.

20. The formation of sexual identity development during adolescence usually involves which of the following?
    i. Forming close friendships with same-sex peers during early adolescence
    ii. Developing intimate relationships with members of the opposite sex during middle adolescence
    iii. Developing emotional and social identities separate from those of families
    iv. Incorporating sexuality successfully into intimate relationships

    a. i, ii, and iii
    b. ii, iii, and iv
    c. ii and iii
    d. i, ii, iii, and iv

21. The development of sexual orientation includes seven developmental milestones during late childhood and through-out adolescence. These milestones do not always occur in the same order or in the same time frame. List these milestones.

22. Intimate relationships are not necessarily characterized by:
    a. concern for each other's well-being.
    b. sharing of sexual intimacy.
    c. a willingness to disclose private, sensitive topics.
    d. sharing of common interests and activities.

23. Changes in family structure and parent employment have resulted in:
    a. adolescents having more time unsupervised by adults.
    b. adolescents having more time for communication and intimacy with parents.
    c. adolescents having less time to spend with peers.
    d. adolescents requiring more supervision by outside family members.

24. Adolescents who feel close to their parents show:
    i. more positive psychosocial development.
    ii. greater behavioral competence.
    iii. less susceptibility to negative peer pressure.
    iv. less tendency to be involved in risk-taking behaviors.

    a. i, iii, and iv
    b. i and ii
    c. iii and iv
    d. i, ii, iii, and iv

25. Describe authoritative parenting and results related to this type of parenting.

26. Internet chatrooms and social networking:
    a. have allowed adolescents a more public arena for developing interpersonal skills.
    b. have decreased the amount of bullying in the school setting.
    c. have increased the development of multitasking and longer attention spans in the adolescent.
    d. have decreased adolescents' risk-taking behaviors.

27. Compared with childhood peer groups, adolescent peer groups are:
    a. more likely to include peers from the opposite sex.
    b. less autonomous.
    c. less likely to influence members' socialization roles.
    d. more likely to require parental supervision.

28. Which of the following statements about adolescents and school is true?
    a. Transition from elementary school to middle school has no negative effects on adolescents.
    b. Teenagers whose grades fall below average spend more time in perceived negative environments and feel alienated from school.
    c. Students who repeat one or more grades are more likely to bring weapons to school.
    d. Students with above-average grades have been identified as more likely to engage in suicide attempts.

29. While Jenny, age 16, is in for her routine checkup, her mother tells the nurse that Jenny wants to get a job at a local fast-food restaurant, where she would work 30 hours a week to earn extra money for clothes. The mother wonders whether this is a good idea. Which one of the following is the nurse's best response?
    a. "Jenny is healthy, and there is no reason she could not take the job."
    b. "All adolescents are preoccupied with clothes, so let her go ahead."
    c. "That sounds like a dead-end job. Why would Jenny want to work there?"
    d. "Working 30 hours a week may take time away from her studies and extracurricular activities and increase fatigue. Looking together at Jenny's future career goals may help identify alternatives."

30. List four primary causes of mortality accounting for 75% of all adolescent deaths.

31. To best effect adolescent health promotion activity, the nurse should incorporate which one of the following in the plan?
    a. The adolescent's definition of health
    b. The adolescent's past health promotion activities
    c. A complete assessment of the adolescent's past medical treatment
    d. A complete physical examination

32. Health concerns consistent with middle adolescence include:
    a. school performance.
    b. emotional health issues.
    c. physical appearance.
    d. future career or employment.

33. School-based health promotion interventions for adolescents do *not* include which of the following?
    a. Classroom health education
    b. Adopting school-level policies
    c. Environmental changes at the school
    d. Mass media production

34. School-linked clinics:
    a. are located on school property and serve adolescent populations from that campus.
    b. do not require parental consent before service can be provided to the adolescent.
    c. provide greater access to adolescents for preventive and primary care services.
    d. have not been widely accepted by the adolescents, since they are not receptive to services offered.

35. Adolescents are more likely to participate in health care services when:
    a. they understand the potentially negative consequences of their health behavior.
    b. they rank confidential care and respect higher than site cleanliness.
    c. they view their health problems as not organic in nature.
    d. they see the health provider as caring and respectful.

36. Factors that best promote adolescent health and well-being include:
    a. the ability of the adolescent to adapt to new persons and situations.
    b. the ability of the adolescent to have universal access to the Internet.
    c. interventions that focus the responsibility for adolescent health to one person or setting.
    d. health promotion efforts aimed at identification of adolescent needs.

37. Effective health education and health care for adolescents does *not* include which one of the following?
    a. Recognizes that adolescents, as they progress through adolescence, can assume additional responsibility for their own health.
    b. Recognizes that the need to maintain privacy and confidentiality decreases as the adolescent ages.
    c. Should meet the physical and emotional needs of the adolescent.
    d. Recognizes that parents need to respect their teenagers' independence and move more toward the role of health consultant.

38. List three strategies that nurses can use in school and clinical settings to promote adolescent self-advocacy skills.

39. During the adolescent health screening interview, the nurse focuses on which of the following to best address injury prevention?
    a. Drownings
    b. Burns
    c. Motor vehicle crashes
    d. Drug use

40. The most appropriate way to prevent firearm injury among adolescents is:
    a. teaching the adolescent proper use of firearms.
    b. counseling the adolescent on nonviolent ways to resolve conflict.
    c. passing laws to prevent parents from having guns.
    d. telling parents to keep guns and ammunition in separate locations within the house.

41. Adolescent girls of low socioeconomic status are particularly at risk for dietary deficiencies of:
       i. calories.
      ii. sodium.
     iii. calcium.
      iv. folic acid.
       v. iron.

    a. i, ii, and iii
    b. ii, iii, iv, and v
    c. iii, iv, and v
    d. i, iii, and v

42. When is a screening hemoglobin or hematocrit recommended for adolescents?
    a. At the first health provider encounter with an adolescent
    b. At the end of pubertal development
    c. At both of the above visits
    d. At neither of the above visits

43. Routine nutrition screening for all adolescents should include:
    a. a complete laboratory evaluation.
    b. questions about meal patterns and consumption of foods.
    c. a complete physical examination.
    d. a complete family history.

44. Which of the following statements as it relates to adolescent physical fitness is true?
    a. Female students are more likely to engage in vigorous physical activity.
    b. High levels of physical activity may increase cardiovascular disease risk factors during adolescence.
    c. Routine exercise has little positive effect on adolescents' risk for depression and emotional stress.
    d. Routine screening of all adolescents should include information about frequency, intensity, and type of physical activity.

45. Which of the following statements as it relates to use of tobacco, alcohol, and cannabis among adolescents is true?
    a. Substance abuse decreases with age, and adolescents between 14 and 15 years of age have the highest use pattern.
    b. The prevalence of binge drinking and tobacco use among high school students is increasing.
    c. Adolescents may use tobacco, alcohol, and marijuana because these substances provide an opportunity to challenge authority, demonstrate autonomy, gain entry into a peer group, or simply relieve the stress of growing up.
    d. Adolescents who begin smoking at a later age are at greater risk for becoming a life-long smoker.

46. Susan, age 15 years, comes to the school-based clinic and complains to the nurse practitioner about a vaginal discharge. After the nurse has established a trusting and confidential relationship, Susan confides that she has been sexually active with three different partners within the past 6 months. She thinks they used condoms every time, but she is not sure. Susan's last period was 4 weeks ago, and she has never had a Pap test. What tests would the nurse assisting the nurse practitioner expect to prepare for?
    i. Pap test
    ii. Gonorrhea test
    iii. Chlamydia test
    iv. Human immunodeficiency virus test
    v. Pregnancy test
    vi. Syphilis test

    a. ii, iii, iv, v, and vi
    b. i, ii, iii, iv, v, and vi
    c. ii, iii, iv, and vi
    d. i and v

47. The troubled adolescent thinking about suicide should be immediately referred for acute intervention when _____
    _____   _____

    _____.

48. Cindy, age 16 years, reports that she has been sexually abused by her uncle. The nurse knows that the adolescent who has been a victim of sexual abuse:
    a. should be informed about the steps in the reporting process before information is disclosed to local authorities.
    b. is more likely to become a runaway.
    c. is more likely to remain in school and form ties with less-threatening families.
    d. will usually attempt suicide within 1 month of reporting the incident.

49. Major risk factors for the development of adult cardiovascular disease can be identified during adolescence. List them.

50. The adolescent with body art:
    a. seeks body art as an expression of personal identity and style and to mark significant life events.
    b. is at lower risk for scarring if the piercing was done on the ear or nose because of the poor blood supply.
    c. should be advised to have the professional use a piercing gun for all piercings.
    d. should be advised that complications of piercing include infection and bleeding, but rarely keloid formation, which occurs most often with tattoos.

51. Sleep patterns among adolescents:
    a. show that teens should get at least 10 hours of sleep nightly.
    b. show that 1 in 8 is regularly sleep deprived.
    c. show that sleep deprivation contributes to school problems.
    d. show that 1 in 4 report use of the Internet as the major reason for lack of sufficient sleep.

52. Which of the following guidelines, if provided to the adolescent about tanning, is correct?
    a. If using self-tanning cream, no further sun protection is required.
    b. Sunscreens should include a sun protective factor (SPF) higher than 15 and an alcohol base with lanolin.
    c. Long-term effects can include premature aging of the skin; increased risk for skin cancer; and, in some adolescents, phototoxic reactions.
    d. Dermatologists recommend tanning machines if used no more often than two times monthly.

53. The nurse, in working with special groups of adolescents, recognizes which of the following statements is true?
    a. Effective health promotion programs for minority adolescents must contain culturally competent information and must be provided by health care professionals with the same cultural background as the adolescent.
    b. Gay and lesbian adolescents programs aimed at "reparative therapy" or treatment designed to alter sexual orientation show no evidence of effectiveness but do show evidence of psychological harm.
    c. Nurses should encourage all gay and lesbian adolescents to disclose their sexual orientation to their families immediately to help eliminate the stress of keeping "the secret."
    d. Rural adolescents' access to health care is the same as for urban areas because of the advantages of Medicaid and incentives offered to physicians to work in these areas.

CRITICAL THINKING—CASE STUDY

Shawna, a 16-year-old, visits the nurse practitioner for a routine checkup. Shawna is an A and B student in school and a member of the girls' drill team. She matured early and started to menstruate at the age of 10. Her menses are now regular. She has a boyfriend and has been dating since the age of 13. Shawna tells the nurse she has no specific concerns.

54. Based on risk factors associated with teens of Shawna's age, the nurse recognizes which one of the following as the most important to discuss with Shawna at this time?
    a. Shawna's perception and concerns about health
    b. Shawna's nutritional habits
    c. Shawna's sexual activity
    d. Shawna's relationship with her family

55. The nurse establishes a trusting relationship with Shawna, who admits to having been sexually active with five boys since she started dating. Besides educating her on the risks for sexually transmitted infections and pregnancy, which one of the following is most important for the nurse to include in her care plan for Shawna at this time?
    a. Discuss with Shawna how she can tell her parents about her sexual activity.
    b. Explore possible reasons for Shawna's behavior with her.
    c. Assess Shawna's immunization status for hepatitis B and human papillomavirus.
    d. Assess how Shawna feels about the possibility of getting pregnant.

56. Mrs. Smith complains to you that her 15-year-old son, Ben, has begun to drift away from the family and that he finds fault with everything she and her husband do. She is worried about the relationship between them and does not understand what she and her husband have done wrong. "Why does Ben seem to suddenly dislike us so much?" Based on your knowledge of adolescent behavior, which one of the following would be the best explanation?
    a. "Ben's behavioral standards are set by his peer group, and he is acting this way because of fear of rejection by this group."
    b. "Ben is defining his moral values, and you and your husband will need to have the same moral values as Ben if you want to continue to be close to him."
    c. "Ben is developing the capacity for abstract thinking and increasing his concern about social issues. He will return to share your views shortly."
    d. "Ben is defining independence-dependence boundaries and beginning to disengage from parents."

57. Christy, age 14, comes to the clinic for a physical examination. It has been longer than 2 years since her last examination. On review of Christy's immunization record, the nurse notes that Christy had a diphtheria-tetanus–acellular pertussis (DTaP) booster at age 4 years and a second measles-mumps-rubella (MMR) vaccine at age 4 years. Past medical history reveals that Christy had been diagnosed with hepatitis A when she was 4 years of age and varicella at age 2 years. Since then, she has been healthy. Which of the following immunizations would you expect Christy to receive today?
    a. Influenza, pneumococcal, and chickenpox vaccines
    b. MMR, hepatitis B, and hepatitis A vaccines
    c. Tdap (acellular pertussis, diphtheria toxoid, and tetanus toxoid), meningococcal, HPV (human papillomavirus), and hepatitis B vaccines
    d. Mantoux tuberculin, hepatitis B, Tdap, and HPV vaccines

58. Carl, age 16 years, has been brought to the clinic after taking some drugs given to him by a friend at school. He is now alert and, after talking to the nurse, confides that he is gay. Carl's parents do not know he is gay. Which one of the following most likely explains Carl's drug-taking behavior?
    a. Carl is suicidal.
    b. Carl is a chronic drug user.
    c. Carl used the drugs as an escape from anxieties and emotional distress related to keeping his sexuality secret.
    d. Carl took the drugs as an attempt to call attention to himself and his gay lifestyle.

Chapter **17** **Health Promotion of the Adolescent and Family**

18 Health Problems of the Adolescent

1. Which one of the following current beliefs about acne formation is true?
   a. Cosmetics containing lanolin and lauryl alcohol are not known to contribute to acne formation.
   b. There is scientific research to support the theory that stress will cause an acne outbreak.
   c. Exposure to oils in cooking grease can be a precursor to acne in adolescents working over fast-food restaurant oils.
   d. Acne usually worsens with dietary intake of chocolates and other foods high in sugars.

2. Nancy, age 16 years, comes to see the nurse because of acne on her face and shoulders. After talking with Nancy, the nurse makes a nursing diagnosis of Knowledge Deficit related to proper skin care. Which one of the following would the nurse include in the instruction plan for Nancy?
   a. Wash the areas vigorously with antibacterial soaps.
   b. Brush the hair down on the forehead to conceal the acne areas.
   c. Avoid the use of all cosmetics.
   d. Gently wash the areas with a mild soap once or twice daily.

3. The practitioner has prescribed tretinoin cream (Retin-A) for Nancy's acne. Nancy has been using the cream for 2 weeks and is concerned she is not improving. Nancy tells the nurse that she has "done everything" that she was told to do and asks, "Why is my acne no better?" The nurse's best reply is:
   a. "Since the medication prevents the formation of new comedones, it will take at least 6 weeks for improvement to be obvious."
   b. "You must not be using the medication right. Show me how you apply it to your face."
   c. "Acne is caused by dirt or oil on the surface of the skin. You will need to increase the number of times you wash these areas each day."
   d. "You will probably need to ask the practitioner about changing your medicine as soon as possible."

4. The nurse is conducting an educational session with Cindy and her parents on medications used for acne. Which of the following is correct information?
   i. Benzoyl peroxide gel has a bleaching effect on bed coverings and towels.
   ii. Topical clindamycin is applied only to the individual lesions.
   iii. Oral contraceptive medications contain estrogen, which will increase acne formation and should be avoided.
   iv. Tretinoin requires that Cindy protect herself from sun exposure.
   v. Oral antibiotics are intended for short-term therapy and are not considered safe for long-term treatment.
   vi. Minocycline is more expensive but less likely to cause gastrointestinal side effects and is effective against severe inflammatory acne.
   vii. Results are better if systemic antibiotics are combined with topical antibiotic creams.
   viii. Resistance to amoxicillin and tetracycline usually develops.

   a. i, iv, and vi
   b. i, ii, iii, and iv
   c. ii, iv, v, vi, and vii
   d. i, v, and viii

5. The proper use of isotretinoin 12-*cis*-retinoic acid (Accutane) for adolescents includes:
   i. reserving its use for severe, cystic acne that has not responded to other treatments.
   ii. limiting treatment to 20 weeks.
   iii. watching for side effects, including mood changes, depression, and suicidal ideation.
   iv. watching for detrimental effects on bone mineralization.
   v. recognizing that it is contraindicated in pregnancy and in sexually active females not using an effective contraceptive method.
   vi. monitoring for elevated cholesterol and triglyceride levels before and during treatment.

a. i, ii, iv, and v
b. i, iii, and v
c. i, ii, iii, v, and vi
d. i, ii, iii, iv, v, and vi

6. Which one of the following is associated with 65% of all penile neoplasias?
   a. Human papillomavirus (HPV) types 6 and 11
   b. HPV type 16
   c. Uncircumcised males
   d. Paraphimosis

7. The adolescent with testicular cancer is most likely to be initially seen with which of the following signs and symptoms?
   a. Tender, painful swelling of the testes
   b. A mass in the posterior aspect of the scrotum that can be transilluminated
   c. A heavy, hard, painless mass palpable on the anterior or lateral surface of the testicle
   d. An asymptomatic scrotal mass that aches, especially after exercise or penile erection

8. In teaching the adolescent male how to perform testicular self-examination, the nurse includes which of the following in the instructions?
   a. Perform the procedure once a month after a warm shower.
   b. A raised swelling palpated on the superior aspect of the testicle indicates an abnormality.
   c. Use the second and third fingers on each hand, holding each testicle between the fingers while palpating it with the other fingers.
   d. The normal testicle will feel soft with a round, smooth contour.

9. The pelvic examination in the adolescent:
   a. should be performed on all females who are sexually active.
   b. should only be conducted when there is a suspicion of a sexually transmitted disease.
   c. is always conducted with a parent or guardian in the room.
   d. should allow for the opportunity to discuss safe sex practices, prevention of sexually transmitted diseases, and postponement of sexual involvement.

10. Match each term with its definition. (Terms may be used more than once.)

    a. Varicocele   e. Paraphimosis
    b. Epididymitis   f. Priapism
    c. Testicular torsion   g. Penile fracture
    d. Gynecomastia

    _____ Breast enlargement that occurs during puberty

    _____ Wormlike mass that is palpated above the testicle and becomes smaller when the adolescent lies down

    _____ Benign and temporary disease that occurs in about 50% of adolescent boys

    _____ Tight foreskin of the penis that cannot be retracted

    _____ Inflammation that is a result of infection, local trauma, or chemical irritant

    _____ Rupture of the corpus cavernosum as a result of trauma to the erect penis

    _____ Marked by the testis hanging free from its vascular structure; results in partial or complete venous occlusion

    _____ Characterized by unilateral scrotal pain, redness, and swelling; may include urethral discharge, dysuria, fever, and pyuria; treated with antibiotics

    _____ Prolonged penile erection

    _____ Manifested by scrotum that is swollen, painful, red, and warm; pain radiating to groin, accompanied by nausea, vomiting, and abdominal pain; typically, an absence of fever and urinary symptoms; immediate surgery required to treat

    _____ The most common treatable cause of male-related impaired fertility

11. Match each term with its definition.

   a. Amenorrhea
   b. Primary amenorrhea
   c. Secondary amenorrhea

   d. Dysmenorrhea
   e. Primary dysmenorrhea

   _____ Pain during or shortly before menstruation

   _____ Associated with ovulatory cycles; usually appears 6 to 12 months after menarche when ovulation is established

   _____ The absence of menstrual flow

   _____ A 6-month or more cessation of menses in a previous menstruating female

   _____ The absence of menses by 16.5 years, regardless of normal growth and development

12. Linda, age 16, started her menses at age 13 years. She comes into the school-based clinic with a history of secondary amenorrhea. Linda is an honor student and a long-distance runner who runs an average of 50 miles per week. The physical examination and laboratory testing results are normal with a negative pregnancy test. Linda's exercise program is thought to contribute to her amenorrhea. Discuss options for management.

13. A treatment of choice for adolescents with dysmenorrhea is:
   a. acetaminophen.
   b. oral contraceptives.
   c. nonsteroidal antiinflammatory drugs.
   d. estrogen-suppression drugs.

14. Match the term with its description.

   a. Syphilis
   b. Premenstrual syndrome
   c. Endometriosis
   d. Dysfunctional uterine bleeding
   e. Vulvovaginal candidiasis
   f. *Trichomonas* vaginitis

   g. Leukorrhea
   h. Bacterial vaginosis
   i. Pelvic inflammatory disease (PID)
   j. Dyspareunia
   k. Abnormal uterine bleeding

   _____ Uterine bleeding that is irregular in amount, duration, or timing and is not related to regular menstrual bleeding

   _____ Condition that has more than 150 associated physical, psychologic, and behavioral symptoms beginning in the luteal phase of the menstrual cycle

   _____ Condition that may be caused by the presence of endometrial tissue outside the uterine cavity

   _____ Abnormal vaginal bleeding, usually associated with anovulation

   _____ Symptoms that include thin, malodorous, "fishy" vaginal discharge; diagnosis confirmed by clue cells on microscopic examination

   _____ Infection of the upper genital tract (endometrium, fallopian tubes, and ovaries), most commonly caused by sexually transmitted bacteria, such as *Neisseria gonorrhoeae, Chlamydia trachomatis*, and a variety of other anaerobic bacteria

   _____ Painful sexual intercourse

   _____ Characterized by a primary lesion, the chancre, which appears 5 to 90 days after infection

   _____ Condition that may manifest with vaginal pruritus and dysuria and is not a sexually transmitted infection (STI); treated with over-the-counter topical antifungal creams; characterized by "cottage cheese–like" discharge

_____ An STI caused by an anaerobic parasitic protozoa

_____ Clear to cloudy vaginal discharge

15. Numerous factors have been identified as predisposing a woman to a vaginal yeast infection. Describe them.

16. In discussing prevention of STIs, the nurse tells the adolescent that which one of the following is most effective?
    a. Birth control pills
    b. Natural skin condoms with nonoxynol-9
    c. Spermicides
    d. Latex condoms

17. Name two STIs for which there is a vaccine.

18. Therapeutic management for chlamydia includes:
    a. doxycycline 100 mg twice daily for 7 days in the pregnant adolescent and her partner.
    b. intramuscular injection of ceftriaxone (Rocephrin) 125 mg for the patient and partner.
    c. intramuscular injection of penicillin 2.4 million international units for the patient and partner.
    d. azithromycin 1 g orally in a single dose for the patient and partner.

19. The nurse is discussing PID with a group of sexually active adolescent females. Which of the following is correct information?
    i. *C. trachomatis* is estimated to cause half of all cases.
    ii. Using IUDs for birth control with more than one sexual partner increases the risk of developing PID.
    iii. Pain is not always found in patients presenting with PID.
    iv. After a single episode of PID, infertility occurs because of tubal scarring.
    v. After a single episode of PID, the risk for ectopic pregnancy increases.
    vi. All pregnant women with PID should be hospitalized and treated with parenteral antibiotics.

    a. i, ii, iii, and vi
    b. ii, v, and vi
    c. i, ii, v, and vi
    d. ii, iv, v, and vi

20. Lesley is a sexually active adolescent. She comes to the clinic with abdominal pain and vaginal bleeding. The nurse recognizes that which of the following must be ruled out immediately?
    a. Ectopic pregnancy
    b. Ovarian cyst
    c. STIs
    d. Endometriosis

21. Human papillomavirus (HPV):
    a. has 10 serotypes associated with causing genital warts.
    b. has lesions that resolve on their own in young women because their immune systems may be strong enough to fight the infection.
    c. has lesions that decrease in size or disappear during pregnancy.
    d. has lesions always visible to the naked eye on the cervix.

22. Herpes simplex virus (HSV):
    a. presents with a less severe clinical course in men than women.
    b. is treated with acyclovir, famciclovir, and valacyclovir for cure of the disease.
    c. is treated with ointments containing cortisone to help inflammation.
    d. requires cesarean birth within 4 hours after labor begins or membranes rupture, if visible lesions are present.

23. Which of the following statements related to human immunodeficiency virus (HIV) is true?
    a. Clinical and epidemiologic studies have shown that increasing levels of CD4 are associated with increased incidence of AIDS-related diseases.
    b. Transmission of the virus from the mother to the infant can occur as early as the first trimester of pregnancy.
    c. The FDA has approved six methods of rapid testing for HIV, requiring vaginal, anal, or oral fluid samples.
    d. Intravenous zidovudine is recommended for all HIV-infected pregnant women during the postpartum period.

24. Indicate whether the following statements are true or false.

    _____ Easy access to cars, unsupervised time at home, and changing family composition have contributed to the incidence of sexual experimentation among adolescents.

    _____ There is evidence that low self-esteem in females and males is associated with sexual intercourse at an earlier age.

    _____ Instruction in the skills needed to resist sexual intercourse has less influence on reducing sexual activity than does providing information on the dangers associated with sexual activity (STIs or pregnancy).

    _____ The less familiar an adolescent is with his or her partner, the more likely he or she is to use contraception during intercourse.

    _____ Contraception use increases among girls as the duration of the relationship increases.

    _____ Adolescents who have at least one supportive parent engage in less risky behavior.

    _____ The pregnancies of adolescents under 15 years old are less frequently complicated by obstetric problems.

    _____ During a second pregnancy for a teenager, obstetric risk and risk to the infant are lower.

    _____ Teens between 12 and 16 years are at high risk for prolonged labor related to fetopelvic incompatibility.

    _____ Pregnant adolescents often have diets deficient in iron, calcium, and folic acid.

    _____ Effective parent-child communication about sexuality can delay the onset of first sexual intercourse.

    _____ The teenage pregnancy rate continues to increase for all age-groups.

25. Ana, age 16, has not had a period for the past 3 months, and her pregnancy test is positive. Which of the following is *not* an appropriate action for the nurse to take at this time?
    a. Inform Ana privately that her test is positive.
    b. Review with Ana facts about the pregnancy, including the duration of pregnancy and anticipated due date.
    c. Understand that Ana's reaction may be one of ambivalence, shock, fear, or apathy.
    d. Arrange for Ana's parents to be present when Ana is given the news.

26. Infants of adolescents are at risk because:
    a. teenage mothers often neglect their infants, leaving them for long periods with grandparents.
    b. teenage mothers supply excessive amounts of cognitive stimulation to their infants.
    c. adolescents often lack knowledge about normal infant growth and development.
    d. adolescents are less likely to treat their infant as love objects or playthings.

27. The first goal in nursing care of the pregnant teenager is:
    a. to arrange for the pregnant teen to register for food supplement programs to ensure proper nutrition.
    b. to assist the pregnant teen in obtaining health care.
    c. to involve the boyfriend and parents in the pregnancy so that the pregnant teen will have support during her pregnancy.
    d. to educate the pregnant teen regarding child care.

28. Postpartum care of adolescents should be directed toward what goal?

29. A drug approved for medical abortion is mifepristone. Which of the following statements about this drug is true?
    a. The drug can be used to provide nonsurgical abortion up to 49 days of pregnancy.
    b. The drug promotes receptor binding of endogenous or exogenous progesterone.
    c. The abortion completion rate is 100% in pregnancies if used correctly.
    d. The drug is administered intramuscularly up to 49 days after the last menstrual period.

30. Amanda comes to the school nurse's office early in the morning, visibly upset. She tells the nurse that she and her boyfriend were having sexual relations last night and the condom broke. Amanda asks the nurse about a new pill she has read about that will keep her from becoming pregnant. She wants the nurse to give her more information about this pill. Which of the following statements made to Amanda provides the best information about levonorgestrel?
    a. "It is available without a prescription and must be taken within 24 hours of the unprotected sexual intercourse."
    b. "It is very effective but has side effects, so you will need to be out of school at least 1 day."
    c. "It contains estrogen, so you will need to have a pregnancy test before it can be administered."
    d. "It is available to women over the counter. It must be taken within 120 hours of the unprotected sexual intercourse."

31. The nurse is conducting a sexual education program. What technique has been found helpful when dealing with the subject of sexual abstinence?

32. Rape victims display a variety of manifestations. Which of the following might the nurse see in 16-year-old Sally as she arrives at the emergency department for treatment after being raped?
    a. Hysterical crying or giggling
    b. Calm and controlled behavior
    c. Anger and rage alternating with helplessness and agitation
    d. All of the above

33. The primary goal of nursing care for the adolescent rape victim is:
    a. not to inflict further stress on the victim.
    b. obtaining a complete history of the incident.
    c. assisting in the physical examination.
    d. notifying the police and the parents of the victim before proceeding with assessment.

34. Match each term to the correct definition.

    a. Overweight   d. Orexigenic
    b. Obesity   e. Anorexigenic
    c. Prader-Willi syndrome   f. Female athlete triad

    _____ Characterized by hypogonadism; slow intellectual development; short stature; they lack the internal mechanism that regulates food satiety and as a result go to great lengths to obtain food

    _____ Produce signals that increase appetite

    _____ Produce signals that promote cessation of appetite

    _____ Characterized by an eating disorder, amenorrhea, and osteoporosis

    _____ Refers to state of weighing more than average for height and body build

    _____ Age- and gender-specific BMI at or above the 95th percentile

35. Increased obesity among children is related to:
    a. high birth weight.
    b. underlying disease.
    c. enzyme abnormalities and metabolic defects.
    d. overeating.

36. Physical inactivity has been linked with overweight children. Which of the following explain this decrease in child-hood activity?
    i. Decrease in physical activity in secondary and elementary schools
    ii. Parental obesity and low levels of physical activity at home
    iii. Increased time spent with television, video games, computers, and the Internet
    iv. Lack of sidewalks, parks, and bike paths in low-income communities

    a. i, ii, and iii
    b. ii and iii
    c. i and iv
    d. i, ii, iii, and iv

37. Which of the following is *not* a complication of obesity in adolescents?
    a. Type 2 diabetes and insulin resistance
    b. Fatty liver disease
    c. Heart failure
    d. Sleep apnea

38. Psychologic and social findings in the obese adolescent include:
    a. negative self-image that persists into adulthood.
    b. decreased practice of unhealthy weight control behaviors as compared to thin adolescents.
    c. increased practice of bullying their classmates.
    d. being less sensitized to obesity and less inclined to incorporate the culture's preference for thinness.

39. Gail, age 14, comes to the health provider's office for a yearly physical. Gail has always been overweight but has gained 50 lb since her last visit and now fits the criteria of obesity. The diagnostic evaluation of Gail should include all of the following *except*:
    a. history regarding the development of obesity.
    b. physical examination to differentiate simple obesity from increased fat that results from organic disease.
    c. family history, especially regarding obesity, diabetes, heart disease, and dyslipidemia.
    d. laboratory studies for anemia.

40. BMI measurement in adolescents:
    a. is currently considered the most reliable method to predict future obesity.
    b. is recommended as the most accurate method for screening for obesity.
    c. is calculated based on skin thickness and muscle mass.
    d. requires determining total body density by total submersion in a water-filled tank.

41. Weight-reduction management in adolescents should include:
    a. significant caloric restriction.
    b. elimination of physical hunger cues.
    c. regular physical activity.
    d. appetite-suppressant drugs.

42. James has kept a diet history for the nurse, and the nurse has carefully reviewed this eating diary. Which one of the following suggestions would best promote healthy eating habits in James?
    a. Limit fast-food consumption to no more than three times a week.
    b. Take second helpings of meat and vegetables only.
    c. Do not skip meals.
    d. Include more low-fat foods.

43. Janie, age 14, wants to discuss with the nurse how to modify her eating habits to reduce her weight. Which one of the following methods does the nurse recognize as *least* helpful in assisting Janie to meet her goals?
    a. Have Janie keep a list of everything she eats.
    b. Request that Janie's parents remind Janie not to eat junk foods.
    c. Establish a system of rewards for changes in eating habits.
    d. Discuss with Janie methods other than eating that can be used to deal with emotional stress.

44. Obesity and overweight nutritional counseling is aimed at preventing an increase in body fat during growth. List the four aspects of changing eating habits that can best accomplish this.

45. The best approach to the management of obesity in children and adolescents is:
    a. prevention.
    b. pharmacologic agents sibutramine and orlistat.
    c. bariatric surgery.
    d. behavior modification.

46. When initiating a treatment plan for obesity, the nurse should do which of the following?
    a. Defer treatment until the family is ready to begin.
    b. Proceed with the plan regardless of the family's readiness if the adolescent is ready.
    c. Understand that the adolescent cannot take personal responsibility for dietary habits and physical activity.
    d. Understand that adolescents who are forced by their parents to seek help can easily become motivated.

47. a. Anorexia nervosa is characterized by:

    b. Bulimia nervosa is characterized by:

48. Cindy, age 16, has been sent to the school nurse because her gym teacher has noticed a marked decrease in Cindy's weight since vacation. Which one of the following does the nurse recognize as a common finding in an adolescent girl with anorexia nervosa?
    a. Wears form-fitting clothes like tank tops and jeans
    b. Has strong peer relationships with classmates and several best friends
    c. Has poor schoolwork performance because of little interest in school
    d. Is present at meals, selects foods, and appears to family and friends to be eating appropriately

49. Karen is suspected of being bulimic. The nurse recognizes which of the following as clinically characteristic of this disease?
    a. Bulimia often begins with decreased dietary intake associated with poor relationships with family members.
    b. Once started, the bingeing decreases in frequency to only about once per day.
    c. Insulin production is decreased because of excessive self-induced vomiting.
    d. Impulse control and satiety regulation are problems in bulimic adolescents.

50. Which of the following diagnostic findings would most likely confirm the diagnosis of bulimia in Karen?
    a. Presence of distinctive lesions on the hands (Russell sign), that is, scars and cuts from repeated abrasions of the skin
    b. Hypertension, weakness, and cool skin
    c. Elevated potassium, magnesium, and erythrocyte sedimentation rate
    d. A heart murmur diagnosed as mitral valve prolapse

51. Adolescents with anorexia nervosa are at risk for refeeding syndrome. Which one of the following best describes refeeding syndrome?
    a. It reduces the risk for osteoporosis and returns the menses to normal.
    b. The risk for heart failure is greatest during the first 2 days of treatment.
    c. It occurs because of shifts in phosphate from extracellular to intracellular spaces in persons with total body phosphorus depletion.
    d. It causes mitral valve prolapse and significant electrolyte imbalance.

52. What are the three main focus goals for the therapeutic management of anorexia nervosa?

53. Cindy has been diagnosed with anorexia nervosa. Her therapeutic management plan includes dietary interventions combined with family psychotherapy. Which one of the following would the nurse recognize as appropriate?
    a. Weight gain is a sign that the patient is not relapsing from the plan.
    b. The patient is only allowed to participate in setting up a food plan as a reward for weight gain.
    c. The plan needs to be firm but flexible.
    d. A reasonable goal for weight gain is about 4 lb/wk.

54. Which of the following is *least* appropriate when developing an outpatient contract between the patient with an eating disorder and the therapist?
    a. Begin the psychotherapy immediately before the contract is developed and before weight gain.
    b. Develop the contract so that the patient's feeling of control and responsibility toward recovery is established.
    c. Specify in the contract the weight at which tube feedings will be implemented.
    d. Specify in the contract when rewards for achievement will be implemented.

55. In treating eating disorders:
    a. weight gain is a reliable sign of positive progress.
    b. when a therapeutic environment is removed, relapses seldom occur.
    c. antianxiety or antidepressant drug use has not been proven effective.
    d. psychotherapy is aimed at resolving adolescent identity crises and distorted body image.

56. Identify the following statements about substance abuse as true or false.

    _____ A person may be physically dependent on a narcotic without being addicted.

    _____ A 2010 survey found that marijuana use and acceptance of marijuana has been on the rise since 2007, while alcohol use has been on the decline since 1980.

    _____ The usual goal for the compulsive drug user is peer acceptance.

    _____ The abuse of prescription and synthetic drugs such as Xanax and oxycodone has increased significantly among adolescents.

    _____ Reports show that adolescents believe that prescription medications, although not taken under practitioner orders, are safer than illicit substances.

    _____ Cough and cold preparations such as NyQuil, Coricidin, and Robitussin were reported in 2006 to be favorite substances abused to get high among persons ages 12 to 25 years of age.

    _____ Cigarette smoking is the chief avoidable cause of death.

    _____ Smokeless tobacco has been proven to be carcinogenic, and regular use can cause dental problems, foul-smelling breath, and tooth erosion or loss.

    _____ Adolescents with alcoholism seldom drink alone.

57. Which one of the following adolescents does the nurse recognize as *least* likely to begin smoking?
    a. Johnny, age 16 years, whose father quit smoking 2 years ago
    b. Karen, age 15 years, whose older sister smokes
    c. Ted, age 17 years, who smoked a cigarette at home in front of his parents
    d. Lilly, age 12, who feels uncomfortable with her early-maturing body

58. The school nurse is planning an educational program centered on smoking prevention for high school adolescents. Which of the following methods does the nurse recognize as the most effective way to present this program?
    a. Focus on the negative, long-term effects of smoking on health.
    b. Teach methods of resistance to peer pressure.
    c. Use peer-led programs that emphasize social consequences.
    d. Use media, videotapes, and films on smoking prevention.

59. Complete the following statements about drug abuse.

    a. The form of cocaine known as the purer and more menacing form is _____.
    b. The physical signs of narcotic abuse are:

    _____

    _____

    c. _____, also known as the "date rape drug," is 10 times more powerful than diazepam and produces short-term memory loss.

    d. _____, with the street names of "crank" and "crystal," produces more stimulation than cocaine, and the user can remain "up" for hours.
    e. Inhalant abuse usually gives the child an inexpensive euphoria but is extremely dangerous and can cause three immediate life-threatening consequences. These consequences are:

    _____

    _____

60. Mark, age 14 years, has been rushed to the emergency department because of illegal drug ingestion at a party. Which of the following are most important for the nurse to collect to assist in the emergency treatment plan?
     i. The type and amount of drug taken
     ii. The time the drug was taken and mode of administration
     iii. Number of times Mark has previously overdosed
     iv. Why the drug was taken

    a. i and ii
    b. i, ii, and iii
    c. i only
    d. i, ii, iii, and iv

61. Match each term with its description.

    a. Suicidal ideation   d. Suicide
    b. Suicide attempt   e. Contagion suicide
    c. Parasuicide

    _____ Behaviors range from gestures to attempts to kill oneself

    _____ Deliberate act of self-injury with death as result

    _____ Deliberate but unsuccessful act of self-injury

    _____ Preoccupation with thoughts about committing suicide

    _____ Phenomenon resulting from excessive media coverage after an adolescent suicide

62. Which one of the following is the most common method of successful suicide among adolescents?
    a. Overdose of drugs
    b. Firearms
    c. Self-inflicted lacerations
    d. Hanging

63. Jim, who has no history of previous suicide attempts, is talking with the school nurse about his feelings of despair and hopelessness about the future. He tells the nurse he would be better off dead. The nurse's best response is which one of the following?
    a. Recognize that Jim is going through a common phase of adolescence.
    b. Recognize that Jim is at low risk for suicide, since he has not previously attempted suicide.
    c. Explain to Jim that suicide never solved anything and that he will feel better tomorrow.
    d. Take Jim seriously, allow time for him to verbalize his feelings, and stay with him until referral.

64. The nurse has been asked to present an educational program on prevention of adolescent stress and suicide. In planning the program, the nurse should include:
    a. the importance of being supportive and establishing positive communication patterns between family and teens.
    b. the precipitating factors for suicide.
    c. effective coping mechanisms and problem-solving skills.
    d. all of the above.

CRITICAL THINKING—CASE STUDY

Kenny, 16 years of age, visits the clinic for follow-up of a recent infection he obtained while on a hunting trip. While talking with the nurse, he tells her that he has recently broken up with his girlfriend after going steady for 11 months. Kenny has a history of having a difficult home situation. His recent school performance has declined, and this has further upset Kenny's parents and their expectations for him. Physical examination of Kenny reveals an expressionless face with a slight smell of alcohol on his breath and signs consistent with depression.

65. The nurse suspects that Kenny might be suicidal. Which factors in the preceding data might support this assumption?
    i. Alcohol consumption
    ii. Recent breakup with girlfriend
    iii. History of difficult home situation
    iv. Depression
    v. Has a gun available to him

    a. i, ii, iii, and iv
    b. ii, iii, and iv
    c. ii, iv, and v
    d. i, ii, iii, iv, and v

66. On questioning by the nurse, Kenny admits to suicidal ideation. What should the nurse first assess to determine risk?
    a. History of suicide attempts within the family
    b. Past methods of coping with stress by the individual
    c. Whether Kenny has a plan for suicide
    d. How Kenny feels about suicide

67. Which one of the following nursing diagnoses would the nurse develop to best deal with Kenny's suicide thoughts?
    a. High Risk for Injury related to feelings of rejection
    b. Sleep Pattern Disturbance related to inability to sleep
    c. Social Isolation related to withdrawal from friends
    d. High Risk for Self-Directed Violence related to excessive alcohol use

68. The most important goal in the nursing management for Kenny at this time should focus on:
    a. reestablishing Kenny's relationship with his girlfriend.
    b. teaching Kenny how to cope with the stress of being an adolescent.
    c. maintaining physical safety for Kenny.
    d. helping Kenny express his emotional pain and regain his ability to perform assigned tasks.

19 Family-Centered Care of the Child with Chronic Illness or Disability

1. Match each term with its description.

   a. Chronic illness
   b. Congenital disability
   c. Family-centered care
   d. Developmental disability
   e. Disability

   f. Normalization
   g. Impairment
   h. Early intervention
   i. Home care
   j. Mainstreaming

   _____ Refers to establishing a normal pattern of living

   _____ A disability that has existed since birth but is not necessarily hereditary

   _____ Includes any systematic and sustained effort to assist young, disabled, and developmentally vulnerable children from birth to 3 years of age

   _____ A condition that interferes with daily functioning for more than 3 months

   _____ Any mental and/or physical disability that is manifested before age 22 years and is likely to continue indefinitely

   _____ A system of care with the goals to normalize the child's life, lessen disruption on the family, and maximize the child's growth and development

   _____ Goal of care is to minimize the manifestatioins of the illness and maximize the child's cognitive, physical, and psychosocial potential

   _____ The process of integrating children with special needs into regular classrooms and child care centers

   _____ A loss or abnormality of a structure or function

   _____ A result of an impairment that could be physical, cognitive, mental, sensory, emotional developmental, or a combination of these

2. Which one of the following diseases is the most common chronic childhood illness?
   a. Asthma
   b. Congenital heart disease
   c. Cancer
   d. Spina bifida

3. Which of the following is an example of how chronic illness and disability affect children's health, functional status, and family functioning?
   a. Families do not bring the disabled child for health care often.
   b. Siblings' routines are completely separated from those of the disabled child.
   c. Parents are usually not able to meet the child's normal developmental needs.
   d. Disabled children are often absent from school.

4. Emphasizing the characteristics that the disabled child has in common with other children, rather than viewing the disabilities within a pathologic framework, best describes which one of the following approaches to care of the disabled child?
   a. Chronologic
   b. Developmental

5. A goal that would be considered inappropriate for family-centered care would be to:
   a. maintain family routine in the hospital.
   b. empower the family members.
   c. support the family during stressful times.
   d. maintain a high level of professional control.

6. The individualized family service plan (IFSP) is:
   a. developed jointly by families and professionals.
   b. a comprehensive insurance plan for families with a disabled child.
   c. developed by a team of professionals for the disabled child.
   d. a plan that finances direct services for the disabled child.

7. When working with people of other cultural backgrounds who are caring for a child with a disability, the nurse should plan care that:
   a. uses a family member to translate into the family's language.
   b. incorporates the generalized culture of the United States.
   c. recognizes that culture fully defines how the child and family will react.
   d. remains consistent with the family's cultural practices when possible.

8. Match each developmental stage with the particular area of development in which a disability poses a challenge or risk.

   a. Infant
   b. Toddler
   c. Preschooler

   d. School-age child
   e. Adolescent

   _____ Self-concept and body image

   _____ Social development

   _____ Attachment

   _____ Mobility

   _____ Participation

9. A strategy that is recommended to promote normalization in children with special needs would be to:
   a. avoid discussing issues of appearance in the adolescent.
   b. focus on the areas of ability and competence.
   c. establish special family rules for the child with a disability.
   d. allow children with special needs to make all decisions about their care.

10. The child who is disabled tends to develop appropriate independence and achievement when the parents:
    a. protect the child from all dangers.
    b. establish reasonable limits.
    c. emphasize the child's limits.
    d. isolate the child to avoid peer rejection.

11. Which one of the following strategies would be *inappropriate* for the nurse to use when teaching families with children who are disabled?
    a. Give information that meets the child's current needs.
    b. Give as much information as possible at the time of diagnosis.
    c. Answer the child's questions openly.
    d. Repeat information as often as needed.

12. The adolescent patient with a disability or chronic illness should be transferred to an adult provider:
    a. when the patient reaches the age of 18 years.
    b. when the patient reaches the age of 16 years.
    c. when the patient knows about the chronic condition and is prepared for the transition.
    d. it is best not to change providers.

13. The purpose of the initial assessment of coping mechanisms in a child who is disabled is for the nurse to:
    a. determine help that the family may want or need.
    b. establish rapport with the child and family.
    c. provide care from stage to stage of development.
    d. provide care from phase to phase of the disorder.

14. Which one of the following statements is *false* about family members' perceptions of a child's illness or disability?
    a. Children may interpret the illness or disability as a punishment.
    b. Family members are usually shocked to learn that their child has a serious illness or disability.
    c. Parents may interpret the illness or disability as a punishment.
    d. Family members usually have no knowledge about the disorder when they learn their child has it.

15. Which of the following statements about the time of diagnosis is *false*?
    a. Parents may not remember all that is said.
    b. Parents remember the tone of the communication.
    c. Parents cannot sense the tone of the communication.
    d. Parents may not hear all that is said.

16. When initially informing the family of a child's serious condition, the nurse should:
    a. explain that, with time, everything will be all right.
    b. accept any emotional reaction without judgment.
    c. decide when and how to tell the child about the diagnosis.
    d. use therapeutic touch to stimulate free expression of feelings.

17. Describe at least three guidelines for the nurse to use when providing ongoing information to the family with a disabled or chronically ill child.

18. Parents in thriving families:
    a. stress normalcy and feel confident.
    b. have an enduring management style.
    c. feel competent but burdened.
    d. feel dominated by the illness.

19. The two most important environments for the child who is disabled or chronically ill are _____ and _____.

20. In adjusting to a child's chronic illness, the father is more likely than the mother to:
    a. suffer from isolation.
    b. use an emotional release.
    c. perceive he is coping poorly.
    d. view the child's temperament as influential.

21. To help siblings prepare for the changes in the disabled child, the nurse should:
    a. wait until questions are asked, since siblings often desire little or no involvement.
    b. recognize that permitting sibling hospital visits will increase stress in the whole family.
    c. reassure siblings that they will continue to be involved in the care whenever possible.
    d. help the sibling realize that the disabled child needs more parental attention.

22. Research indicates that, compared with their peers, siblings of a child with a disability exhibit:
    a. greater independence.
    b. more maturity.
    c. an increased sense of responsibility.
    d. all of the above.

23. Which one of the following characteristics would most likely indicate that a sibling of a child with a disability is having difficulty?
   a. Sharing
   b. Withdrawal
   c. Competing
   d. Compromising

24. Describe how an extended family member may be a source of stress to the parents of the disabled or chronically ill child.

25. Identify each of the following coping behaviors as an approach behavior or an avoidance behavior.

   a. _____ A father stops at a friend's house and talks about his child's poor prognosis.

   b. _____ A father's alcohol use increases to the point of being excessive.

   c. _____ A mother tells the nurse that she is afraid to tell her child about his or her poor prognosis.

   d. _____ A mother never carries a glucose source for her toddler who takes insulin for type 1 diabetes mellitus.

   e. _____ A mother begins to cry in the nurse's office at school, saying that she always gets depressed at the beginning of the new year.

   f. _____ A father asks the nurse to explain a diagnosis again.

   g. _____ A mother asks her neighbor to watch her older child for a few hours while she is at the clinic.

26. Corbin and Strauss's chronic illness trajectory model is based on the idea that the:
   a. family understands the meaning of the illness situation.
   b. course of the illness changes over time.
   c. family member roles do not change with illness.
   d. coping patterns for the illness can be learned.

27. Nursing interventions that can encourage and empower families include:
   a. fostering normalization.
   b. teaching coping skills.
   c. assisting to define social support networks.
   d. all of the above.

28. If a family member reacts to the diagnosis of a chronic illness with denial, the nurse would recognize that denial is:
   a. an abnormal response to grieving this type of loss.
   b. preventing treatment and rehabilitation.
   c. necessary to prevent disintegration.
   d. necessary for the child's optimum development.

29. In regard to denial, it is imperative that health professionals:
   a. actively attempt to remove the denial behaviors.
   b. repeatedly give blunt explanations.
   c. label denial as maladaptive.
   d. understand the concept of denial.

30. Hope in the chronically ill child's family would be considered:
   a. a way to absorb stress in a manageable way.
   b. negative coping with a serious diagnosis.
   c. a maladaptive mechanism for dealing with the inevitable death.
   d. to have the same meaning for the nurse and the family.

31. Describe at least two effective methods of support that would help families manage their emotional response to the diagnosis of a disability or chronic illness in their child.

32. A strategy for the nurse to encourage parents to express their feelings about the diagnosis of a chronic illness in their child would be to:
    a. tell them that what they are going through is completely understandable.
    b. help them focus on their emotions.
    c. explain the policies and procedures regarding visiting hours.
    d. review the disease process with them.

33. Parents who provide adequate physical care but detach themselves emotionally from the child characterizes the type of parental reaction known as:
    a. overprotection.
    b. denial.
    c. gradual acceptance.
    d. rejection.

34. The nurse's response to anger in parents of a disabled child should be:
    a. reciprocal anger.
    b. disapproval.
    c. acceptance.
    d. avoidance.

35. List at least five characteristics of parental overprotection.

36. Nurses who provide support to parents of a child with a disability should develop an attitude that has all of the following characteristics *except* the belief that:
    a. every person has burdens to bear.
    b. trust is a foundation for good communication.
    c. parents are experts about their own child.
    d. parents and professionals are colleagues.

37. When the parents of a child with special needs experience chronic sorrow, the process:
    a. of grief is pronounced and self-limiting.
    b. involves social reintegration after grieving.
    c. is characterized by realistic expectations.
    d. is interspersed with periods of intensified grief.

38. Which one of the following stressors can usually be predicted for a child with special needs?
    a. The approximate cost of the yearly medical bills
    b. The future needs for residential care
    c. The types of schooling and vocational training that will be needed
    d. The stress of developmental milestones and the start of school

39. The adjustment of the family to caring for and living with the child with special needs is greatly influenced by the:
    a. functional burden.
    b. severity of the condition.
    c. complexity of the care.
    d. resources required for care.

40. The effectiveness of the family's support system depends on the:
    a. ability to match the best source of support for each need.
    b. diversity of the family's social network.
    c. extended family and their availability.
    d. extended family and their resources.

41. Which of the following is *not* necessarily a criterion to consider when selecting parents to offer support to other parents of children with disabilities?
    a. The parents should possess advocacy and problem-solving skills.
    b. The parents should have a child with the same diagnosis.
    c. The parents should have a nonjudgmental approach to problem solving.
    d. The parents should be good listeners.

42. Out-of-home placement of a child with a disability:
    a. may be the best option if the integrity of the family unit is in jeopardy.
    b. occurs if coping strategies are not employed within the home.
    c. is becoming increasingly difficult to accomplish.
    d. demonstrates that the family is maladjusted.

43. The program formerly known as Crippled Children's Services, which provides financial assistance for children with many disabling conditions, is now called:
    a. Programs for Children with Special Needs.
    b. National Information Center for Children and Youth with Disabilities.
    c. Association for the Care of Children's Health.
    d. Alliance for Health, Physical Education, Recreation and Dance.

CRITICAL THINKING—CASE STUDY

Jerome is a 15-month-old infant who was born prematurely and was discharged from the hospital at age 3 months after multiple invasive procedures, including intubation, ventilation, and surgery. He is delayed in his motor development, but other areas of development are progressing as would be expected for a prematurely born infant of his age. Jerome has recently been diagnosed with cerebral palsy. He is at the physician's office for a routine health check. His mother is with him.

44. To assess the family's adjustment to the diagnosis, the nurse would gather more information. One area that could be deferred to a later date would be the assessment of the family's:
    a. goals for the future.
    b. available support system.
    c. coping mechanisms.
    d. perception of the disorder.

Jerome's mother has returned to work part-time as a partner in a computer consulting firm. Jerome's father is a marketing consultant in the food industry and travels frequently. The parents, who are in their late thirties, have hired a woman whom they trust with Jerome's many needs to come into the home. Jerome, who is an only child, goes out of the home several times a week for therapy.

45. Based on the information given, select the best nursing diagnosis for Jerome.
    a. Risk for Injury
    b. Dysfunctional Family Processes
    c. Delayed Growth and Development
    d. Disturbed Body Image

46. With the selected diagnosis in mind, what is the expected outcome with the highest priority for Jerome?
    a. Jerome will attain the physical development that is appropriate for any 15-month-old.
    b. Jerome will attain psychosocial and cognitive development that is appropriate for any 15-month-old.
    c. Jerome will attain physical, psychosocial, and cognitive development that is appropriate for his age and abilities.
    d. Jerome's parents will set realistic goals for themselves and Jerome.

47. An intervention that would address the issues involved with altered family process related to the birth of Jerome and the complexity of his care after birth would be to:
    a. teach safety precautions.
    b. help the family achieve a realistic view of Jerome's capabilities and limitations.
    c. stress the importance of sound health practices and frequent health supervision.
    d. encourage responsible use of equipment and appliances.

48. Between now and Jerome's next visit at 24 months of age, the nurse should provide anticipatory guidance to the parents about Jerome's growth toward developing:
    a. a sense of trust and attachment.
    b. mastery of self-care skills.
    c. a sense of body image.
    d. independence.

20 Family-Centered Palliative Care

1. Match each term with its description.

   a. Burnout
   b. Hospice
   c. Drug tolerance
   d. Addiction

   e. Palliative care
   f. DNR
   g. The Compassionate Friends
   h. Principle of Double Effect

   _____ Ethical standard that supports the use of interventions that have the intention of relieving pain and suffering even though there is a foreseeable possibility that death may be hastened.

   _____ Psychologic dependence on the side effects of a drug; usually not a factor in pain management of terminally ill children

   _____ Active total care of patients whose disease is not responsive to curative treatment

   _____ One of the reasons for administering high doses of opioids for pain control in order to maintain the same level of pain relief

   _____ A community health care organization that specializes in the care of dying patients and their families; combines the philosophy of dying as a natural process with palliative care

   _____ A state of physical, emotional, and mental exhaustion that occurs as a result of prolonged involvement with individuals in situations that are emotionally demanding; an occupational hazard to which nurses are susceptible

   _____ An indication to withhold cardiopulmonary resuscitation in response to cardiac arrest; "do not resuscitate"; no code

   _____ An international organization for bereaved parents and siblings

2. In children 1 to 19 years of age, the most frequent causes of death are:
   a. accidents/trauma, infectious illness, and suicide.
   b. injuries/trauma, cancer, and congenital anomalies.
   c. accidents/trauma, homicide, suicide, and cancer.
   d. prematurity, congenital birth defects, and infectious illness.

3. List three strategies nurses can use to communicate with families of children with life-threatening illness.

4. Which one of the following regarding palliative care is *false*?
   a. Serves to hasten death
   b. Provides pain and symptom management
   c. Promotes optimal functioning and quality of life
   d. Addresses issues faced by the family regarding death and dying

5. Pediatric nurses report that a common obstacle to the provision of good palliative care is:
   a. parents who do not understand the concept of palliative care.
   b. communication with practitioners is inadequate.
   c. uncertainty about the goals of care.
   d. the cost of providing palliative care is excessive.

150

6. List and discuss two common ethical dilemmas encountered in caring for the terminally ill child.

7. A nurse is about to present facts to parents about the possible death of their child. In this case, which of the following techniques would be most effective in promoting communication?
   a. Acknowledging denial in the parents whenever it occurs
   b. Using only medical terms for all explanations
   c. Using body language to communicate caring
   d. Recognizing feelings and reactions but not acknowledging them

8. When communicating with dying children, the nurse should remember that:
   a. older children tend to be concrete thinkers.
   b. when children can recite facts, they understand the implications of those facts.
   c. if children's questions direct the conversation, the assessment will be incomplete.
   d. games, art, and play provide a good means of expression.

9. When assisting parents in supporting their dying child, the nurse should stress the importance of honesty; if parents are honest and openly discuss their fears, the child is more likely to:
   a. discuss his or her fears.
   b. ask fewer distressing questions.
   c. lose his or her sense of hope.
   d. do all of the above.

10. Fear of the unknown is one of the greatest threats to seriously ill children of which age-group?
    a. Toddlers
    b. Preschoolers
    c. School-age children
    d. Adolescents

11. Separation is one of the greatest threats to seriously ill children of which age-group?
    a. Toddlers
    b. Preschoolers
    c. School-age children
    d. Adolescents

12. Fear of punishment is one of the greatest threats to seriously ill children of which age-group?
    a. Toddlers
    b. Preschoolers
    c. School-age children
    d. Adolescents

13. The perceived inability to use their parents for emotional support is one of the greatest threats to seriously ill children of which age-group?
    a. Toddlers
    b. Preschoolers
    c. School-age children
    d. Adolescents

14. Which one of the following age-groups is most likely to suffer negative reactions to an altered body image as a result of a life-threatening illness?
    a. Young children
    b. School-age children
    c. Adolescents
    d. All age-groups are affected equally.

15. Describe at least three benefits of implementing the hospice concept in the child's home environment.

16. Which one of the following interventions is most important for the dying child?
    a. Emotional support
    b. Preparing parents to deal with fears
    c. Relief from pain
    d. Control of pain

17. When the parent of a child who is dying tells the nurse the child is in pain, even when the child appears comfortable, the nurse should be sure that:
    a. as-needed pain control measures are instituted.
    b. pain control is administered on a regular preventive schedule.
    c. parents understand that pain is a physical process.
    d. parents understand that the child is probably in less pain than the parents think.

18. Interventions to help the family prepare for the care of a terminally ill child include:
    a. educating the family about complications of overfeeding or overhydration.
    b. providing a supply of medications to alleviate discomfort.
    c. encouraging fun and memorable activities.
    d. all of the above.

19. The sibling of a dying child may feel:
    a. displaced.
    b. isolated.
    c. resentful.
    d. all of the above.

20. List at least five physical signs of approaching death.

21. Methods to support grieving families at the time of death and in the grieving period after death include:
    a. encouraging family members to avoid upsetting each other by keeping their feelings to themselves.
    b. consoling with phrases such as "I know how you feel."
    c. emphasizing that the painful grieving usually lasts less than a year.
    d. allowing the family time to stay with the child after the death.

22. List at least three behaviors that are characteristic in children as death approaches.

23. Complicated grief reactions:
    a. usually takes about a year.
    b. are accompanied by support of the family at the funeral.
    c. may extend over years.
    d. can be eliminated if the family is well prepared.

24. Which one of the following strategies would be best for the nurse to use to support the family's spiritual needs when their child's death is imminent and a clergy member is unavailable?
    a. Pray appropriately with the family.
    b. Implement relaxation techniques.
    c. Make an appointment for the family to speak with an expert.
    d. Review the physical signs of death with the family.

25. When a child dies suddenly, which one of the following interventions would be *least* beneficial?
    a. Avoid having the family view the body of a disfigured child.
    b. Inform the family of what to expect when they see the disfigured body of their child.
    c. Offer the parents the opportunity to see the child's body even after resuscitation was performed.
    d. Arrange to have a health care worker with bereavement training meet with the family.

26. Identify each of the following statements as true or false.

    _____ Children with cancer, chronic disease, or infection or who have suffered prolonged cardiac arrest are excellent candidates for organ donation.

    _____ The nurse should never inquire whether organ donation was discussed with the child but should allow the family to come forward with this information on their own.

    _____ If organs are donated, the family will most likely need to choose a closed-casket funeral service.

    _____ Most families choose not to donate organs because of the high cost.

    _____ Many body tissues and organs can be donated, but their removal may cause mutilation of the body.

27. In regard to whether a child should attend the funeral of a loved one, the nurse should consider:
    a. the child's age.
    b. that it will be a frightening experience.
    c. his or her responsibility to protect the child from distressing events.
    d. that attending the funeral may be beneficial to the child.

28. Current research supports the notion that:
    a. involvement in the experiences of the dying sibling is beneficial.
    b. siblings of children who died in the hospital reported readiness for the death.
    c. protecting the sibling of the dying child from the death rituals is beneficial.
    d. it is better for the sibling to remember the dying child as he or she was when alive.

29. Which one of the following techniques would be considered an example of the most therapeutic communication to use with the bereaved family?
    a. Cheerfulness
    b. Interpretation
    c. Validating loss
    d. Reassurance

30. Which one of the following helping statements would be *least* therapeutic for the nurse to use with the bereaved family?
    a. "You can stay with him and hold him if you wish."
    b. "It must be painful for you to return to the doctor's office without her."
    c. "Fortunately his suffering is over now."
    d. "You have been through a very difficult time."

31. Which one of the following symptoms would be considered normal grief behavior?
    a. Depression
    b. Anger
    c. Hearing the dead person's voice
    d. All of the above

32. The resolution of grief usually:
    a. occurs in sequential phases.
    b. is completed in about 2 years.
    c. is completed in about 3 years.
    d. is a timeless process that is never completed.

33. Reorganization after the death of a child means that the:
    a. loved one is forgotten.
    b. pain is gone.
    c. survivors have "let go."
    d. survivors have recovered from their loss.

34. List at least three of the reactions that nurses have when caring for a child with a terminal illness.

35. Intervening therapeutically with terminally ill children and their families requires:
    a. only self-awareness.
    b. nursing practice that is based on a theoretical foundation.
    c. years of experience.
    d. personal experience with death.

CRITICAL THINKING—CASE STUDY

Julie is a 6-year-old child with leukemia. She has undergone a bone marrow transplant with associated complications and has had several remissions. After the last remission, she deteriorated rapidly. Her parents tell the nurse that they believe Julie is now in the final stages of her illness. Her parents also express their feelings of discouragement and depression.

36. How should the nurse approach the parents in regard to their feelings about Julie's impending death?
    a. The nurse should begin by assessing the reason for the depression.
    b. The nurse should be certain that Julie's parents know that repeated relapses with remissions are associated with a better prognosis.
    c. The nurse should begin to help the parents work through their depression.
    d. The nurse should use heavy sedation to help Julie and her parents cope with this phase.

37. As Julie's parents express their concerns, it becomes clear that pain control is a fear for Julie and her parents. What strategy should the nurse use to help them deal with this fear?
    a. The nurse should assure the parents that all of Julie's pain will be eliminated.
    b. The nurse should use heavy sedation to help Julie and her parents cope with this phase.
    c. A regular preventive medication schedule should be adopted as pain develops.
    d. The pain medications should be given only intravenously when Julie is near death.

38. After Julie's death in late December, which one of the following evaluation strategies is most likely to help support and guide the family through the resolution of their loss?
    a. A written questionnaire
    b. A telephone call placed in early January
    c. A meeting with the family at the time of death
    d. A telephone call placed in early February

39. Which one of the following would be the best expected outcome for the nursing diagnosis of Fear/Anxiety when planning care for Julie in this terminal stage?
    a. Julie will discuss her fears without evidence of stress.
    b. Julie will exhibit no evidence of loneliness.
    c. Julie's parents are actively involved in Julie's care.
    d. Julie's parents demonstrate ability to provide care for her.

21 The Child with Cognitive, Sensory, or Communication Impairment

1. List five causes of cognitive impairment and cite one example of each.

2. Identify the standardized test most commonly used in infants to evaluate cognitive ability.

3. List four measures for the prevention of cognitive impairment.

4. The American Association on Intellectual and Developmental Disabilities definition of intellectual disability includes:
   a. significant limitations in intellectual functioning and adaptive behavior.
   b. an emphasis on function.
   c. only intelligence and no other criteria.
   d. an age limit of 16.

5. List at least four early signs that are suggestive of cognitive impairment.

6. When teaching a child with a cognitive impairment, the nurse's best strategy to present symbols in an exaggerated, concrete form is:
   a. singing.
   b. memorizing.
   c. verbal explanation.
   d. ignoring the child.

7. Define the term *fading*.

8. Define the term *shaping*.

9. Acquiring social skills for the child who is intellectually disabled includes:
   a. learning acceptable sexual behavior.
   b. being exposed to strangers.
   c. learning to greet visitors appropriately.
   d. all of the above.

10. Which of the following strategies would best help the intellectually disabled child acquire social skills?
    a. Use discipline and negative reinforcement.
    b. Provide information about the importance of socialization skills.
    c. Use active rehearsal with role-playing and practice sessions.
    d. Use all of the above.

11. Define task analysis and describe its use when teaching a child who is intellectually disabled.

12. The primary purpose of record keeping for 7 days before toilet training an intellectually disabled child is to:
    a. determine the child's patterns of behavior and parents' response.
    b. determine the amount of urinary output and usual times the child urinates.
    c. assess the child's physical and psychologic readiness to use the toilet.
    d. determine all of the above.

13. Describe the conditions necessary for a child with cognitive impairment to begin learning how to dress.

14. The mutual participation model of care for the child who is cognitively impaired and needs hospitalization would include:
    a. isolating the child from others to avoid conflicts.
    b. allowing parents to room in and participate in the care.
    c. having the parents perform all activities of daily living.
    d. having the nurse perform all activities of daily living.

15. Another name for trisomy 21 is:
    a. phenylketonuria.
    b. Turner syndrome.
    c. Down syndrome.
    d. galactosemia.

16. Testing of the parents is necessary to identify the carrier and offer genetic counseling when Down syndrome is caused by:
    a. mosaicism.
    b. translocation.
    c. maternal age over 40.
    d. paternal age over 40.

17. List five physical features that are found in the infant with Down syndrome.

18. Decreased muscle tone in the infant with Down syndrome:
    a. indicates inadequate parenting.
    b. is a sign of infant detachment.
    c. compromises respiratory expansion.
    d. predisposes the infant to diarrhea.

19. Children with Down syndrome may have a number of associated anomalies. List the most common congenital anomalies found in these children.

20. Fragile X syndrome is:
    a. the most common inherited cause of cognitive impairment.
    b. the most common inherited cause of cognitive impairment next to Down syndrome.
    c. caused by an abnormal gene on chromosome 21.
    d. caused by a missing gene on the X chromosome.

21. In regard to Fragile X syndrome, the fragile site is caused by:
    a. 5 to 40 repeats of nucleotide base pairs.
    b. gene mutation.
    c. infection.
    d. advanced maternal age.

22. List 5 behavioral features common to children with Fragile X syndrome.

23. The correct term to use for a person whose hearing disability precludes successful processing of linguistic information through audition without the use of a hearing aid is:
    a. deaf-mute.
    b. slight to moderate hearing loss.
    c. severe to profound hearing loss.
    d. deaf and dumb.

24. Conductive hearing loss in children is most often a result of:
    a. the use of tobramycin and gentamicin.
    b. the high noise levels from ventilators.
    c. congenital defects.
    d. recurrent serous otitis media.

25. Sensorineural hearing loss occurs as a result of:
    a. kernicterus.
    b. use of tobramycin and gentamicin.
    c. congenital defects of inner ear structures.
    d. all of the above.

26. At what decibel level would a hearing loss be considered profound?
    a. Less than 30 dB
    b. 41-60 dB
    c. 61-80 dB
    d. More than 81 dB

Chapter **21** **The Child with Cognitive, Sensory, or Communication Impairment**

27. One behavior associated with hearing impairment in the infant is:
    a. a monotone voice.
    b. consistent lack of the startle reflex to sound.
    c. a louder than usual cry.
    d. inability to form the word "da-da" by 6 months.

28. In assessing a child for the development of a hearing impairment, the nurse would look for:
    a. a loud monotone voice.
    b. stuttering.
    c. unusual shyness.
    d. attentiveness, especially when someone is talking.

29. All of the following strategies will enhance communication with a child who is hearing impaired *except*:
    a. touching the child lightly to signal the presence of a speaker.
    b. speaking at eye level or moving to a 45-degree angle.
    c. using facial expressions to convey the message better.
    d. moving and using animated body language to communicate better.

30. To best promote socialization for the child with a hearing aid, teachers should:
    a. discourage hearing-impaired children from playing together.
    b. use frequent group projects to promote communication.
    c. use audiovisual-assisted instruction as much as possible.
    d. minimize background noise.

31. Care for the hearing-impaired child who is hospitalized should include:
    a. supplementing verbal explanations with tactile and visual aids.
    b. communicating only with parents to ensure accuracy.
    c. discouraging parents from rooming in.
    d. sending nonvocal communication devices home to avoid loss.

32. Which of the following situations would be considered abnormal?
    a. A neonate who lacks binocularity
    b. A toddler whose mother says he looks cross-eyed
    c. A 5-year-old who has hyperopia
    d. Presence of a red reflex in a 7-year-old

33. If a child has a penetrating injury to the eye, the nurse should:
    a. apply an eye patch.
    b. attempt to remove the object.
    c. irrigate the eye.
    d. use strict aseptic technique to examine the eye.

34. Match each type of visual impairment with its description or characteristics.

    a. Astigmatism   d. Strabismus
    b. Anisometropia   e. Cataract
    c. Amblyopia   f. Glaucoma

    _____ Increased intraocular pressure

    _____ Squint or cross-eye; malalignment of eyes

    _____ Different refractive strength in each eye

    _____ Unequal curvatures in refractive apparatus

    _____ Opacity of crystalline lens

    _____ Lazy eye; reduced visual acuity in one eye

35. List at least eight strategies the nurse can use during hospitalization of a child who has lost his or her sight.

36. Which of the following statements is correct about eye care and sports?
    a. Glasses may interfere with the child's ability in sports.
    b. Face mask and helmet should be required gear for softball.
    c. Contact lenses provide less visual acuity than glasses for sports.
    d. It is usually difficult to convince children to wear their glasses to play sports.

37. The method of communication used with combined auditory and visual impairments that involves spelling into the child's hand is called:
    a. finger spelling.
    b. the Tadoma method.
    c. blindism.
    d. the tapping method.

38. To help families with children who are hearing and vision impaired, the nurse should teach the parents to establish communication by:
    a. always placing the child in the same place in the room to help identify surroundings.
    b. selecting a cue that is always used to help the child discriminate one person from another.
    c. limiting the cues that are sent and received.
    d. limiting stimulation to allow the child to feel safe.

39. Which one of the following examples would be most indicative of a language disorder?
    a. A 22-month-old child who has not uttered his first word
    b. A 38-month-old who has not uttered his first sentence
    c. An 18-month-old who uses short "telegraphic" phrases
    d. A 4-year-old who stutters

40. Which of the following statements about stuttering is correct?
    a. Stuttering is normal in the school-age child.
    b. Stuttering occurs because children do not know what they want to say.
    c. Undue emphasis on a stutter may cause an abnormal speech pattern.
    d. Chances for reversal of stuttering are good until about age 3 years.

41. One of the clinical manifestations associated with the speech sounds known as articulation errors is the:
    a. omission of consonants at the end of words.
    b. deviation in pitch or quality of the voice.
    c. pauses within a word.
    d. frequent use of circumlocutions.

42. Diagnostic criteria for autism spectrum disorders (ASD) include symptoms related to:
    a. social interactions.
    b. impairments in communication.
    c. repetitive behavior patterns.
    d. all of the above.

43. Strategies to use when caring for the hospitalized child with autism include:
    a. maintaining direct eye contact when explaining procedures.
    b. using holding and touch to comfort the child.
    c. decreasing stimulation.
    d. all of the above.

44. The parents of a child who is stuttering should be encouraged to:
    a. have the child start again more slowly.
    b. give the child plenty of time.
    c. show concern for the hesitancy.
    d. reward the child for proper speech.

45. Detecting communication disorders during early childhood:
    a. adversely affects the child's social relationships.
    b. increases the child's difficulty with academic skills.
    c. increases the child's ability to correct deficit skills.
    d. adversely affects the child's emotional interactions.

46. Following assessment and detection of a language problem, the nurse should advise the family to:
    a. wait and see what happens.
    b. wait because the child will grow out of it.
    c. obtain a specialized evaluation.
    d. repeat words so that the child will learn more language.

CRITICAL THINKING—CASE STUDY

Paula Larson, a 9-month-old infant with Down syndrome (DS) who is also blind and hearing impaired, is admitted to the hospital with pneumonia. She holds her head steady but cannot sit without support or pull up on the furniture. Paula squeals and laughs but does not imitate speech sounds or have any words, not even "da-da" or "ma-ma." She can shake a rattle but cannot pass a block from one hand to the other. She smiles spontaneously and holds her own bottle, but she does not play "pattycake" or wave "bye-bye."

Along with the developing developmental deficits, Paula has a congenital heart anomaly and has been hospitalized many times for pneumonia and bronchiolitis. Paula's parents knew that she would be born with DS. They have chosen to care for Paula at home. Paula's care has become increasingly time-consuming. During the admission assessment interview, Mr. and Mrs. Larson state they are both exhausted.

47. The nurse determines that Paula's developmental lag is *least* pronounced in the area of:
    a. gross motor skills.
    b. language skills.
    c. fine motor skills.
    d. personal-social skills.

48. Paula's parents have cared for her at home since her birth. Mrs. Larson expresses concern that she is not doing a good enough job and that perhaps it is time to consider placement out of the home for Paula. The nurse responds based on the knowledge that:
    a. the potential for development varies greatly in DS.
    b. every available source of assistance to help Mr. and Mrs. Larson with the care of Paula should be explored.
    c. the nurse's responses may influence Mr. and Mrs. Larson's decisions.
    d. all of the above are true.

49. Which one of the common nursing diagnoses used in planning care for intellectually disabled children should take priority in Paula's current situation?
    a. Altered Growth and Development
    b. Interrupted Family Processes
    c. Anxiety related to the hospitalization
    d. Impaired Social Interaction

50. Mr. and Mrs. Larson make the decision to explore residential care for Paula. The best expected outcome during this time for Paula would be for the parents to:
    a. demonstrate acceptance of Paula.
    b. express feelings and concerns regarding the implications of Paula's birth.
    c. make a realistic decision based on Paula's needs and capabilities as well as their own.
    d. identify realistic goals for Paula's future home care.

160

22 Family-Centered Care of the Child During Illness and Hospitalization

1. The following terms are related to children's reactions to hospitalization. Match each term with its description.

   a. Separation anxiety
   b. Family-centered care
   c. Protest
   d. Despair

   e. Detachment
   f. Play
   g. Sense of helplessness
   h. Self-care

   _____ The practice of activities that individuals initiate and perform on their own behalf to maintain life, health, and well-being

   _____ The philosophy of care that recognizes the integral role of the family in a child's life and acknowledges the family as an essential part of the child's care and illness experience

   _____ Reactions that parents may have following the realization of their child's illness; they may resist admitting to such feelings because they expect others to disapprove of behavior that is less than perfect

   _____ Well-recognized technique for emotional release, allowing children to reenact frightening or puzzling hospital experiences; use of puppets and replicas or actual hospital equipment to allow children to act out the situations

   _____ Also called "denial," the uncommon third phase of separation anxiety, in which superficially the child appears to have finally adjusted to the loss; behavior that is a result of resignation and not a sign of contentment

   _____ The phase of separation anxiety in which the child stops crying, is much less active, and withdraws from others

   _____ A phase of separation anxiety in which children react aggressively, cry loudly, scream for parents, refuse the attention of anyone else, and are inconsolable in their grief

   _____ Most common stressor in hospitalized children from infancy through preschool

2. Separation anxiety would be most expected in the hospitalized child at age:
   a. 3 to 6 months.
   b. 12 to 24 months.
   c. 3 to 6 years
   d. 7 to 12 years.

3. One difference between toddlers and school-age children in their reactions to hospitalization is that most school-age children:
   a. experience more separation anxiety.
   b. show less fright or overt resistance to pain.
   c. may react more to separation from school friends.
   d. may throw temper tantrums.

4. A toddler is most likely to react to short-term hospitalization with feelings of loss of control that are manifested by:
   a. regression.
   b. withdrawal.
   c. formation of new superficial relationships.
   d. self-assertion and anger.

5. Which one of the following is *not* considered to be a major stressor of hospitalization in the young child?
   a. Separation
   b. Loss of control
   c. Bodily injury
   d. School absence

6. Describe at least one of the possible psychologic benefits a child might gain from hospitalization.

7. Which one of the following factors, according to Craft's 1993 framework, would be considered most likely to negatively influence the reactions of siblings to the hospitalized child?
   a. The sibling is an adolescent.
   b. Care providers are not relatives.
   c. The sibling has received information about the ill child.
   d. The ill child is cared for in the home.

8. List five functions of play in the hospital.

9. List three strategies nurses can use to minimize stressors for the parents of the hospitalized child.

10. To help the parents deal with issues related to separation while their child is hospitalized, the nurse should *not* suggest:
    a. using associations to help the child understand time frames.
    b. ways to explain departure and return.
    c. quietly leaving while the child is distracted or asleep.
    d. short, frequent visits over an extended stay if rooming in is impossible.

11. Strategies used to minimize the hospitalized child's feelings of loss of control include attempts to:
    a. alter the child's schedule to match the hospital schedule.
    b. establish a daily schedule for the hospitalized child.
    c. eliminate rituals that have been used at home.
    d. perform all of the above.

12. Strategies to minimize the effects of separation in school-age children and adolescents include:
    i. allowing visits from peers
    ii. allowing children to wear their own clothes
    iii. bringing favorite items from home, such as a laptop or stuffed animal
    iv. enforcing strict rules and routines regarding diagnostic procedures
    v. asking the family to leave the room when the physician enters

    a. i, ii, and iv
    b. i, ii, and iii
    c. iv and v

13. When performing a painful procedure on a child, to minimize fear of bodily injury, the nurse should attempt to:
    a. perform the procedure in the playroom.
    b. standardize techniques from one age group to the next.
    c. perform the procedure quickly with the parent present.
    d. have the parents leave during the procedure.

14. After administering an intramuscular injection, the nurse would best reassure the young child with poorly defined body boundaries by:
    a. telling the child that the bleeding will stop after the needle is removed.
    b. using a large bandage to cover the injection site.
    c. using a small bandage to cover the injection site.
    d. using a bandage but removing it a few hours after the injection.

15. Which of the following reactions to surgery is most typical of an adolescent's reaction of fear of bodily injury?
    a. Concern about the pain
    b. Concern about the procedure itself
    c. Concern about the scar
    d. Understanding explanations literally

16. When helping parents select activities for the convalescing hospitalized child, the nurse should recommend:
    a. simpler activities than would normally be chosen.
    b. new toys and games to help distract the child.
    c. challenging new games to keep the child engaged.
    d. games that can be played with adults.

17. List at least two ways that drawing or painting can be used by the nurse in caring for the hospitalized child.

18. Preparation for hospitalization reduces stress in which of the following age-groups?
    a. Adolescence
    b. Toddlerhood
    c. Preschool
    d. All of the above

19. Questions related to activities of daily living at the time of admission are:
    a. inappropriate and should be saved for later.
    b. directed toward evaluation of the child's preparation for hospitalization.
    c. asked directly and in the order provided on the assessment form.
    d. designed to help the nurse develop appropriate routines for the hospitalized child.

20. Describe at least three strategies that can be used in the intensive care unit to support the child and family.

21. The advantages of a hospital unit specifically for adolescents include:
    a. exclusive group membership.
    b. fewer preparation requirements.
    c. increased socialization with peers.
    d. all of the above.

22. The question "How does your child act when annoyed or upset?" would be asked on admission to assess the child's:
    a. health perception–health management pattern.
    b. cognitive-perceptual pattern.
    c. activity-exercise pattern.
    d. self-perception/self-concept pattern.

23. The question "How does your child usually handle problems or disappointments?" would be asked on admission to assess the child's:
    a. role-relationship pattern.
    b. sexuality-reproductive pattern.
    c. coping–stress tolerance pattern.
    d. value-belief pattern.

24. The benefit(s) of the ambulatory/outpatient setting is reduction of:
    a. stressors.
    b. infection risk.
    c. cost.
    d. all of the above.

25. Discharge instructions from the ambulatory setting should include all of the following *except*:
    a. guidelines for when to call.
    b. dietary restrictions.
    c. activity restrictions.
    d. referral to a home health agency.

26. When caring for the child in isolation, the nurse should:
    a. spend as little time as possible in the room.
    b. teach the parents to care for the child to decrease the risk for spreading infection.
    c. let the child see the nurse's face before donning the mask.
    d. perform all of the above.

27. The most ideal way to support parents when they first visit the child in the intensive care unit is:
    a. for the nurse to accompany them to the bedside.
    b. to use picture books of the unit in the waiting area.
    c. to limit the visiting hours so that parents are encouraged to rest.
    d. to expect parents to stay with their child continuously.

28. Transfer from the intensive care unit to the regular pediatric unit can be best facilitated by:
    a. discussing the details of the transfer at the bedside, where the child can listen.
    b. establishing a schedule that mimics the child's home schedule.
    c. assigning a primary nurse from the regular unit who visits the child before the transfer.
    d. explaining to the family that there are fewer nurses on the regular unit.

CRITICAL THINKING—CASE MANAGEMENT

Peter Chen is a 9-year-old child who is admitted to the pediatric unit for an appendectomy. He is in the third grade and is very active in after-school activities. Recently he began to take karate lessons, and he also plays baseball. Peter loves school, particularly when he is able to read. He awakens every morning at 6 AM to read, and reading is the last thing he does before he falls asleep at night.

Peter's parents are with him during the admission interview. His mother works, but she has made arrangements to take some time off after surgery and during his hospital stay to be available to him.

29. Based on the preceding information, the nurse should expect:
    a. a normal response to hospitalization.
    b. more anxiety than would normally be seen.
    c. difficulty with the parents.
    d. cultural factors to take precedence.

30. The nurse identifies which of the following nursing diagnoses after surgery for Peter?
    a. Powerlessness related to the environment
    b. Activity Intolerance related to pain or discomfort
    c. Anxiety/Fear related to distressing procedures
    d. Any of the above would be appropriate

31. One reasonable expected outcome for Peter's diagnosis of Powerlessness would be?
    a. Peter will tolerate increasing activity.
    b. Peter will remain injury-free.
    c. Peter will play and rest quietly.
    d. Peter will help plan his care and schedule.

32. Which one of the following interventions would be best for the nurse to incorporate into Peter's plan related to the diagnosis of Activity Intolerance?
    a. Organize activities that allow for rest periods
    b. Keep side rails up.
    c. Choose an appropriate roommate.
    d. Assist with dressing and bathing.

23 Pediatric Nursing Interventions and Skills

1. The following terms are related to general hygiene and care. Match each term with its description.

   a. Pressure ulcers
   b. Pressure reduction device
   c. Pressure relief device
   d. Friction
   e. Shear

   f. Epidermal stripping
   g. Set point
   h. Fever
   i. Hyperthermia
   j. Chill phase

   k. Plateau
   l. Defervescence
   m. Reactive hyperemia

   _____ Flush; the earliest sign of tissue compromise and pressure-related ischemia

   _____ Hyperpyrexia; an elevation in set point such that the body temperature is regulated at a higher level; may be arbitrarily defined as temperature above 38° C (100° F)

   _____ The point in the febrile state in which shivering and vasoconstriction generate and conserve heat and raise the central temperatures to a level of the new set point

   _____ The point during the febrile state in which the temperature stabilizes at the higher range

   _____ Can develop when the pressure on the skin and underlying tissues is greater than the capillary closing pressure, causing capillary occlusion; results in tissue anoxia and cellular death; most commonly occurs over a bony prominence

   _____ The result of the force of gravity pulling down on the body and friction of the body against a surface; occurs, for example, when a patient is in the semi-Fowler position and begins to slide to the foot of the bed

   _____ A product used to decrease the pressure that occurs with a regular hospital bed or chair; usually consists of an overlay that is placed on top of the regular mattress

   _____ Occurs when the surface of the skin rubs against another surface, such as the sheets on a bed

   _____ A product that maintains pressure below the level that would cause capillary closing; usually consists of a high-technology bed used for patients who have multiple problems and cannot be turned effectively

   _____ A situation in which body temperature exceeds the set point; usually occurs when the body or external conditions create more heat than the body can eliminate, such as in heat stroke, aspirin toxicity, or hyperthyroidism

   _____ The point when the temperature is greater than the set point or when the pyrogen is no longer present

   _____ Results when the epidermis is unintentionally torn away when tape is removed

   _____ The temperature around which body temperature is regulated by a thermostat-like mechanism in the hypothalamus

2. An informed consent is required for:
   a. an emergency appendectomy.
   b. a cutdown for intravenous medications.
   c. release of medical information.
   d. all of the above.

3. When parents are divorced, who is eligible to consent to medical treatment of the child?
   a. Usually, the custodial parent consents.
   b. Only the noncustodial parent may consent.
   c. Both parents must consent.
   d. The child is the responsible party.

4. The statutes for the mature minor doctrine vary from state to state. Based on the doctrine, a minor may be permitted to consent for:
    a. treatment for any kind of health problem.
    b. routine physical examinations only.
    c. treatment for sexually transmitted infections.
    d. minor surgery.

5. Although statutes vary from state to state, minors are usually recognized as having the legal capacity of an adult in all matters after they:
    a. have acquired a sexually transmitted infection.
    b. use contraceptives.
    c. use drugs or alcohol.
    d. become pregnant.

6. When preparing a child for a procedure, the nurse should:
    a. use abstract terms.
    b. teach based on the child's developmental level.
    c. use phrases with dual meanings.
    d. introduce anxiety-laden information first.

7. If a child needs support during an invasive procedure, the nurse should:
    a. insist that the parents participate in distraction techniques.
    b. instruct parents to stand quietly in back of the room and maintain eye contact with the child.
    c. respect parents' wishes and coach the parents about what to do.
    d. instruct parents to stay close by to console the child immediately after the procedure.

8. To prepare a toddler for an invasive procedure, the best strategy for the nurse to use would be to:
    a. give one direction at a time.
    b. prepare the child a day in advance.
    c. set up the equipment while the child watches.
    d. expect the child to sit still and cooperate.

9. Which of the following words or phrases is considered nonthreatening to a small child?
    a. "A little stick"
    b. "An owie"
    c. Die
    d. Deaden

10. Which of the following strategies is a powerful coping method that can be used with a small child during painful procedures?
    a. Ask the child whether he or she wants to take the pain medicine.
    b. Administer medication in the playroom.
    c. Give a comprehensive explanation of what will occur.
    d. Use distraction techniques for a painful procedure.

11. List at least five strategies the nurse can use to support the child during and after a procedure.

12. Describe at least one play activity for each of the following procedures.

    a. Ambulation:

    b. Range-of-motion exercises:

c. Injections:

d. Deep breathing:

e. Extending the environment:

f. Soaks:

g. Fluid intake:

13. The most effective method of preoperative preparation for a child is:
    a. consistent supportive care.
    b. systematic preparation at specific stress points.
    c. offering parents the option of attending the induction of anesthesia.
    d. a single session of preparation.

14. One strategy to provide atraumatic care for pediatric patients undergoing surgery is:
    a. restrict fluids in infants for at least 10 hours.
    b. always use a face mask during induction.
    c. allow child to wear underpants or pajama bottoms into surgery.
    d. remove parents from the child's sight.

15. To prepare a breast-fed infant physically for surgery, the nurse would expect to:
    a. permit breastfeeding up to 4 hours before surgery.
    b. withhold breastfeeding from midnight the night before surgery.
    c. permit breastfeeding up to 6 hours before surgery.
    d. replace breast milk with formula and permit feeding up to 2 hours before surgery.

16. With the concept of atraumatic care in mind, preoperative sedation in children is best accomplished by:
    a. intramuscular opioids.
    b. intravenous midazolam.
    c. intravenous opioids.
    d. oral midazolam.

17. Early symptoms of malignant hyperthermia include:
    a. anemia.
    b. enlarged lymph nodes.
    c. tachycardia.
    d. hypertension.

18. A change in vital signs of the young child in the postanesthesia recovery room that demands immediate attention is:
    a. increased temperature.
    b. tachypnea.
    c. muscle rigidity.
    d. all of the above.

19. Which one of the following would provide the best pain control for a child who is recovering from a tonsillectomy?
    a. Administration of an opioid analgesic IM on an as-needed (PRN) basis
    b. Administration of an opioid analgesic every 4 hours for 24 hours by mouth (as tolerated)

20. Noncompliant families:
    a. share typical characteristics.
    b. have less education than compliant families.
    c. often have complex medical regimens.
    d. often have an increased loss of control.

21. An example of an organizational strategy to improve compliance would be for the nurse to:
    a. incorporate teaching principles that are known to enhance understanding.
    b. encourage the family to adapt hospital medication schedules to their home routine.
    c. evaluate and reduce the time the family waits for their appointment.
    d. all of the above are organizational strategies.

22. In planning strategies to improve the child's compliance with the prescribed treatment, the nurse knows that:
    a. an every-8-hour schedule should be implemented.
    b. an every-6-hour schedule should be implemented.
    c. the child may not be able to swallow pills.
    d. the family usually does not remember or understand the instructions given.

23. General guidelines for care of a child's skin includes:
    a. covering the fingers of the extremity used for an intravenous line.
    b. lifting the child under the arms to transfer the child from the bed to a stretcher.
    c. placing a pectin-based skin barrier directly over excoriated skin.
    d. keeping the skin moist at all times.

24. Which of these is not usually a factor in the development of a pediatric pressure ulcer?
    a. Shear
    b. Skin moisturizer
    c. Moisture
    d. Chemical factors
    e. Friction

25. To prevent skin injuries from shear, the nurse should avoid:
    a. using sheepskin over the elbows.
    b. pulling the patient up in bed without a lift sheet.
    c. pulling the patient up in bed with a lift sheet.
    d. using Montgomery straps.

26. When bathing an uncircumcised boy over the age of 3 years, the nurse should:
    a. gently remind the child to clean his genital area.
    b. not retract the foreskin.
    c. gently retract the foreskin.
    d. avoid cleansing between the skinfolds of the genital area.

27. To prevent a child with diarrhea from becoming dehydrated the nurse should:
    a. use gentle persuasion.
    b. force fluids.
    c. awaken the child to offer fluids.
    d. allow only high-quality, nutritious liquids.

28. The best example of adequate documentation of a child's food intake would be:
    a. "Child ate one bowl of cereal with milk."
    b. "Child ate an adequate breakfast."
    c. "Child ate 80% of the breakfast served."
    d. "Parent states that child ate an adequate breakfast."

29. During the chill phase of the febrile state:
    a. heat is generated and conserved.
    b. the temperature stabilizes at a higher range.
    c. a crisis of the temperature is occurring.
    d. the temperature is greater than the set point.

30. The most effective intervention for the treatment of fever in a 4-year-old child is to administer:
    a. a tepid sponge bath.
    b. ibuprofen.
    c. an alcohol sponge bath.
    d. acetaminophen.

31. The best intervention for the treatment of hyperthermia in a 4-year-old child is to administer:
    a. a tepid sponge bath.
    b. acetaminophen.
    c. an alcohol sponge bath.
    d. aspirin.

32. List four essential teaching points the nurse should cover when providing anticipatory guidance for a family who asks about the danger of fever in a child.

33. The best way to identify children at risk for falls in the hospital setting is to perform a _____ _____ _____ on admission and _____.

34. What is a choke tube test and for whom is the test performed?

35. Standard Precautions involve the use of personal protective equipment such as gloves, gown, and mask to prevent contamination from:
    a. blood.
    b. body fluids.
    c. mucous membranes.
    d. all of the above.

36. To prevent spread of illnesses from one patient to another after procedures, the most important strategy the nurse can use is to:
    a. follow disease-specific infection control guidelines.
    b. wear vinyl gloves.
    c. avoid wearing nail polish.
    d. wash the hands routinely after each patient contact.

37. After mouth or lip surgery, the nurse would choose to restrain the small child using:
    a. arm and leg restraints.
    b. elbow restraints.
    c. a jacket restraint.
    d. a mummy restraint.

38. The best strategy to use when performing venipuncture on a toddler is to:
    a. give simple instructions for the child to hold still.
    b. extend the neck and maintain head alignment to expose the jugular vein.
    c. place the child prone with legs in a frog position to expose groin the area.
    d. hold the child's upper body to prevent movement.

39. The best positioning technique for a lumbar puncture in a neonate is a:
    a. side-lying position with neck flexion.
    b. sitting position.
    c. side-lying position with modified neck extension.
    d. side-lying position with knees to chest.

40. An 18-month-old child hospitalized with RSV is in a crib with side rails up, but he is very mobile and the mother says he has climbed out of his crib at home. The best way to provide a safe environment for this toddler is to:
    a. place him in a Posey vest.
    b. use a papoose board to keep him from climbing out of the bed.
    c. place a crib top on the crib.
    d. use bilateral elbow restraints.

41. A 14-year-old boy is admitted to the ER and placed on a suicide watch, as he told his mother he would kill himself if she went out drinking again. This is his second or third threat in as many weekends, and the ER staff is acquainted with the family situation. The adolescent is placed in a locked room with a nonbreakable glass window in the wood door. A hospital security guard is positioned at the door. The practitioner asks the nurse if he thinks body restraints are necessary to protect the child. The nurse's priority intervention would be to:
    a. immediately place the boy in a Posey vest.
    b. talk with the boy and assess his mental status with focus on risk for self-harm.
    c. ask the mother for permission to administer sedation to the adolescent to prevent him from harming himself.
    d. None of the above would be appropriate.

42. The most frequently used site for bone marrow aspiration in children is the:
    a. femur.
    b. sternum.
    c. tibia.
    d. iliac crest.

43. When necessary, suprapubic aspiration may be used:
    a. to access the bladder through the urethra.
    b. to obtain a sterile urine specimen from an infant.
    c. even though it may increase the risk for contamination.
    d. to prevent complications associated with urinary catheterization.

44. To collect a blood culture specimen from a central venous line or peripheral lock, research suggests that the nurse:
    a. use the first sample of blood.
    b. discard the first sample of blood.
    c. irrigate the device with D_5W first.
    d. use a heparinized collection tube.

45. Of the following heelsticks techniques, the one that would be most important to use to avoid the complication of necrotizing osteochondritis would be to:
    a. warm the site.
    b. cleanse the site with alcohol.
    c. puncture no deeper than 2 mm.
    d. use the inner aspect of the heel.

46. To obtain a sputum specimen to test for tuberculosis in an infant, the nurse may need to:
    a. stimulate the infant's cough reflex.
    b. obtain mucus from the throat.
    c. insert a suction catheter into the back of the throat.
    d. perform gastric lavage.

47. The most accurate method for determining the safe dosage of a chemotherapy medication for a child is to use:
    a. the body surface area formula.
    b. Clark's rule.
    c. Wright's rule.
    d. milligrams per kilogram.

48. To safely administer 1 teaspoon of medication at home, the parent should use the:
    a. household soup spoon.
    b. disposable calibrated syringe.
    c. hospital's molded plastic cup.
    d. household teaspoon.

49. All of the following techniques for medication administration in the infant are acceptable *except*:
    a. adding the medication to the infant's formula.
    b. allowing the infant to sit in the parent's lap during administration.
    c. allowing the infant to suck the medication from a nipple.
    d. inserting a needleless syringe into the side of the mouth while the infant nurses.

50. According to recent research, the following intramuscular injection site is associated with fewer local and systemic reactions:
    a. Deltoid muscle
    b. Vastus lateralis
    c. Dorsogluteal
    d. Ventrogluteal

51. When administering intravenous medication to an infant, the nurse should:
    a. check site for patency before each dose.
    b. administer medications along with blood products.
    c. combine antibiotics to avoid fluid overload.
    d. use the maximum dilution of the drug permitted by the manufacturer.

52. When administering medications to a child through a gastric tube, the nurse should:
    a. use oily medications to ease passage through the tube.
    b. mix the medication with the enteral formula.
    c. use a syringe with the plunger in place to administer the drug.
    d. flush the tube well between each medication administration.

53. The rectal route of medication administration is used in children when the child:
    a. is not responding to oral antiemetic preparations.
    b. needs a reliable route of administration.
    c. is constipated.
    d. all of the above.

54. To instill eye drops in an infant whose eyelids are clenched shut, the nurse should:
    a. apply finger pressure to the lacrimal punctum.
    b. place the drops in the nasal corner where the lids meet and wait until the infant opens the lid.
    c. administer the eye drops before nap time.
    d. use any of the above techniques.

55. During continuous enteral feedings, the nurse should:
    a. use the same pole as used for the intravenous line.
    b. use a burette to calibrate the feeding times.
    c. give the infant a pacifier for sucking.
    d. all of the above.

56. To avoid multiple needle punctures for chemotherapy administration and blood draws, the _____ _____ provides access for such procedures.

57. A child with cerebral palsy and feeding difficulties related to poor oral motor function may benefit from being given enteral nutrition at night through a(n) _____ _____ _____.

58. To prevent an ostomy pouch from being pulled off, a young child may need to:
    a. wear one-piece outfits.
    b. use an alcohol-based skin sealant.
    c. use a rubber band to help the appliance fit.

CRITICAL THINKING—CASE STUDY

Janis is an 8-year-old child admitted to the hospital with suspected appendicitis. Her parents have been divorced for 4 years, and her mother accompanies her to the hospital. Janis has a sister who is 7 years old.

59. Based on Janis's developmental characteristics, the nurse's plan for preparing the girl for surgery should include:
    a. an emphasis on privacy.
    b. the correct scientific medical terminology.
    c. ways to help Janis accept new authority figures.
    d. teaching sessions that last no longer than 5 minutes.

60. One of the nursing diagnoses identified by the nurse for Janis is Risk for Injury related to the surgical procedure and anesthesia. During the assessment interview, which of the following sets of facts would be most pertinent to this diagnosis?
    a. The nurse auscultated vesicular breath sounds.
    b. Janis's mother tells the nurse that the child's father is 27 years old and in good health but had some heart problems related to anesthesia after a minor surgical procedure last year.
    c. Janis's mother tells the nurse not to expect the child's father to participate in the preoperative preparation because he lives in another state.
    d. The nurse determines that the child has moist mucous membranes and no tenting of the skin.

61. The nursing diagnosis of Anxiety related to the surgery and hospitalization is identified by the nurse. Which of the following strategies is the best one for the nurse to incorporate into the surgical care plan to address this diagnosis?
    a. Encourage Janis's mother to be present as much as possible.
    b. Administer analgesics around the clock.
    c. Teach Janis to use the incentive spirometer.
    d. Help Janis ambulate as early as possible.

62. Which of the following findings represents the most appropriate measurable data to evaluate the care plan in regard to the nursing diagnosis of Risk for Fluid Volume Deficit?
    a. The child has vesicular breath sounds.
    b. The child's father, who is 27 years old and in good health, had some heart problems with anesthesia after a minor surgical procedure last year.
    c. The child's father lives in another state.
    d. The child has moist mucous membranes and no tenting of the skin.

24 The Child with Fluid and Electrolyte Imbalance

1. Match each term with its description or function.

   a. Total body water
   b. Intracellular fluid
   c. Extracellular fluid
   d. Renin-angiotensin system
   e. Dehydration
   f. Aldosterone
   g. Antidiuretic hormone
   h. Intravascular fluid
   i. Interstitial
   j. Transcellular fluid
   k. Insensible water loss

   l. Third-spacing
   m. Edema
   n. Ascites
   o. Pulmonary edema
   p. Oral rehydration solution
   q. Shock
   r. Near-infrared spectroscopy (NIRS)
   s. Colloids
   t. Enteral nutrition
   u. Entonox

   _____ Constitutes about half of the total body water at birth; fluid outside the cell

   _____ Fluid within the cells

   _____ Constitutes 45% to 75% of body weight

   _____ Placement of a small-bore feeding tube into the duodenum

   _____ Short-term analgesic; mixture of gases in a fixed ratio of 50% nitrous oxide and 50% oxygen; used in burn therapy to control procedural pain

   _____ Enhances sodium reabsorption in renal tubules

   _____ Released from the posterior pituitary gland in response to increased osmolality and decreased volume of intravascular fluid

   _____ Diminished blood flow to the kidneys stimulates secretion, which reacts with plasma globulin to generate a vasoconstrictor

   _____ Occurs whenever the total output of fluid exceeds the total intake

   _____ Fluid loss through the skin and respiratory tract

   _____ Pooling of body fluids in a body space

   _____ Abnormal accumulation of fluid within the interstitial tissue and subsequent tissue expansion

   _____ Used to treat infants with dehydration

   _____ Surrounding the cell and the location of most extracellular fluid

   _____ Accumulation of fluid in the abdomen

   _____ Fluid contained within the body cavities (e.g., cerebrospinal fluid)

   _____ Occurs when there is an increase in the interstitial volume

   _____ Fluid contained within the blood vessels

   _____ Protein containing fluid often administered to children in shock

   _____ Noninvasive measure of regional tissue oxyhemoglobin saturation that is used in severe illness to predict catastrophic cerebral events and monitor oxygenation and perfusion

   _____ Circulatory failure results in cellular dysfunction and eventual organ failure

2. The nurse would expect which of the following conditions to produce an increased fluid requirement?
   a. Heart failure
   b. High intracranial pressure
   c. Mechanical ventilation
   d. Tachypnea

3. The nurse recognizes which of the following individuals as having the *least* water content in relation to weight?
   a. Obese adolescent female
   b. Thin adolescent female
   c. Obese adolescent male
   d. Thin adolescent male

4. Infants and young children are at high risk for fluid and electrolyte imbalances. Which one of the following factors contributes to this vulnerability?
   a. Decreased body surface area
   b. Lower metabolic rate
   c. Mature kidney function
   d. Increased extracellular fluid volume

5. Chloe, age 4 weeks, is brought to the clinic by her mother. When asking about Chloe's feeding schedule, the nurse learns that the mother has been adding twice the required amount of dry formula powder to water in Chloe's bottles for the past 2 days. The mother thinks that this will help Chloe gain weight faster. Which of the following does the nurse recognize as true about this practice?
   a. The infant's kidneys are functionally mature at birth and able to handle this concentration of formula.
   b. The infant's kidneys are functionally immature at birth, and this concentration of formula can cause Chloe to be dehydrated.
   c. The infant's kidneys are functionally immature at birth, and this concentration of formula will cause Chloe to become overhydrated.
   d. The infant's kidneys are functionally mature at birth, but because of her greater body surface area and longer gastrointestinal tract, Chloe would need the formula diluted.

6. What is the chief solute in extracellular fluid (ECF) and the primary determinant of ECF?
   a. Potassium
   b. Calcium
   c. Sodium
   d. Water

7. _____ dehydration occurs when electrolyte and water deficits are present in balanced proportion.

8. _____ dehydration occurs when the electrolyte deficit exceeds the water deficit. There is a greater proportional loss of extracellular fluid, and plasma sodium concentration is usually _____ than 130 mEq/L.

9. _____ dehydration results from water loss in excess of electrolyte loss. This is often caused by a large _____ of water and/or a large _____ of electrolytes. Plasma sodium concentration is _____ than 150 mEq/L.

10. In infants and young children, the most accurate means of describing dehydration or fluid loss is:
    a. as a percentage.
    b. by milliliters per kilogram of body weight.
    c. by the amount of edema present or absent.
    d. by the degree of skin elasticity.

11. An infant with moderate dehydration has what clinical signs?
    a. Mottled skin color, decreased pulse and respirations
    b. Decreased urinary output, tachycardia, and fever
    c. Tachycardia, oliguria, capillary filling within 2 to 4 seconds
    d. Tachycardia, bulging fontanel, decreased blood pressure

12. Diagnostic evaluation of dehydration to initiate a therapeutic plan includes:
    i. serum electrolytes.
    ii. acid-base imbalance determination.
    iii. physical assessment to determine degree of dehydration.
    iv. type of dehydration based on pathophysiology.

    a. i and ii
    b. i, ii, and iii
    c. i, ii, iii, and iv
    d. iii and iv

13. Which of the following instructions for treating the child with mild dehydration is *not* correct?
    a. Administer 2 to 5 ml of oral rehydration solution (ORS) by syringe or small medication cup every 2 to 3 minutes until the child is able to tolerate larger amounts.
    b. Oral administration of ondansetron (Zofran) to the child with acute gastroenteritis and vomiting may prevent the need for intravenous (IV) therapy.
    c. ORS management consists of replacement of fluid loss over 4 to 6 hours.
    d. ORS should not be started until after all vomiting has stopped.

14. Johnny, age 13 months, is being admitted for parenteral fluid therapy because of excessive vomiting. The nurse would recognize which one of the following as most essential in implementing care for Johnny?
    a. Give Johnny oral fluids until the parenteral fluid therapy can be established.
    b. Question the physician's order for parenteral fluid therapy of 0.9% sodium chloride.
    c. Withhold the ordered potassium additive until Johnny's renal function has been verified.
    d. Replace half of Johnny's estimated fluid deficit over the first 24 hours of parenteral fluid therapy.

15. Rapid fluid replacement is contraindicated in which one of the following types of dehydration?
    a. Isotonic
    b. Hypotonic
    c. Hypertonic

16. Water intoxication can occur in children from:
    i. excessive intake of electrolyte-free formula.
    ii. administration of inappropriate hypotonic solutions.
    iii. dilution of formula with water.
    iv. isotonic dehydration.
    v. vigorous hydration with water following a febrile illness.
    vi. fluid shifts from intracellular to extracellular spaces.

    a. i, ii, iii, and iv
    b. i, ii, iii, and v
    c. ii, iii, and iv
    d. ii, iii, v, and vi

17. Severe generalized edema in all body tissues is called _____.

18. Edema formation can be caused by which one of the following?
    a. Decreased venous pressure
    b. Alteration in capillary permeability
    c. Increased plasma proteins
    d. Increased tissue tension

19. How does the nurse assess for pitting edema?
    a. Measure abdominal girth.
    b. Observe for fluid retention in the lower extremities.
    c. Press fingertip against bony prominence for 5 seconds.
    d. Observe for loss of normal skin creases.

20. To obtain relevant information from the parents of a child with fluid and electrolyte disturbances, the nurse should question the parents about:
    a. the type and amount of the child's intake and output.
    b. the child's general appearance.
    c. the child's weight over the past month.
    d. whether they have taken the child's temperature within the past 24 hours.

21. Joan, age 3 years, is admitted for fluid and electrolyte disturbances. The nurse's assessment should include:
    i.   general appearance observation.
    ii. vital signs.
    iii. intake and output measurements.
    iv. daily weights.
    v.   review of laboratory results.

    a. i, ii, iii, and iv
    b. ii, iii, and iv
    c. iii, iv, and v
    d. i, ii, iii, iv, and v

22. Which symptoms would the nurse expect in a child with hypocalcemia?
    a. Abdominal cramps, oliguria
    b. Tingling of nose, ears, fingertips and toes, neuromuscular irritability, tetany
    c. Thirst, low urine specific gravity
    d. Flushed, mottled extremities and weight gain

23. Fill in the blanks to identify the type of shock described in each of the following statements.

    a. _____ shock follows a reduction in circulating blood volume, plasma volume, or extracellular fluid loss.

    b. _____ shock results from impaired cardiac muscle function resulting in reduced cardiac output.

    c. _____ shock results from a vascular abnormality that produces maldistribution of blood supply throughout the body.

    d. _____ type of distributive shock is characterized by a hypersensitivity reaction, causing massive vasodilation and capillary leak.

    e. _____ type of distributive shock is characterized by decreased cardiac output and derangements in the peripheral circulation in response to a severe, overwhelming infection.

    f. _____ type of distributive shock is characterized by massive vasodilation resulting from the loss of sympathetic nervous system tone, which can occur with spinal cord injuries.

24. Clinical manifestations of lowering blood pressure, pronounced tachycardia, narrowed pulse pressure, poor capillary filling, and increased confusion would suggest which of the following?
    a. Compensated shock
    b. Hypotensive (decompensated shock)
    c. Irreversible shock

25. List the three major efforts in the treatment of shock.

26. The position of choice for the child in shock is:
    a. Trendelenburg.
    b. head-down with feet straight.
    c. flat with the legs elevated.
    d. semi-Fowler.

27. Which of the following drugs used to improve cardiac function in the pediatric patient with shock also improves renal function?
    a. Dopamine
    b. Lasix
    c. Vasopressin
    d. Epinephrine

28. The nurse, caring for a pediatric patient with septic shock, knows that therapeutic goals associated with tissue perfusion include:
    i. capillary refill < 2 seconds
    ii. arterial pressure 65-70 mm Hg
    iii. urinary output > 0.5 ml/kg/hr
    iv. CVP 8-12 mm Hg

    a. i, ii, iii, and iv
    b. i, ii, and iii
    c. i and iii
    d. ii, iii, and iv

29. Match each stage of septic shock with its characteristics.

    a. Hyperdynamic stage
    b. Normodynamic stage
    c. Hypodynamic stage

    _____ Progressive deterioration of cardiovascular function, hypothermia, cold extremities, weak pulses, hypotension

    _____ Warm, flushed skin with normal blood pressure, chills, fever, and normal urinary output

    _____ Duration of only a few hours; cool skin, normal pulses and blood pressure, decreased urinary output, and depressed mental state

30. What is the primary goal in treating any pediatric patient with allergies?
    a. Have Benadryl available for use immediately for any contact
    b. Obtaining a thorough and complete health history
    c. Prevention of a reaction
    d. Prevention of anaphylaxis

31. Which of the following describes the most common initial signs of anaphylaxis?
    a. Cutaneous signs of flushing and urticaria and complaint of feeling warm
    b. Bronchiolar constriction with wheezing
    c. Vasodilation and hypotension
    d. Laryngeal edema and stridor

32. Toxic shock syndrome (TSS) is caused by the toxins produced by:
    a. *C. difficile* bacteria
    b. human papillomavirus
    c. *Streptococcus* bacteria
    d. *Staphylococcus* bacteria

33. The sudden development of high fever, vomiting and diarrhea, profound hypotension, shock, oliguria, and an erythematous macular rash with subsequent desquamation are clinical signs of:
    a. anaphylaxis
    b. irreversible shock
    c. *C. difficile* infections
    d. toxic shock syndrome

34. What should be included in the teaching plan for adolescent females to prevent toxic shock syndrome associated with tampon use?

35. Burn injuries are attributed to what five causes?

36. The most common burn among young children is caused by:
    a. playing with matches.
    b. heaters such as kerosene or wood burning.
    c. careless smoking.
    d. scald burns, as with hot water or grease.

37. The standard adult "rule of nines" cannot be used to determine the total body surface area of a burn in a child because:
    a. the child has different body proportions than the adult.
    b. the child has different fluid body weight than the adult.
    c. the child's trunk and arm proportions are larger than the adult's.
    d. as the infant grows, the percentage allotted for the head increases while the percentages for the arms decrease.

38. Brock, 12 years old, has burns involving the epidermis and part of the dermis. Blister and edema formation are present, and the burns are extremely sensitive to temperature changes, exposure to air, and light touch. Brock has:
    a. superficial first-degree burns.
    b. partial-thickness second-degree burns.
    c. full-thickness third-degree burns.
    d. full-thickness fourth-degree burns.

39. The severity of burn injury is determined by which of the following?
    i. Pain associated with the burn, measured on a scale of 0 to 10
    ii. Percentage of body surface area burned
    iii. Level of consciousness of the victim
    iv. Depth of the burn
    v. Vital sign measurements
    vi. The causative agent

    a. i, ii, and iv
    b. i, ii, iii, and v
    c. iv, v, and vi
    d. ii, iv, and vi

40. The expected predominant symptom of a superficial burn is:
    a. pain.
    b. significant tissue damage.
    c. absence of protective functions of the skin.
    d. blister formation.

41. In conducting the physical examination of a pediatric burn patient, how would the nurse best assess to see whether circulation to the area is intact?
    a. Touch the area to see if pain is felt.
    b. Test injured surfaces for blanching and capillary refill.
    c. Inspect the burns for eschar formation.
    d. Watch for edema of the affected part.

42. Which one of the following pediatric patients is at higher risk for complications from burn injury?
    a. The 12-month-old infant who pulled a pan of hot water over on his chest
    b. The 12-month-old infant who is burned on his chest by gasoline
    c. The 9-month-old infant who is burned on the hands and feet with scalding water
    d. The 12-year-old child who is burned on one side of the face as a result of playing with cigarettes

43. Jordan, age 12 years, has suffered severe burns, and now his chest appears constricted. The nurse should prepare for:
    a. intubation.
    b. chest tube insertion.
    c. escharotomy.
    d. hydrotherapy.

44. Systemic response to thermal injury would include:
    a. hypoglycemia.
    b. increased capillary permeability.
    c. myoglobinuria.
    d. decreased metabolic rate.

45. Decrease in cardiac output in the postburn period is caused by which of the following?
    a. Circulating myocardial depressant factor
    b. Fluid losses through denuded skin
    c. Vasodilation and increased capillary permeability
    d. All of the above

46. In the first few days after a major thermal burn injury, the nurse observes oliguria. What is the most likely cause for this finding?
    a. Acute renal failure
    b. Inadequate fluid replacement
    c. BUN and creatinine elevations
    d. All of the above

47. After severe burns, changes in the gastrointestinal system include all the following *except*:
    a. ischemia that can produce ulcer formation, enterocolitis, and intestinal perforation.
    b. disruption of the GI mucosal integrity, which allows sepsis to occur.
    c. a greatly accelerated metabolic rate.
    d. blood glucose levels are decreased as a result of insulin resistance.

48. Systemic responses to severe burns may include:
    i. blood flow decreases to the gastrointestinal system by one third even though cardiac output is maintained by resuscitation fluids.
    ii. adrenal activity decreases.
    iii. hematocrit decreases.
    iv. loss of circulating red blood cells.
    v. metabolic acidosis.

    a. ii, iii, and iv
    b. i, iv, and v
    c. i, iii, and v
    d. ii and iv

49. Kenny, age 5, is brought to the emergency department for severe burns on his anterior trunk and neck. Singed nasal hair and some minor burns are evident on physical examination. What immediate complication should be watched for?
    a. Inhalation injury
    b. Facial deformities
    c. Bacterial pneumonia
    d. Carbon monoxide inhalation

50. A common cause of respiratory failure in the pediatric population after severe burns is:
    a. bacterial pneumonia.
    b. pneumothorax.
    c. pulmonary edema.
    d. restriction of chest wall as a result of edema and inelastic eschar formation.

51. A gram-negative organism that is commonly found on the burn wound surface on the third day after burn and is responsible for wound sepsis is:
    a. *C. difficile*
    b. *Pseudomonas aeruginosa.*
    c. group B streptococci.
    d. *Haemophilus influenzae.*

52. What should be included in the plan for emergency care of the burned child?
    a. Apply large amounts of cold water over denuded areas.
    b. Apply ointments to the burned area.
    c. Remove jewelry and metal.
    d. Apply neutralizing agents to the skin of chemical burn areas.

53. Bobby, age 2 years, has suffered a minor burn injury. Expected management would include:
    a. redressing the wound with a gauze dressing every 3 days.
    b. soaking stuck dressings in hydrogen peroxide before removal.
    c. watching wound margins for redness, edema, or purulent drainage.
    d. administering narcotics for pain.

54. Which of the following is the best method to establish an adequate airway for a burned pediatric patient exhibiting changes in sensorium, air hunger, nasal flaring, and grunting?
    a. 100% oxygen administration
    b. intubation
    c. administration of bronchodilators
    d. suctioning to remove secretions

55. In major burn injuries of children weighing less than 30 kg (66 lb), adequate fluid replacement during the emergent phase is best assessed by which one of the following?
    a. Urinary output of 30 ml/hr
    b. Urinary output of 0.5 to 1 ml/kg/hr
    c. Increasing hematocrit
    d. Normal blood pressure

Chapter **24**   **The Child with Fluid and Electrolyte Imbalance**

56. To maintain adequate nutrition and promote healing in the child with a major burn injury, the nurse would recommend which one of the following nutrition plans?
    a. Diet high in proteins and calories
    b. Diet high in calories and low in proteins
    c. Diet high in fats and carbohydrates
    d. Diet high in vitamins A and D

57. Topical antimicrobial agents in burn therapy:
    a. eliminate organisms from the wound.
    b. effectively inhibit bacterial growth.
    c. encourage strains of resistant bacteria.
    d. are not used because they diffuse through eschar.

58. Which of the following is a temporary graft obtained from human cadavers and used in burn treatment?
    a. Allograft
    b. Xenograft
    c. Autograft
    d. Isograft

59. Which of the following statements about Integra, an artificial skin used in burn treatment, is correct?
    a. It is applied only to full-thickness burns.
    b. The second layer is pulled off after the dermis is formed.
    c. It replaces the need for additional skin grafting.
    d. It prepares the burn wound to accept an ultrathin autograft.

60. In caring for the donor site following split-thickness skin graft, the nurse expects:
    a. the dressing to be changed daily.
    b. the dressing not to be changed for 10 to 14 days.
    c. the area to be washed daily with soap and water.
    d. the application of an antibiotic ointment daily.

61. Johnny, age 8 years, suffered partial-thickness second-degree burns of his chest, abdomen, and upper legs while on a recent camping trip. He is scheduled for hydrotherapy each morning for 20 minutes followed by debridement. The best nursing action to assist Johnny at this time is to:
    a. ensure that pain medication is given before treatment.
    b. hold Johnny's breakfast until he returns from treatment.
    c. offer sedation after the procedure to promote rest.
    d. reassure Johnny that hydrotherapy and debridement are not painful.

62. Which of the following nursing diagnoses would be recognized as the highest priority during the management phase of his illness?
    a. Impaired Gas Exchange related to inhalation injury
    b. High Risk for Altered Nutrition: Less Than Body Requirements related to loss of appetite
    c. Fluid Volume Deficit related to edema associated with burn injury
    d. High Risk for Infection related to denuded skin, presence of pathogenic organisms, and altered immune response

63. A burn pediatric patient is in the rehabilitative phase of care. Which of the following statements about scar tissue during this period is correct?
    a. Scar tissue that is raised, red, and firm is considered inactive.
    b. Uniform pressure applied to the scar increases the blood supply and forces the collagen into a more normal alignment.
    c. Continuous pressure to areas of scarring can be achieved by elastic pressure garments and help to prevent scarring.
    d. When pressure to the scar is removed, blood supply to the scar slowly increases; therefore, elastic pressure garments can be removed frequently without scar formation.

64. Prevention of burn injury in children includes education of parents and caregivers. Which of the following is *not* included in the educational program?
    a. Stressing the importance of adequate supervision and establishment of a safe play area in the home
    b. Teaching children at an early age how to "stop, drop, and roll" to extinguish a fire
    c. Placing microwave ovens higher than children's faces
    d. Setting hot water heater thermostats no higher than 54° C (130° F)

CRITICAL THINKING—CASE STUDY

Jennifer, age 4 months, is admitted to the hospital because of dehydration caused by diarrhea. Her mother has been giving her electrolyte-free solutions for volume replacement. Parenteral fluids have been ordered for Jennifer.

65. What type of dehydration does Jennifer most likely have?
    a. Isotonic
    b. Hypertonic
    c. Hypotonic
    d. Water intoxication

66. Which of the following data about Jennifer should the nurse obtain during the admission history?
    a. Type and amount of food and fluid intake
    b. Urinary output amount or frequency
    c. Number and consistency of stools in the past 24 hours
    d. All of the above

67. Which of the following observations does the nurse recognize as the best indicator that Jennifer's dehydration is becoming more severe?
    a. Jennifer's cry is whining and low-pitched.
    b. Jennifer's pulse is slightly increased.
    c. Jennifer's appetite is diminished.
    d. Jennifer is becoming more irritable and lethargic.

68. A priority goal in the management of acute diarrhea is:
    a. determining the cause of the diarrhea.
    b. preventing the spread of the infection.
    c. rehydrating the child.
    d. managing the fever associated with the diarrhea.

69. The nurse's most critical responsibility when administering IV fluids to Jennifer is to:
    a. prevent IV infiltration.
    b. ensure sterility.
    c. prevent cardiac overload.
    d. maintain the fluid at body temperature.

25 The Child with Renal Dysfunction

1. Identify the following statements as true or false.

_____ The primary responsibility of the kidney is to maintain the composition and volume of body fluids in excess of body needs.

_____ The kidney functions in the production of erythropoietin and thus in the formation of red blood cells.

_____ Renin is secreted by the kidney in response to reduced blood volume, decreased blood pressure, or increased secretion of catecholamines.

_____ Approximately half of the total cardiac output makes up the blood flow to the kidneys.

_____ Protein is a normal finding in urine because it is too large a molecule to be reabsorbed in the proximal tubule.

_____ Glucose is reabsorbed in the proximal tubule and returned directly to the blood.

_____ Because there is a limit to the concentration gradient against which sodium can be transported out, when larger than normal amounts of sodium remain in the tubules, water is obliged to remain with the sodium.

_____ An end product of protein metabolism is urea.

_____ The newborn is unable to dispose of excess water and solute rapidly or efficiently because glomerular filtration and absorption do not reach adult values until the child is between 1 and 2 years of age.

_____ The loop of Henle, the site of the urine-concentrating mechanism, is short in the newborn, thus reducing the ability to reabsorb sodium and water and produce concentrated urine.

_____ Newborn infants are unable to excrete a water load at rates similar to those of older persons.

_____ *Escherichia coli* is responsible for 85% of urinary tract infections.

_____ Extrinsic factors that can cause functional bladder neck obstruction and contribute to urinary stasis are pregnancy and chronic and intermittent constipation.

_____ Research studies conducted on cranberry products have proven their effectiveness in prevention of urinary tract infections.

_____ Renal or bladder ultrasound is an invasive procedure that allows visualization of the renal pelvis.

2. What are the three factors that must function normally for urinary continence to be achieved and maintained?

3. Jordan is a 2-year-old who has had a clean-catch urinalysis done as part of a diagnostic work-up. The results of Jordan's urinalysis are listed below. Identify whether each result is normal (mark with an N) or abnormal (mark with an A).

_____ +1 glucose

_____ Specific gravity 1.020

_____ RBC 3-4

_____ WBC greater than 10

_____ Occasional casts

_____ Negative protein

_____ Positive nitrites

184

4. Match each term with its description.

a. Bacteriuria
b. Efflux
c. Reflux
d. Glomerular filtration rate
e. Creatinine
f. Cystitis
g. Urethritis
h. Pyelonephritis

i. Urosepsis
j. Vesicoureteral reflux
k. Azotemia
l. Chronic renal function
m. Uremia
n. Auria
o. Familial nephritis (Alport syndrome)

_____ Backward flow of urine

_____ Inflammation of the bladder

_____ Inflammation of the upper urinary tract and kidneys

_____ Retrograde flow of bladder urine into the ureters

_____ Accumulation of nitrogenous waste within the blood resulting in elevated blood urea nitrogen (BUN) and creatinine levels

_____ Forward movement of urine from kidney to bladder

_____ Measure of the amount of plasma from which a substance is cleared in 1 minute; generally accepted as the best overall index of kidney function

_____ Febrile urinary tract infection coexisting with systemic signs of bacterial illness; blood culture reveals presence of urinary pathogen

_____ An end product of protein metabolism in muscle

_____ Inflammation of the urethra

_____ Presence of bacteria in the urine

_____ Toxic symptoms caused by retention of nitrogenous products in the blood

_____ Begins when the diseased kidneys can no longer maintain the normal chemical structure of body fluids under normal conditions

_____ Hereditary disease characterized by sensorineural deafness, ocular disorders, and chronic kidney disease caused by mutations in the type IV collagen

_____ No urinary output for 24 hours

5. The nurse, in preparing the child for a diagnostic test, explains that which one of the following tests provides direct visualization of the bladder through a small scope?
   a. Cystoscopy
   b. Voiding cystourethrogram
   c. Intravenous pyelogram
   d. Renal biopsy

6. Preprocedural preparation of the child who is scheduled to have a cystourethrography includes:
   a. keeping the child NPO (nothing by mouth) for 8 hours before the test.
   b. assessing for an allergy to iodine.
   c. administering a Fleet enema before the examination.
   d. preparing the child for catheterization.

7. Which of the following is the most important nursing intervention to prevent urinary tract infections in pediatric patients?
   a. Teach parents of pediatric patients ways to prevent constipation by encouraging a diet high in fiber and fluids and ways to prevent stool and urine withholding by encouraging good toilet habits.
   b. Teach parents of pediatric patients the importance of administering prescribed medications for infection including dosage and scheduling.
   c. Teach parents of pediatric patients the signs and symptoms of urinary tract infections.
   d. Teach parents the proper collection techniques for urine samples.

185

8. Which one of the following does *not* predispose the patient to urinary tract infections?
   a. The short urethra in the young girl
   b. Urinary stasis
   c. Urinary reflux
   d. Lowering of urine pH

9. Symptoms of urinary tract infection often observed in children over age 2 years include:
   i. incontinence in a child previously toilet trained.
   ii. abdominal pain.
   iii. strong or foul odor to the urine.
   iv. frequency of urination.
   v. diarrhea.

   a. i, ii, and iii
   b. iii and iv
   c. iii, iv, and v
   d. i, ii, iii, and iv

10. Three-year-old Ivy is brought to the clinic because of a suspected urinary tract infection. Which of the following is the correct method for collecting the urine specimen?
   a. Encourage large amounts of water because Ivy is unable to void at this time.
   b. Set Ivy on the toilet facing the tank to decrease likelihood of contamination.
   c. Wait until the first morning voided specimen can be collected.
   d. Bag Ivy with the bag covering the entire perineal area.

11. The treatment goals for children with urinary tract infections include:
   a.

   b.

   c.

12. Which symptom suggests pyelonephritis in a 3-year-old child?
   a. Flank pain and tenderness
   b. Foul-smelling urine
   c. Dysuria or urgency
   d. Enuresis or daytime incontinence

13. The nurse is asked to obtain a urine specimen from 5-year-old Anne. Which of the following is the correct procedure?
   a. Place a urine bag on Anne to collect the next specimen.
   b. Obtain a catheterized specimen.
   c. Encourage Anne to drink large volumes of water in an attempt to obtain a specimen.
   d. Obtain a midstream specimen, preferably the first morning specimen.

14. Justin, age 8 years, has been diagnosed with pyelonephritis. The nurse would expect medical management to include all of the following *except*:
   a. admission to the hospital with intravenous antibiotics administered for the first 48 hours.
   b. blood and urine cultures obtained on admission.
   c. urine cultures repeated after therapy.
   d. administration of nitrofurantoin.

15. Common antiinfective agents used for urinary tract infections in children include all of the following *except*:
   a. quinolones.
   b. penicillins.
   c. sulfonamides.
   d. cephalosporins.

16. The nurse is developing a preventive teaching plan for Tracy, a sexually active 16-year-old who has been diagnosed with a urinary tract infection. Which of the following should be included in the plan?
    a. Promote perineal hygiene by wiping back to front.
    b. Urinate as soon as possible after intercourse.
    c. Douche as soon as possible after intercourse to flush out bacteria.
    d. Eliminate all carbonated and caffeinated beverages because they irritate the bladder.

17. Vesicoureteral reflux (VUR) is closely associated with which one of the following?
    a. Acute glomerulonephritis
    b. Nephrotic syndrome
    c. Renal scarring and kidney damage
    d. High alkaline content in the urine

18. Medical management for vesicoureteral reflex (VUR) consists of continuous antibiotic prophylaxis (CAP).
    a. What is the rationale behind CAP use in VUR patients?

    b. Why is amoxicillin used only for infants less than 2 months of age with VUR?

19. Acute poststreptococcal glomerulonephritis (APSGN):
    i. is the less common of the noninfectious renal diseases in children.
    ii. can occur at any age but primarily affects school-age children, the peak age of onset being 6 to 8 years.
    iii. is an immune complex disease related to a reaction that occurs as a by-product from certain strains of group A β-hemolytic streptococcus.
    iv. follows a latent period of 1 to 2 weeks between the infection of the throat or 3 to 4 weeks between skin infection and the onset of symptoms for APSGN.
    v. most commonly occurs in fall and spring.

    a. i, ii, iii, iv, and v
    b. ii, iii, and iv
    c. i, iii, and iv
    d. ii, iii, and v

20. Which of the following clinical manifestations are associated with acute glomerulonephritis?
    a. Normal blood pressure, generalized edema, oliguria
    b. Periorbital edema, hypertension, dark-colored urine
    c. Fatigue, elevated serum lipid levels, elevated serum protein levels
    d. Temperature elevation, circulatory congestion, normal BUN and creatinine serum levels

21. The major complications that may develop during the acute phase of glomerulonephritis are:

22. Nursing interventions in caring for the child with acute glomerulonephritis include:
    a. enforced bed rest.
    b. daily weights.
    c. keeping the child NPO.
    d. a high-sodium diet.

23. Chronic glomerulonephritis (CGN) describes a variety of different disease processes that may be distinguished from one another by:
    a. renal biopsy.
    b. cystoscopy.
    c. blood cultures.
    d. serologic tests, including ASO titers.

24. Which of the following diagnostic findings would suggest failing renal function?
    a. Decreased creatinine and elevated BUN
    b. Elevated BUN, creatinine, and uric acid levels
    c. Elevated potassium, phosphorus, and calcium
    d. Proteinuria and decreased creatinine and BUN

25. Clinical manifestations of nephrotic syndrome include:
    a. hyperlipidemia, hypoalbuminemia, edema, and proteinuria.
    b. hematuria, hypertension, periorbital edema, flank pain.
    c. oliguria, hypolipidemia, and hyperalbuminemia.
    d. hematuria, generalized edema, hypertension, and proteinuria.

26. Which child is most at risk for minimal-change nephrotic syndrome?
    a. A 4-year-old recovering from viral upper respiratory tract infection
    b. A 7-year-old after a group A β-hemolytic streptococcus throat infection
    c. A 6-year-old with acquired immunodeficiency syndrome (AIDS)
    d. A 2-year-old who recently received several bee stings

27. The diet requirement for minimal-change nephrotic syndrome includes:
    a. water restriction.
    b. low-protein diet in both acute and remission stages.
    c. salt restriction during periods of edema and while on corticosteroid therapy.
    d. high-protein diet during both acute and remission stages.

28. In addition to the usual vaccinations, children with nephrotic syndrome should receive what vaccinations?

29. Therapeutic management in nephrotic syndrome includes the administration of prednisone. The nurse teaches which of the following as correct administration guidelines?
    a. Corticosteroid therapy is begun after BUN and serum creatinine elevation.
    b. Prednisone is administered orally once daily for 3 weeks.
    c. The drug is given daily for 4 to 6 weeks, then decreased in dosage and given on alternate days for 2 to 5 months with taper.
    d. The drug is discontinued as soon as the urine is free from protein.

30. Drug side effects associated with cyclophosphamide (Cytoxan) are:
    i. leukopenia.
    ii. azoospermia.
    iii. effects on gonadal function in females.
    iv. hypertension.
    v. cognitive impairment.

    a. i, ii, and iii
    b. i, iv, and v
    c. ii, iii, and v
    d. i, ii, iii, iv, and v

31. Which one of the following urine tests is conducted daily while the child is receiving medicine for nephrotic syndrome?
    a. Glucose
    b. Specific gravity
    c. Albumin
    d. pH

32. Which of the following statements about renal tubal disorders is *false*?
    a. Renal tubal disorders can be either congenital or acquired.
    b. Renal tubal disorders are primarily metabolic disorders.
    c. Renal tubal disorders present with clinical manifestations of edema and hypertension with elevated blood urea nitrogen.
    d. Renal tubal disorders present with abnormal urinalysis.

33. A syndrome of sustained metabolic acidosis in which there is impaired reabsorption of bicarbonate or excretion of net hydrogen ion but in which glomerular function is normal is termed:
    a. Renal tubular acidosis
    b. Nephrogenic diabetes insipidus
    c. Hemolytic uremic syndrome
    d. Unexplained proteinuria

34. A disorder associated with a defect in the ability to concentrate urine in which the distal tubules and collecting ducts are insensitive to the action of antidiuretic hormone or its exogenous counterpart, vasopressin, is termed:
    a. Renal tubular acidosis
    b. Nephrogenic diabetes insipidus
    c. Hemolytic uremic syndrome
    d. Unexplained proteinuria

35. Multiple cases of hemolytic uremic syndrome caused by enteric infection of the *E. coli* O157:H7 serotype have been traced to:
    i. undercooked meat, especially ground beef.
    ii. unpasteurized apple juice.
    iii. alfalfa sprouts.
    iv. public pools.
    v. unwashed grapes.

    a. i, iv, and v
    b. i and ii
    c. i, ii, iii, and iv
    d. ii, iii, and v

36. Diagnostic evaluation results for hemolytic uremic syndrome include which of the following?
    a. Proteinuria, hematuria, urinary cast, elevated BUN and serum creatinine, low hemoglobin and hematocrit, and a high reticulocyte count
    b. High potassium, low sodium, high hemoglobin and hematocrit, and proteinuria
    c. High number of urinary casts, low serum BUN and creatinine, and decreased sedimentary rates
    d. Urine negative for protein but positive for red blood cells, normal hemoglobin and hematocrit, and elevated serum BUN and creatinine levels

37. In evaluation of the child with possible renal trauma, which one of the following is usually indicative of kidney damage?
    a. Flank pain and hematuria
    b. Dysuria, proteinuria, and nausea
    c. Abdominal ascites, nausea, and hematuria
    d. Proteinuria and bladder spasms

38. What is the most frequent cause of prerenal failure in infants and children?
    a. Nephrotoxic agents
    b. Obstructive uropathy
    c. Dehydration related to diarrhea and vomiting
    d. Burn shock

39. The primary manifestation of acute renal failure is:
    a. edema.
    b. oliguria.
    c. metabolic acidosis.
    d. weight gain and proteinuria.

40. The most immediate threat to the life of the child with acute renal failure is:
    a. hyperkalemia.
    b. anemia.
    c. hypertension crisis.
    d. cardiac failure from hypovolemia.

41. Which drug therapy is used in the removal of potassium from the body?
    a. Mannitol
    b. Sodium bicarbonate
    c. Kayexalate
    d. Calcium gluconate

42. The major nursing task in the care of the infant or child with acute renal failure is:

43. Which one of the following manifestations of chronic renal failure can have the most social consequences for the developing child?
    a. Anemia
    b. Growth retardation
    c. Bone demineralization
    d. Septicemia

44. Dietary regulation in the child with chronic renal failure includes:
    a. increasing dietary phosphorus.
    b. providing protein of high biologic value in the diet.
    c. continuous restricting of potassium.
    d. adding vitamin A, E, and K supplements.

45. The treatment for the pediatric patient with anemia related to chronic renal failure includes all of the following *except*:
    a. ferrous sulfate supplements.
    b. ascorbic acid supplements.
    c. vitamin B_{12} supplements.
    d. administration of erythropoietin.

46. Measures aimed at helping control the calcium/phosphorus imbalance for osteodystrophy in chronic renal failure include all the following *except*:
    a. increase in milk products to help control dietary phosphorus.
    b. calcium carbonate preparations given with meals to bind phosphorus if the child is hyperphosphatemic or mildly hypocalcemic.
    c. appropriate therapy with vitamin D is instituted when serum phosphate levels are normal.
    d. monitoring serum calcium levels frequently during periods when drugs are being changed or regulated.

47. Bobby, age 12 years, has been diagnosed with chronic renal failure since the age of 6 years. He has reached end-stage renal failure. Which one of the following nursing care management interventions should *not* be included in Bobby's care plan?
    a. Assist Bobby in adjusting to the fact that he will always be different from his peers. He will be shorter, more tired at times, and unable to participate in all activities.
    b. Prepare Bobby for acceptance of the need for dialysis.
    c. Explain to Bobby that he will no longer be able to go to school.
    d. Assist the parents in exploring the financial drain the disease will have on the family resources and provide information on assistance that is available.

48. Complete the following statements as they relate to dialysis for renal care.

    a. The three methods of dialysis are: _____.

    b. The three absolute indications for dialysis are: _____ _____.

    c. The major complication associated with peritoneal dialysis is: _____.

    d. _____ is a type of dialysis ideal for use in children with fluid overload from surgical procedures who do not have severe biochemical abnormalities; removes excess fluid from patients with severe oliguric fluid overload.

49. Amy, age 14 years, is scheduled to receive hemodialysis. She will need to have a vein and artery surgically connected for blood access. Which one of the following is the correct name for this type of blood access?
    a. Graft
    b. Fistula
    c. Percutaneous catheter

50. Johnny, age 12, had a renal transplant 5 months ago. He now comes to the hospital outpatient clinic with fever, tenderness over the graft area, decreased urinary output, and slightly elevated blood pressure. The nurse's priority at this time is:
    a. to recognize that Johnny is probably undergoing acute rejection and to notify the physician immediately.
    b. to recognize that this is an episode of increased inflammation within the donor kidney because Johnny has probably been noncompliant with his immunosuppressant drugs. The nurse should educate Johnny regarding drug compliance and notify Johnny's physician when he makes rounds.
    c. to obtain a urine specimen for culture and sensitivity and a blood count to quickly identify Johnny's infection before alerting the physician.
    d. to recognize that Johnny is in chronic rejection and that no present therapy can halt the progressive process.

51. Match each term with its description.

    a. Phimosis   f. Hydronephrosis
    b. Cryptorchidism   g. Balanitis
    c. Hypospadias   h. Oligohydramnios
    d. Epispadias   i. Renal colic
    e. Hydrocele   j. Anorchism

    _____ Prevents retraction of the foreskin

    _____ Absence of testes

    _____ Fluid in the processus vaginalis

    _____ Failure of one or both testes to descend

    _____ Condition in which urethral opening is located below the glans penis or along the ventral surface of penile shaft

    _____ Defect of urinary system characterized by failure of urethral canalization

    _____ Distention of the renal pelvis and calyces

    _____ Characterized by discomfort in the flank, lower abdomen, or lower back

    _____ Inflammation or infection of the phimotic foreskin

    _____ Decreased amount of amniotic fluid

52. Which of the following statements about undescended testes is *false*?
   a. In the case of retractile testes, the parents may report intermittently observing the testes in the scrotum, interspersed with periods when they cannot be palpated or observed.
   b. Retractile testes and true undescended testes both will need surgical correction.
   c. Surgical repair of undescended testes is done to prevent damage to the undescended testicle, decrease incidence of malignancy, avoid trauma and torsion, and close the processus vaginalis.
   d. True undescended testes rarely descend spontaneously after 1 year of age.

53. Which of the following discharge instructions should *not* be included for the child who is post hypospadias repair and still has a catheter or stent?
   a. Position the urine bag below the waist.
   b. The child is allowed to take a tub bath daily.
   c. An antibacterial ointment may be applied to the penis.
   d. Avoid straddle toys, sandboxes, and rough activities.

54. In caring for the infant with exstrophy, which of the following is *incorrect*?
   a. Staged repair is started during the neonatal period, perferably within the first 1 to 2 days of life.
   b. Until closure is performed, the bladder is covered with clear plastic wrap or a thin film dressing.
   c. Petroleum jelly is used to keep the area moist and prevent breakdown.
   d. After closure, the infant is monitored for urinary output and signs of urinary tract infection.

55. The child with obstruction of the renal pelvis or ureter is most likely to present with which of the following clinical manifestations?
   a. Poor force of urinary stream or intermittency of voided stream.
   b. Nocturia, urgency to urinate, and pain in the lower abdomen.
   c. Pain in the flank and lower back or abdomen that is not relieved by changes in position.
   d. Fever, chills, vomiting, and proteinuria.

CRITICAL THINKING—CASE STUDY

Dean, age 3 years, is brought to the clinic by his mother. He has a history of a recent fever of 37.8° C (100.2° F), sore throat, and slight cough approximately 8 days ago that lasted about 3 days. Yesterday morning, Dean's mother noticed "puffiness around his eyes" when he got up and then "swelling of his lower legs and scrotal area." Dean's appetite and activity level have decreased. This morning, Dean's mother noticed that his urine was "darker in color" and "seemed to be less than usual." Physical examination of Dean reflects a child who does not appear acutely ill but who is irritable and seems fatigued, with pale skin color. His blood pressure, pulse, and temperature are within normal limits. He has generalized edema. Laboratory findings of Dean's urine specimen include large amounts of protein and microscopic hematuria. Serum protein levels are very low, with elevated lipid levels.

56. Based on the information given, the nurse would suspect that Dean has developed which one of the following conditions?
   a. Acute poststreptococcal glomerulonephritis
   b. Minimal-change nephrotic syndrome
   c. Acute renal failure
   d. Hemolytic uremic syndrome

57. Dean is diagnosed by the health care provider as having nephrotic syndrome. Identify goals for restoring renal function in Dean.
   i. Urine is protein free.
   ii. Edema is resolved.
   iii. Acute infection is prevented.
   iv. Fluid and electrolyte balance are restored.
   v. Nutritional needs have returned to a state of positive nitrogen balance.

   a. i, ii, and iii
   b. i, ii, and iv
   c. ii, iii, and iv
   d. i, ii, iii, iv, and v

192

58. Which one of the following nursing diagnoses is of *least* benefit in planning for Dean's care?
    a. Impaired Skin Integrity related to edema, lowered body defenses
    b. Altered Nutrition: Less Than Body Requirements related to decreased appetite
    c. Altered Patterns of Elimination related to obstruction
    d. Fluid Volume Excess related to fluid accumulation in tissues and third space

59. Which nursing intervention is appropriate for Dean's nursing diagnosis of Impaired Skin Integrity?
    a. Administer corticosteroids on time with careful monitoring for infections.
    b. Monitor for complications, strict intake and output, daily checks of urine for protein, daily weight, and abdominal girth.
    c. Enforce bed rest during the edema phase of the disease.
    d. Support scrotum on small pillow.

60. Dean has progressed well and is being discharged. What teaching interventions will be necessary to prepare the family for discharge?

61. Darlene, age 15 years, has been diagnosed with chronic renal failure. She is being discharged and will need peritoneal dialysis at home. Describe the teaching interventions the nurse would include in the discharge plan for Darlene.

62. The nurse has developed the nursing diagnosis of Altered Nutrition: Less Than Body Requirements related to the restricted diet based on Darlene's diagnosis of chronic renal failure. Discuss expected nursing interventions to be used with this nursing diagnosis.

63. BUN and serum creatinine are both blood tests for renal function. Which one, if elevated, would be the best indicator of renal dysfunction? Why?

Copyright © 2015 by Mosby, an imprint of Elsevier Inc. All rights reserved.
Copyright © 2011, 2007, 2003 by Mosby, Inc., an affiliate of Elsevier Inc. All rights reserved.

193

Chapter **25** **The Child with Renal Dysfunction**

26 The Child with Gastrointestinal Dysfunction

1. Which one of the following is *not* a function of the gastrointestinal (GI) system?
   a. Process and absorb nutrients necessary to support growth and development
   b. Maintain thermoregulatory functions
   c. Perform excretory functions
   d. Maintain fluid and electrolyte balance

2. Identify the following as true or false.

   _____ At birth, the term infant has the ability to move food particles from the front of the mouth to the back of the mouth.

   _____ The infant has no voluntary control of swallowing for the first 3 months.

   _____ The chewing function is facilitated by eruption of the primary teeth.

   _____ The primary purpose of saliva in the newborn is to moisten the mouth and throat.

   _____ The infant's stomach is smaller in capacity but faster to empty than the child's stomach.

   _____ The infant's stomach at birth has an elongated shape.

3. Correctly answer each of the following.
   a. The three processes necessary for the body to convert nutrients into forms it can use are:

   _____

   _____

   _____

   b. The five types of GI secretions involved in chemical digestion are:

   _____

   _____

   _____

   c. The principal absorption site in the GI system is:

   _____

   _____

   _____

4. What are the five most important basic nursing assessments included in a thorough GI assessment?

5. Acute diarrhea:
   a. can be caused by celiac disease.
   b. can be related to hyperthyroidism.
   c. can be caused by viral, bacterial, and parasitic pathogens.
   d. is an increase in stool frequency and increased water content with a duration of more than 14 days.

6. Chronic diarrhea:
   a. can be caused by viral, bacterial, and parasitic pathogens.
   b. is an increase in stool frequency and increased water content with a duration of more than 14 days.
   c. is a leading cause of illness in children younger than 5 years of age.
   d. is often associated with upper respiratory or urinary tract infections.

7. What type of diarrhea occurs in the first few months of life, persists for longer than 2 weeks with no recognized pathogens, and is refractory to treatment?

8. Which one of the following is most likely to cause acute diarrhea?
   a. Food allergy
   b. Malabsorption syndromes
   c. Parasitic infections
   d. Immunodeficiency

9. Which one of the following is most likely to develop acute diarrhea?
   a. The 2-month-old infant who attends daycare each day
   b. The 18-month-old infant who stays at home each day with his mother
   c. The 6-year-old child who attends public school
   d. The 24-month-old infant with two older brothers, ages 5 years and 8 years

10. Identify the following statements as true or false.

    _____ Rotavirus is the most important cause of serious gastroenteritis among children and the most common cause of diarrhea-associated hospitalizations.

    _____ Forceful vomiting in infants is associated with pyloric stenosis.

    _____ Chronic and intermittent episodes of vomiting in children may indicate malrotation, whereas vomiting on a specific day at a specific time is not likely to be a result of organic disease.

    _____ Antibiotics are seldom associated with diarrhea in children because of their lower specific gravity.

    _____ *Clostridium difficile* produces a protective mechanism against diarrhea because it alters the intestinal flora, increasing absorption surfaces.

    _____ Infants are more susceptible to frequent and severe bouts of diarrhea because their immune system has not been exposed to many pathogens and has not acquired protective antibodies.

    _____ Continuing to feed breast milk to an infant during diarrhea illness results in reduced severity and duration of the illness.

11. Which one of the following is *not* a serious and immediate physiologic disturbance associated with severe diarrheal disease?
    a. Dehydration
    b. Acid-base imbalance
    c. Circulatory status impairment
    d. Decreased growth rate

12. Johnny, age 2 years, is diagnosed with uncomplicated diarrhea with no signs of dehydration. Diagnostic evaluation should include which one of the following?
    a. Cultures of the stool
    b. Presence of associated symptoms
    c. Complete blood count
    d. Urine specific gravity

13. Listed below are subjective and objective findings associated with diarrhea. For each finding, identify the suspected cause of diarrhea.

a. _____ Administration of cefaclor for 1 month for recurrent ear infections

b. _____ Neutrophils or red blood cells in the stool

c. _____ Watery, explosive stools

d. _____ Foul-smelling, greasy, bulky stools

e. _____ High numbers of eosinophils in the stools

14. Which of the following laboratory values, often found in acute diarrhea with dehydration, will return to normal after hydration of the patient?
    a. Elevated hemoglobin, hematocrit, blood urea nitrogen (BUN), and creatinine
    b. Decreased hemoglobin, hematocrit, BUN, and creatinine
    c. Red blood cells in stool
    d. Decreased white blood cell count, decreased hemoglobin, elevated BUN, and creatinine

15. What are the four major goals in the management of acute diarrhea?

16. What is the most appropriate therapeutic management for rehydration of Jenny, age 8 months, who has been diagnosed with acute diarrhea and has evidence of mild dehydration?
    a. Beginning oral rehydration therapy of 40 to 50 ml/kg within 4 hours
    b. Restarting lactose-free formula
    c. Encouraging oral intake of clear fluids, such as fruit juices and gelatin
    d. Feeding the BRAT diet, which consists of bananas, rice, apples, and toast or tea

17. Early reintroduction of nutrients (normal diet) in the patient with diarrhea:
    a. is delayed until after the diarrhea has stopped except in the case of breast-fed infants.
    b. has adverse effects and actually prolongs diarrhea.
    c. should be limited to formula-fed infants being given lactose-free formula.
    d. has no adverse effects, lessens the severity and duration of the illness, and improves weight gain when compared to gradual reintroduction of foods.

18. Which of the following dietary instructions given by the nurse to the parents of a pediatric patient with acute diarrhea without dehydration is correct?
    a. Follow the BRAT diet for the first 24 hours.
    b. Give clear fluid diet for the first 24 hours.
    c. Give fluids and a normal diet during diarrhea illness.
    d. Keep the patient NPO (nothing by mouth) until stool output slows.

19. Which one of the following nursing interventions is *not* appropriate for 6-month-old Terry, admitted to the pediatric unit with acute diarrhea and vomiting?
    a. Ongoing assessment of Terry's intake and output and physical appearance
    b. Education of the parents about the necessity of administering oral rehydration solution
    c. Rectal temperatures at least every 4 hours to monitor fever elevations
    d. Gentle cleansing of perianal areas and application of protective topical ointments

20. Prevention measures for diarrhea in children include all of the following *except*:
    a. wash hands, utensils, and work area with hot, soapy water after contact with raw meat.
    b. proper disposal of soiled diapers.
    c. during travel to areas where water may be contaminated, allow the child to drink only bottled water from the container through a straw supplied from home.
    d. administration of vaccines and medications to prevent traveler's diarrhea before travel.

196

21. The major emphasis of nursing care for the vomiting infant or child is:
    a. determining prior treatments used for the vomiting.
    b. preventing the spread of the infection.
    c. managing the fever associated with the vomiting.
    d. observing and reporting vomiting behavior and associated symptoms.

22. The nurse is preparing Dottie, age 7, for an upper GI endoscopy. Which one of the following does the nurse recognize as *not* being an appropriate preparation for this test?
    a. Bowel cleansing with magnesium citrate or GoLYTELY
    b. Keeping Dottie NPO (nothing by mouth) for 8 hours before the procedure
    c. Giving Dottie sedation before the procedure is begun
    d. Explaining to Dottie in advance about the procedure by use of pictures or play with dolls and demonstration

23. Jenny, an 8-year-old, has been brought to the clinic with continuing pain in the epigastric region of the abdomen. The medical provider has ordered *Helicobacter pylori* testing. Which of the following tests does the nurse recognize as being the most accurate method to determine active infection?

    a. Serology test
    b. C urea breath test
    c. Esophagus manometry
    d. Occult blood guaiac test

24. Match each term with its description.
    a. Pica

    i. Dysphagia
    j. Occult blood guaiac test
    k. Stool for O&P (ova and parasites)
    l. Constipation
    m. Paralytic ileus
    n. Atresia

    b. Failure to thrive
    c. Regurgitation
    d. Projectile vomiting
    e. Encopresis
    f. Hematemesis
    g. Hematochezia
    h. Melena

    _____ Detects presence of blood in the stool

    _____ Vomiting of bright red blood as a result of bleeding in the upper GI tract or from swallowed blood from the upper respiratory tract

    _____ Passage of bright red blood from the rectum

    _____ Passage of dark-colored "tarry" stools

    _____ Impaired motility of the GI tract

    _____ Eating disorder in which there is compulsive eating of both food and nonfood substances

    _____ A decrease in bowel movement frequency or trouble defecating for more than 2 weeks

    _____ Absence of a normal opening or normally patent lumen

    _____ Accompanied by vigorous peristaltic waves

    _____ Outflow of incontinent stool, causing soiling

    _____ Deceleration from normal pattern of growth or growth below the 5th percentile

    _____ Difficulty swallowing

    _____ Aids in the diagnosis of parasitic infections

    _____ A backward flowing such as the return of gastric contents into the mouth

Chapter **26 The Child with Gastrointestinal Dysfunction**

25. Pica should be considered in which of the following children coming to the health clinic?
    a. Seven-year-old with nausea and vomiting for the past 3 days
    b. Four-year-old with history of celiac disease being seen with anemia and abdominal pain
    c. Two-year-old who is still drinking from a bottle and is seen with anemia
    d. Four-month-old who is crying, is irritable, and has reddish stools

26. Lance, a 2-year-old, has been brought to the clinic because his parents are afraid he swallowed a small button battery from his father's watch, which he was playing with. The nurse recognizes which one of the following as the most appropriate nursing action at this time?
    a. Reassure the parents that Lance has probably not swallowed the battery because he has no symptoms, he is playing in the examination room, and his lung fields are clear.
    b. Explain to the parents that Lance will probably be allowed to normally pass the battery through the GI system because Lance has been able to eat and drink normally since the event.
    c. Start immediate teaching of Lance's parents on how to assess Lance's environment for hazardous objects, and how to assess Lance's toys and other items he might play with for safety.
    d. Explain to Lance's parents that x-ray examination will be conducted to verify that Lance has swallowed the battery, and the battery will need to be removed immediately to prevent local damage.

27. Constipation in infancy:
    a. may be due to normal developmental changes.
    b. may be related to dietary practices.
    c. is found more often in breast-fed infants.
    d. may be due to environmental stressors.

28. After fecal impaction is removed, maintenance therapy for constipation may include laxative use. Why is polyethylene glycol considered safe to use for pediatric patients?
    a. Decreases fluid in the colon
    b. Increases fluid in the colon
    c. Increases peristaltic stimulation
    d. Increases osmotic pressure and acidification of the colon contents

29. The nurse is counseling the mother of 12-month-old Brian on methods to prevent constipation. Which one of the following methods would be contraindicated for Brian?
    a. Add bran to Brian's cereal.
    b. Increase Brian's intake of water.
    c. Add prunes to Brian's diet.
    d. Add popcorn to Brian's diet.

30. Sally, age 5, has been diagnosed with chronic constipation. Management includes:
    a. decreasing the water and increasing the milk in Sally's diet.
    b. an organized approach of at least 6 to 12 months of treatment to be effective.
    c. daily use of rectal stimulation to promote stool passage.
    d. having Sally sit on the toilet each day until she has a bowel movement.

31. Which of the following is a congenital anomaly that results in mechanical obstruction from inadequate motility of part of the intestine?
    a. Intussusception
    b. Short-bowel syndrome
    c. Crohn disease
    d. Hirschsprung disease

32. To confirm the diagnosis of Hirschsprung disease, the nurse prepares the child for which one of the following tests?
    a. Barium enema
    b. Upper GI series
    c. Rectal biopsy
    d. Esophagoscopy

33. The nurse would expect to see what clinical manifestations in the child diagnosed with Hirschsprung disease?
    a. History of bloody diarrhea, fever, and vomiting
    b. Irritability, severe abdominal cramps, fecal soiling
    c. Decreased hemoglobin, increased serum lipids, and positive stool for O&P
    d. History of constipation; abdominal distention; and passage of ribbonlike, foul-smelling stools

34. The transfer of gastric contents into the esophagus is termed:
    a. esophageal atresia.
    b. Meckel diverticulum.
    c. gastritis.
    d. gastroesophageal reflux (GER).

35. In preschool children, GER may manifest with:
    a. symptoms of heartburn and reswallowing.
    b. intermittent vomiting.
    c. respiratory conditions such as bronchospasm and pneumonia.
    d. failure to thrive, bleeding, and dysphagia.

36. Which of the following information given to the parents about administration of a proton pump inhibitor for the treatment of GER is correct?
    a. The medication is administered on a full stomach.
    b. The medication is administered 30 minutes before breakfast.
    c. The medication will be immediately effective in suppressing acid formation.
    d. Side effects of the drug include increased fatigue, dry mouth, and bloating.

37. The nurse instructs the parents of a 4-month-old with GER to include which one of the following in the infant's care?
    a. Stop breastfeeding, since breast milk is too thin and easily leads to reflux.
    b. Rescheduling of the family's routine to accommodate more frequent feeding times.
    c. Increase the infant's intake of fruit and citrus juices.
    d. Try to increase feeding volume right before bedtime, because this is the time when the stomach is more able to retain foods.

38. The child with irritable bowel syndrome is most likely to present with:
    a. history of alternating diarrhea and constipation, recurrent abdominal pain, and bloating.
    b. alternating patterns of constipation and bloody diarrhea with little flatulence.
    c. history of parasitic infections, poor nutrition, and low abdominal pain.
    d. history of colic, laxative abuse, and growth retardation.

39. What are the classic first symptoms of appendicitis?

40. Which one of the following would alert the nurse to possible peritonitis from a ruptured appendix in a child suspected of having appendicitis?
    a. Colicky abdominal pain with guarding of the abdomen
    b. Periumbilical pain that progresses to the lower right quadrant of the abdomen with an elevated white blood cell count
    c. Low-grade fever of 38° C (100.6° F) with the child demonstrating difficulty walking and assuming a side-lying position with the knees flexed toward the chest
    d. Temperature of 38.8° C (102° F), rigid guarding of the abdomen, and sudden relief from abdominal pain

41. a. What is the name given to the most intense site of pain in appendicitis?

    b. Where is this site located?

c. What is the term used to describe pain elicited by deep percussion and sudden release, indicating the presence of peritoneal irritation?

42. The clinical manifestations expected with Meckel diverticulum include which of the following?
a. Fever, vomiting, and constipation
b. Weight loss, hypotension, and obstruction
c. Painless rectal bleeding, abdominal pain, or intestinal obstruction
d. Abdominal pain, bloody diarrhea, and foul-smelling stool

43. A common feature of inflammatory bowel diseases (IBD) in pediatric patients is:
a. growth failure.
b. chronic constipation.
c. obstruction.
d. burning epigastric pain.

44. Describe the pathophysiologic differences between Crohn disease (CD) and ulcerative colitis (UC).

45. Which of the following is used to visualize the surface of the GI tract to diagnose the extent of inflammation and narrowing in IBD?
a. Upper GI series
b. Magnetic resonance imaging
c. Endoscopy
d. Ultrasound

46. IBD can be treated with immunomodulators such as 6-mercaptopurine and azathioprine. When the patient is receiving these drugs, the nurse knows that which of the following adverse effects can occur?
a. Anemia
b. Malignancy
c. Peripheral neuropathy
d. Decreased serum calcium levels, leading to osteoporosis

47. The pediatric nurse knows that the child diagnosed with IBD needs nutritional support that includes:
a. avoiding all foods high in fat.
b. supplementation with multivitamins, iron, and folic acid.
c. meal planning for three large meals daily.
d. using bran as a source for high fiber.

48. The most reliable way to detect peptic ulcer disease in children is:
a. fiberoptic endoscopy.
b. an upper GI series.
c. C urea breath test.
d. complete blood count with differential, erythrocyte sedimentation rate, and stool analysis.

49. Billy, age 14, has an ulcer involving the mucosa of the stomach that has resulted from prolonged use of nonsteroidal antiinflammatory agents. The best term to describe the ulcer Billy has is:
a. secondary duodenal ulcer.
b. primary duodenal ulcer.
c. secondary gastric ulcer.
d. primary gastric ulcer.

50. Which one of the following is *not* thought to contribute to peptic ulcer disease?
    a. *H. pylori*
    b. Alcohol and smoking
    c. Caffeine-containing beverages and spicy foods
    d. Psychologic factors such as stressful life events

51. Triple-drug therapy is the recommended treatment regimen for *H. pylori*. Identify three examples of drug combinations used in triple therapy.

52. Common therapeutic management of peptic ulcer disease includes histamine receptor antagonists. Which of the following medications is an example of this drug class?
    a. Bismuth subsalicylate
    b. Famotidine (Pepcid)
    c. Omeprazole (Prilosec)
    d. Sulfasalazine

53. Justin, age 1 month, is brought to the clinic by his mother. The nurse suspects pyloric stenosis. Which of the following symptoms would support this theory?
    a. Diarrhea
    b. Projectile vomiting
    c. Fever and dehydration
    d. Abdominal distention

54. Preoperatively, the nursing plan for suspected pyloric obstruction should include which of the following?
    i. Observation for dehydration
    ii. Keeping body temperature below 37.7° C (100° F)
    iii. Parental support and reassurance
    iv. Observation for coughing and gagging after feeding
    v. Observation of quality of stool

    a. i, ii, iii, iv, and v
    b. i, iii, and iv
    c. iii, iv, and v
    d. i, iii, and v

55. An invagination of one portion of the intestine into another is called:
    a. intussusception.
    b. pyloric stenosis.
    c. tracheoesophageal fistula.
    d. Hirschsprung disease.

56. Al, age 5 months, is suspected of having intussusception. What clinical manifestations would he most likely have?
    a. Crampy abdominal pain, inconsolable crying, a drawing up of the knees to the chest, and passage of red, currant jelly–like stools
    b. Fever; diarrhea; vomiting; lowered white blood cell count; and tender, distended abdomen
    c. Weight gain, constipation, refusal to eat, and rebound tenderness
    d. Abdominal distention, periodic pain, hypotension, and lethargy

57. Which of the following usually indicates that the intussusception has reduced itself?
    a. Passage of a normal brown stool
    b. Increase in appetite
    c. Hyperactive bowel sounds
    d. Normal complete blood count

58. Al's intussusception is reduced without surgery. The nurse should expect care for Al after the reduction to include:
    a. administration of antibiotics.
    b. enema administration to remove remaining stool.
    c. observation of stools.
    d. rectal temperatures every 4 hours.

59. Abnormal rotation of the intestine is called _____. When the intestine completely

    twists around itself, it is termed _____.

60. Symptoms in celiac disease include stools that are:
    a. fatty, frothy, bulky, and foul smelling.
    b. currant jelly–appearing.
    c. small, frothy, and dark green.
    d. white with an ammonia-like smell.

61. The most important therapeutic management for the child with celiac disease is:
    a. eliminating corn, rice, and millet from the diet.
    b. adding iron, folic acid, and fat-soluble vitamins to the diet.
    c. eliminating wheat, rye, barley, and oats from the diet.
    d. educating the child's parents about the short-term effects of the disease and the necessity of reading all food labels for content until the disease is in remission.

62. The prognosis for children with short-bowel syndrome has improved as a result of:
    a. dietary supplement of vitamin B_{12}.
    b. improvement in surgical procedures to correct the defect.
    c. improved home care availability.
    d. total parenteral nutrition and enteral feeding.

63. Jerry, a 4-year-old, is brought to the emergency department by his parents, who say he vomited a large amount of bright red blood. Jerry is pale, is cool to the touch, and has increased respiratory rate and heart rate. The nurse expects priority care at this time to include:
    a. administration of intravenous fluids, usually normal saline or lactated Ringer solution.
    b. stool testing for blood by Hemoccult.
    c. insertion of a nasogastric tube for ice-water lavage.
    d. preparation for tracheostomy.

64. Match each type of viral hepatitis with its description. (Types may be used more than once.)

    a. Hepatitis A (HAV)   d. Hepatitis D (HDV)
    b. Hepatitis B (HBV)   e. Hepatitis E (HEV)
    c. Hepatitis C (HCV)

    _____ Spread directly or indirectly by fecal-oral route with a routine vaccination available

    _____ Virus with incubation period of 15 to 50 days; average 28 days

    _____ Formerly known as non-A, non-B, with transmission through the fecal-oral route or with contaminated water

    _____ About 85% of persons infected develop chronic disease.

    _____ Occurs rarely in children and must occur in those already infected with HBV

    _____ Often becomes a chronic condition and can cause cirrhosis

    _____ HBsAg has been detected in breast milk, but no increased risk of transmission has been found, and breastfeeding is currently recommended after infant immunization

    _____ Universal vaccination recommended for all newborns

    _____ Does not cause chronic liver disease, is not a chronic condition, and has no carrier state; however, can be a devastating disease among pregnant women, with an unusually high fatality rate.

65. Sandy, age 2, is brought to the clinic by her mother because a toddler who attends Sandy's daycare center has been diagnosed with hepatitis A. Sandy's mother is concerned that Sandy might develop the disease. Which one of the following serum laboratory tests would indicate to the nurse that Sandy has immunity to hepatitis A?
    a. Anti-HAV IgG
    b. Anti-HAV IgM
    c. HAsAg
    d. HAcAg

66. Which of the following would indicate the patient has been immunized with HBV vaccine?
    a. Anti-HBs
    b. Anti-HBs and anti-HBc
    c. HBsAg
    d. Anti-HBc

67. Sandy's testing reflects that she has not had hepatitis A. Because her exposure to hepatitis A occurred within the past 2 weeks, the nurse would expect the physician to order which one of the following for prophylactic administration?
    a. Hepatitis B immune globulin (HBIG)
    b. HBV vaccine
    c. Standard immune globulin (IG)
    d. HAV vaccine

68. The best definition of biliary atresia is:
    a. jaundice persisting beyond 2 weeks of age with elevated direct bilirubin levels.
    b. progressive inflammatory process causing intrahepatic and extrahepatic bile duct fibrosis.
    c. absence of bile pigment.
    d. hepatomegaly and palpable liver.

69. Which one of the following would *not* be expected in the child diagnosed with cirrhosis?
    a. Hepatosplenomegaly
    b. Elevated liver function tests
    c. Decreased ammonia levels
    d. Ascites

70. Brian, 16 years old, has been diagnosed with cirrhosis. The health care practitioner has ordered daily administration of lactulose. What is the rationale for the use of this drug?
    a. Decreases ascites
    b. Decreases bleeding from the esophageal varices
    c. Decreases the formation of ammonia
    d. Improves absorption of fat-soluble vitamins

71. The nurse observes frothy saliva in the mouth and nose of the neonate, as well as frequent drooling. When fed, the infant swallows normally, but suddenly the fluid returns through the infant's nose and mouth. The nurse should suspect what medical condition?
    a. Esophageal atresia
    b. Cleft palate
    c. Anorectal malformation
    d. Biliary atresia

72. Preoperative care of the neonate with esophageal atresia and tracheoesophageal fistula includes all of the following *except*:
    a. keep NPO.
    b. accumulated secretions are suctioned frequently from the mouth and pharynx.
    c. feed through the gastrostomy tube.
    d. position neonate in the supine position with the head elevated on an inclined plane of 30 degrees.

73. Preoperative care of the neonate with either gastroschisis or omphalocele includes all of the following *except*:
    a. protect the exposed bowel from injury.
    b. adequate thermoregulation.
    c. fluid management.
    d. mechanical ventilation.

74. Match each term with its description. Terms may be used more than once.

    a. Umbilical hernia
    b. Incarcerated hernia
    c. Inguinal hernia
    d. Femoral hernia

    e. Rectal atresia
    f. Rectal stenosis
    g. Persistent cloaca

    _____ The hernia is constricted and cannot be reduced manually

    _____ Complete obstruction; inability to pass stool

    _____ May resolve spontaneously by 3 to 5 years of age; needs surgical repair if persists beyond this age

    _____ Taping or strapping the abdomen to flatten the protrusion does not aid in resolution

    _____ Painless inguinal swelling that varies in size; disappears during rest and is reducible by gentle compression

    _____ May manifest as a recurrent hernia following inguinal hernia repair; occurs more often in girls than boys

    _____ Complex anorectal malformation in which the rectum, vagina, and urethra drain into a common channel opening into the perineum

    _____ May not become apparent until late in infancy, when the infant has a history of difficulty stooling, abdominal distention, and ribbonlike stools

CRITICAL THINKING—CASE STUDY

Danny, age 17, is a junior in high school. He comes to the clinic with complaints of right lower abdominal pain and slight fever.

75. What questions should be included in the history of present illness and associated symptoms if appendicitis is suspected?

76. Danny should be advised to avoid which of the following until seen by the physician?
    a. All activity
    b. All laxatives
    c. Ice to the abdomen
    d. All of the above

77. Danny is admitted to the hospital with a diagnosis of acute appendicitis. The nurse should institute which one of the following independent nursing actions?
    a. Allow clear liquids only.
    b. Start intravenous fluids with antibiotics.
    c. Insert a nasogastric tube and connect to suction.
    d. Monitor closely for progression of symptoms.

78. What laboratory blood evaluation and results would the nurse expect to see in a patient with acute appendicitis?

79. Danny is now 2 hours postoperative. During surgery, his appendix was found to have ruptured before surgery. A priority nursing diagnosis at this time would be:
   a. high risk for spread of infection related to rupture.
   b. pain related to inflamed appendix.
   c. altered growth and development related to hospital care.
   d. anxiety related to knowledge deficit regarding disease.

80. Which of the following is the most critical outcome for Danny after surgery?
   a. Danny's peritonitis has resolved as evidenced by no fever, lack of elevated white blood cell count, and a wound that is clean and healing.
   b. Danny's pain is relieved as evidenced by no verbalization of pain and the fact that Danny is resting quietly.
   c. Danny and his family demonstrate understanding of hospitalization.
   d. Danny is able to express feelings and concerns.

27 Overview of Oxygen and Carbon Dioxide Exchange

1. Of the following respiratory system structures, the one that does *not* distribute air is the:
   a. bronchiole.
   b. alveolus.
   c. bronchus.
   d. trachea.

2. The general shape of the chest at birth is:
   a. relatively round.
   b. flattened from side to side.
   c. flattened from front to back.
   d. the same shape as an adult's.

3. The infant relies primarily on:
   a. mouth breathing.
   b. intercostal muscles for breathing.
   c. diaphragmatic abdominal breathing.
   d. thoracic respiratory muscles.

4. Gas exchange occurs in the:
   a. bronchi.
   b. alveoli.
   c. trachea.
   d. all of the above.

5. Match the following terms with the appropriate description.

   a. Compliance
   b. Pneumothorax
   c. Pleural effusion
   d. Hydrothorax
   e. Hemothorax
   f. Empyema (pyothorax)
   g. Resistance
   h. Surfactant

   i. Oxyhemoglobin dissociation curve
   j. Alveolar surface tension
   k. Clubbing
   l. Retractions
   m. Grunting
   n. Tachypnea
   o. Nasal flaring

   p. Atelectasis
   q. Hypoxemia
   r. Wheezing
   s. Head bobbing
   t. End-tidal carbon monoxide monitoring

   ___C___ The disease state in which there is fluid in the space between the visceral and the parietal pleura

   ___E___ The disease state in which there is blood in the space between the visceral and the parietal pleura

   ___G___ Determined primarily by airway size; caused during breathing by the chest wall, lungs, and flow in the airways; determined by flow rate velocity, gas viscosity, length of the airway, and airway diameter

   ___M___ Body's attempt to increase end-expiratory pressure and prolong gas exchange; in older children represents chest pain

   ___S___ A sign of dyspnea in the infant who is sleeping or exhausted

   ___R___ A continuous musical sound heard from vibrations in narrowed airways; noise is made by air moving through the constricted airways

   ___D___ The disease state in which there is serum in the space between the visceral and the parietal pleura

_____F_____ The disease state in which there is pus in the space between the visceral and the parietal pleura

_____A_____ The process of elasticity of the lungs, which allows the lungs to expand and recoil; complemented by the concept of resistance, which affects the flow through the airways

_____B_____ The disease state in which there is air in the space between the visceral and the parietal pleura

_____H_____ A lipoprotein at the air-fluid interface that allows alveolar expansion and prevents alveolar collapse

_____J_____ One of the major factors determining compliance; lowered by surfactant

_____L_____ Sinking in of soft tissues relative to the cartilaginous and bony thorax; noted in some pulmonary disorders

_____N_____ Rapid ventilations; observed with anxiety, elevated temperature, severe anemia, and metabolic acidosis

_____K_____ Proliferation of tissue at the terminal phalanges; associated with chronic hypoxia; does not reflect disease progression

_____Q_____ Reduced blood oxygenation

_____H_____ The nonlinear relationship between Pao_2 and Sao_2; influences oxygen binding and release by hemoglobin into tissues

_____O_____ Reduces nasal resistance and maintains airway patency

_____I_____ Measures exhaled carbon dioxide and provides real-time evidence of ventilation

_____P_____ Collapsed alveoli; may occur as a result of the washing out of nitrogen from the alveoli by the high concentrations of oxygen; more likely to occur in persons with low tidal volume and retention of secretions

6. Because of the position of the diaphragm in the newborn:
   a. there is additional abdominal distention from gas and fluid in the stomach.
   b. the diaphragm does not contract as forcefully as that of an older infant or child.
   c. diaphragmatic fatigue is uncommon.
   d. lung volume is increased.

7. List four anatomic factors that significantly affect the development of respiratory disorders in infants.

8. As the child grow, chest wall compliance:
   a. increases.
   b. decreases.

9. As the child grows, elastic recoil of the lungs:
   a. increases.
   b. decreases.

10. Room air (ambient air) consists of:
    a. 7% oxygen.
    b. 21% oxygen.
    c. 50% oxygen.
    d. 79% oxygen.

11. A child with anemia tends to be fatigued and breathes faster, since the majority of oxygen is carried through the blood as:
    a. a solute dissolved in the plasma and the water of the red blood cells.
    b. bicarbonate and hydrogen ions.
    c. carbonic acid.
    d. oxyhemoglobin.

12. Retraction is defined as:
    a. the sinking in of soft tissues during the respiratory cycle.
    b. proliferation of the tissue near the terminal phalanges.
    c. an increase in the end-expiratory pressure.
    d. contraction of the sternocleidomastoid muscles.

13. In a child, cough may be absent in the early stages of:
    a. cystic fibrosis.
    b. measles.
    c. pneumonia.
    d. croup.

14. Match each pulmonary function parameter with its description and its significance. Each parameter is used twice.
    a. Forced vital capacity (FVC), or peak flow
    b. Tidal volume (TV or V_T)
    c. Functional residual volume (FRV); functional residual capacity (FRC)

Description

___B___ Volume of air remaining in lungs after passive expiration

___C___ Maximum amount of air that can be expired after maximum inspiration

___A___ Amount of air inhaled and exhaled during any respiratory cycle

Significance

___C___ Allows for aeration of alveoli; increased in hyperinflated lungs of obstructive lung disease

___B___ Information needed to determine rate and depth of artificial ventilation; multiplied by respiratory rate to provide minute volume

___A___ Reduced in obesity and obstructive airway disease

15. Of the following arterial blood gas results, which value would indicate acidosis in an 8-year-old child?
    a. pH of 7.32
    b. pH of 7.47
    c. PCO_2 of 44 mm Hg
    d. PaO_2 of 75 mm Hg

16. Respiratory regulation in acid-base balance influences ___Carbon___ ___dioxide___ regulation.

17. The condition in which the body attempts to return an abnormal pH to normal is called ___Compensation___.

18. List the normal value for each of the below laboratory data in a 2-year-old child.
    pH: 7.35 - 7.45

    PCO_2: 35 - 45

    HCO_3^-: 22 - 26

    BE (base excess):

19. Hypoventilation will result in which imbalance?
    a. Respiratory alkalosis
    b. Respiratory acidosis
    c. Metabolic acidosis
    d. Metabolic alkalosis

20. Diabetic ketoacidosis will most likely result in which of the following imbalances?
    a. Respiratory acidosis
    b. Respiratory alkalosis
    c. Metabolic acidosis
    d. Metabolic alkalosis

21. A child with prolonged diarrhea will likely lose _____ _____, which will result in _____

    _____.

22. A child with salicylate intoxication (ingestion) and hyperventilating will likely lose large amounts of _____

    _____, which will result in _____ _____.

23. An infant with prolonged vomiting from undiagnosed pyloric stenosis will likely lose large amounts of _____

    _____, which will result in _____ _____.

24. Stridor in children is usually associated with:
    a. upper airway obstruction.
    b. lower airway obstruction.

25. A child is to undergo a bronchoscopy. The nurse is aware that this procedure is often performed to:
    a. remove an aspirated foreign object.
    b. identify a structural abnormality in the trachea.
    c. perform bronchial lavage.
    d. do all of the above.

26. The primary physiologic factor that influences the accuracy of a pulse oximetry reading is:
    a. child's body temperature.
    b. pulsatile blood flow.
    c. percentage of oxygen being administered.
    d. method of oxygen administration.

27. The nurse is called to see a 3-month-old infant who has been diagnosed with respiratory syncytial virus and is on continuous pulse oximetry. The pulse oximeter is reading 87% and a heart rate of 80 beats per minute. The nurse auscultates the apical pulse and obtains a rate of 100 beats per minute. These findings would indicate that:
    a. the infant needs immediate medical attention.
    b. the pulse oximeter sensor (electrode) is functioning properly.
    c. the pulse oximeter sensor (electrode) is unreliable and must be repositioned.
    d. the infant needs to have the supplemental oxygen increased.

28. Oxygen delivered to infants is best tolerated when it is administered by:
    a. an oxygen mask.
    b. nasal cannula.
    c. delivery of oxygen directly into the incubator.
    d. partial rebreathing mask.

29. In children, oxygen-induced carbon dioxide narcosis is encountered most frequently with which one of the following disorders?
    a. Prematurity
    b. Asthma
    c. Cystic fibrosis
    d. Congenital heart disease

30. For a 6-year-old child who needs intermittent delivery of an aerosolized medication, the nurse should consider using a:
    a. hand-held nebulizer.
    b. metered-dose inhaler with a spacer device.
    c. humidified mist tent with low-flow oxygen.
    d. metered-dose inhaler without a spacer device.

31. Postural drainage is best when performed:
    a. before meals but after other respiratory therapy.
    b. after meals but before other respiratory therapy.
    c. before meals and before other respiratory therapy.
    d. after meals and after other respiratory therapy.

32. When performing postural drainage, the nurse uses special modifications of the usual techniques for:
    a. infants.
    b. children with head injuries.
    c. children in traction.
    d. all of the above.

33. The best method to stimulate deep breathing in a child is to:
    a. encourage the child to cover the mouth and suppress his or her cough.
    b. encourage the child to cough repeatedly.
    c. use games that extend expiratory time and pressure.
    d. leave some balloons at the bedside for the child to blow up.

34. To avoid barotrauma when using the bag-valve-mask device, the nurse should:
    a. use the type without a reservoir.
    b. use the type with a pop-off valve.
    c. use a low oxygen concentration.
    d. hyperextend the infant's neck.

35. Identify the child most likely to require endotracheal intubation:
    a. 2-year-old child with mild croup
    b. 3-month-old child with respiratory failure
    c. 8-year-old child with mild exercise-induced (bronchospasm) asthma
    d. 5-year-old child with bronchitis

36. The most severe complication that can occur during the intubation procedure is:
    a. infection.
    b. sore throat.
    c. hoarseness.
    d. hypoxia.

37. Research has shown that routine instillation of normal saline in the intubated infant or child may cause:
    a. hypoxemia.
    b. tracheomalacia.
    c. pneumothorax.
    d. ventilator-associated pneumonia.

38. The mnemonic DOPE may be used when caring for a child with an endotracheal tube and mechanical ventilation. Describe the meaning of each letter in this mnemonic.
    D:

    O:

    P:

    E:

39. List four basic assessments for a child who is being mechanically ventilated.

40. List the two primary purposes for the insertion of a chest tube in a child.

41. Describe the chambers as well as the purpose of each chamber in a closed chest drainage system of a child with a pneumothorax.

42. A tracheotomy may be performed in a child for all of the following *except*:
    a. subglottic stenosis.
    b. tracheomalacia.
    c. epiglottitis.
    d. short-term mechanical ventilation.

43. Tracheostomy stoma care should include:
    a. daily cleaning with warm soap and water.
    b. weekly cleaning with hydrogen peroxide.
    c. cleaning every 12 hours with saline.
    d. daily cleaning with hydrogen peroxide.

44. After the initial postoperative change, the tracheostomy tube is usually changed:
    a. weekly by the surgeon.
    b. weekly by the nurse or family.
    c. monthly by the surgeon.
    d. monthly by the nurse or family.

45. Describe three factors in the home environment that need to be considered when discharging a child with a tracheostomy.

46. A tracheostomy with a speaking valve:
    a. decreases secretions.
    b. decreases the child's sense of taste and smell.
    c. limits gas exchange.
    d. has no effect on the ability to swallow.

47. The pediatric nurse knows that the early subtle indication of hypoxia in an older child is:
    a. peripheral cyanosis.
    b. central cyanosis.
    c. hypotension.
    d. mood changes and restlessness.

48. The utmost priority in the nursing care of the child in respiratory failure should focus on:
    a. anticipation of respiratory failure and determining course of action.
    b. placing the child in a prone position to maximize ventilation.
    c. placing the child on a cardiorespiratory monitor.
    d. performing high-quality CPR.

CRITICAL THINKING—CASE STUDY

A 3-year-old boy, Charlie, is admitted to the ED with suspected toxic ingestion. He requires oxygen and has a peripheral IV in his left hand for the infusion of a normal saline bolus. His status is labile and he has been irritable at times, unresponsive to his caretaker's voice commands, and responds to painful stimuli. Respirations are labored and at a rate of 20 per minute; heart rate 112 per minute; he has marked retractions.

49. What would be the best method to deliver oxygen to this child?

50. How should the nurse best monitor Charlie's oxygenation status?

51. What assessment parameters should the nurse obtain in regard to Charlie's respirations?

Charlie's respiratory rate deteriorates, he is intubated, and plans are made to transfer him to the pediatric intensive care unit.

52. Charlie's arterial blood gas results are as follows: pH 7.32; PCO_2 56; HCO_3^- 22. What acid-base imbalance do these ABGs represent?

resp. acidosis

53. Charlie is transported to the PICU; upon arrival, his color is cyanotic, pulse oximeter reading is 69%, and heart rate is 67 per minute. What should the nurse perform to ascertain the cause of these findings?

28 The Child with Respiratory Dysfunction

1. The following terms are related to respiratory tract infection. Match each term with its description.

   a. Antigenic shift
   b. Antigenic drift
   c. Strep throat
   d. Acute rheumatic fever
   e. Acute glomerulonephritis
   f. Adenoids
   g. Waldeyer tonsillar ring
   h. Palatine tonsils

   i. Pharyngeal tonsils
   j. Lingual tonsils
   k. Tubal tonsils
   l. Tonsillectomy
   m. Adenoidectomy
   n. Epstein-Barr
   o. Heterophil antibody test
   p. Spot test (Monospot)

   _____ One of the more serious sequelae of strep throat; an inflammatory disease of the heart, joints, and central nervous system

   _____ Adenoids; located above the palatine tonsils on the posterior wall of the nasopharynx

   _____ One of the more serious sequelae of strep throat; an acute kidney infection

   _____ Removal of the adenoids; recommended for those children in whom hypertrophied adenoids obstruct nasal breathing

   _____ The mass of lymphoid tissue that encircles the nasal and oral pharynx

   _____ Faucial tonsils; located on either side of the oropharynx, behind and below the pillars of the fauces; usually visible during oral examination; removed during tonsillectomy

   _____ A slide test of high specificity for the diagnosis of infectious mononucleosis

   _____ Removal of the palatine tonsils; indicated for massive hypertrophy that results in difficulty breathing or eating

   _____ Also known as the pharyngeal tonsils

   _____ Major changes in viruses that occur at intervals of years (usually 5 to 10)

   _____ A virus; the principal cause of infectious mononucleosis

   _____ Group A β-hemolytic streptococcus (GABHS) infection of the upper airway

   _____ Located at the base of the tongue

   _____ Minor variations in viruses that occur almost annually

   _____ Determines the extent to which the patient's serum will agglutinate sheep red blood cells; used to diagnose infectious mononucleosis (titer of 1:160 required for diagnosis); rapid, sensitive, inexpensive, and easy to perform

   _____ Found near the posterior nasopharyngeal opening of the eustachian tubes; not a part of the Waldeyer tonsillar ring

2. The largest percentage of respiratory tract infections in children is caused by:
   a. pneumococci.
   b. viruses.
   c. streptococci.
   d. *Haemophilus influenzae.*

3. The most likely reason that the respiratory tract infection rate increases drastically in the age range from 3 to 6 months is that the:
   a. infant's exposure to pathogens is greatly increased during this time.
   b. viral agents that are mild in older children are severe in infants.
   c. maternal antibodies have disappeared, and the infant's own antibody production is immature.
   d. diameter of the airways is smaller in the infant than in the older child.

4. A febrile seizure is *least* likely to be associated with:
   a. fever in a 2-year-old child.
   b. a family history of febrile seizures.
   c. fever in an 8-year-old child.
   d. fever in an 18-month-old child with otitis media.

5. When giving tips for how to increase humidity in the home of a child with a respiratory tract infection, the nurse should emphasize that the primary concern is to ensure that the child has:
   a. a steam vaporizer.
   b. a warm humidification source.
   c. a safe humidification source.
   d. a cool humidification source.

6. For an older child who can tolerate decongestants and who is having difficulty breathing through his stuffy nose, the nurse should recommend:
   a. dextromethorphan nose drops.
   b. phenylephrine nose drops.
   c. dextromethorphan cough squares.
   d. steroid nose drops.

7. List three reasons infants and small children can become easily dehydrated when they have an upper respiratory tract infection.

8. Children with nasopharyngitis may be treated with:
   a. decongestants.
   b. antihistamines.
   c. expectorants.
   d. cough suppressants.

9. The best technique to use to prevent spread of nasopharyngitis is:
   a. antibiotic administration.
   b. to avoid contact with infected persons.
   c. mist vaporization.
   d. to ensure adequate fluid intake.

10. Group A β-hemolytic streptococci infection is usually a:
    a. serious infection of the upper airway.
    b. common cause of pharyngitis in children over the age of 15 years.
    c. brief illness that leaves the child at risk for serious sequelae.
    d. disease of the heart, lungs, joints, and central nervous system.

11. The standard effective treatment for GABHS is:
    a. intravenous antibiotic administration.
    b. oral or intramuscular antibiotic administration.
    c. nebulized racemic epinephrine.
    d. warm saline gargles.

12. The American Academy of Pediatrics recommends that health care providers base their diagnosis of group A β-hemolytic streptococcus on:
    a. antibody responses.
    b. antistreptolysin O responses.
    c. complete blood count.
    d. throat culture.

13. Offensive mouth odor, persistent dry cough, and a voice with a muffled nasal quality are commonly the result of:
    a. pneumonia.
    b. otitis externa.
    c. tonsillitis.
    d. otitis media.

14. In the postoperative period following a tonsillectomy, the child should be:
    a. placed in Trendelenburg position.
    b. encouraged to cough and deep breathe.
    c. suctioned vigorously to clear the airway.
    d. observed for subtle signs of hemorrhage.

15. Pain medication for the child in the postoperative period following a tonsillectomy should be administered:
    a. rectally at regular intervals.
    b. orally only as requested.
    c. orally or intravenously at regular intervals.
    d. rectally or intravenously as needed.

16. Of the following foods, the most appropriate to offer first to an alert child in the postoperative period following a tonsillectomy would be:
    a. ice cream.
    b. red gelatin.
    c. flavored ice pops.
    d. flavored yogurt.

17. An early indication of hemorrhage in a child who has had a tonsillectomy is:
    a. frequent swallowing.
    b. decreasing blood pressure.
    c. restlessness.
    d. bradycardia.

18. There is evidence that _____ may not be metabolized effectively in some small children after tonsillectomy or adenoidectomy, possibly causing life-threatening adverse events or death.
    a. acetaminophen
    b. morphine
    c. codeine
    d. oxycodone

19. In about half of all cases of infectious mononucleosis, there will be:
    a. skin rash.
    b. otitis media.
    c. splenomegaly.
    d. failure to thrive.

20. Diagnosis of infectious mononucleosis is established when the:
    a. red blood cell count is depressed.
    b. leukocyte count is depressed.
    c. heterophil agglutination test is positive.
    d. heterophil agglutination test is negative.

21. Infectious mononucleosis is usually a:
    a. disease complicated by pneumonitis and anemia.
    b. self-limiting disease.
    c. disabling disease.
    d. difficult and prolonged disease.

22. Clinical manifestations of influenza usually include all of the following *except*:
    a. nausea and vomiting.
    b. fever and chills.
    c. sore throat and dry mucous membranes.
    d. photophobia and myalgia.

23. Most antiviral influenza medications must be administered within _24_ to _48_ hours of the onset of symptoms in order to be effective.

24. The prevention of influenza in children 6 months to 18 years of age is primarily based on:
    a. administration of antiviral medications.
    b. yearly immunization with influenza vaccine.
    c. strict avoidance of infected persons.
    d. yearly administration of *Haemophilus influenzae* type B vaccine.

25. Which of the following is *not* an influenza vaccine?
    a. *Haemophilus influenzae* type B (Hib) vaccine
    b. Live attenuated influenza vaccine
    c. Inactivated influenza vaccine
    d. Intradermal influenza vaccine

26. The infant is predisposed to developing otitis media because the eustachian tubes:
    a. lie in a relatively horizontal plane.
    b. have a limited amount of lymphoid tissue.
    c. are long and narrow.
    d. are underdeveloped.

27. In addition to acute pain, the clinical manifestations of otitis media include:
    a. purulent discharge in the external auditory canal.
    b. clear discharge in the external auditory canal.
    c. enlarged axillary lymph nodes.
    d. enlarged cervical lymph nodes.

28. An otoscopic examination in a child with OM would reveal:
    a. bulging tympanic membrane.
    b. a light reflex.
    c. orange tympanic membrane.
    d. mobile tympanic membrane.

29. Of the following antibiotics, the one that would most likely be prescribed for uncomplicated otitis media would be:
    a. tetracycline.
    b. amoxicillin.
    c. gentamicin.
    d. methicillin.

30. To help alleviate the discomfort and fever of acute otitis media, the parents are advised to administer:
    i. acetaminophen or ibuprofen (as age permits).
    ii. antihistamines (as age permits).
    iii. benzocaine ear drops.
    iv. decongestants (as age permits).

    a. i and iii
    b. ii and iv
    c. ii, iii, and iv
    d. i and iv

31. Recurrent otitis media with effusion after a total of 4 to 6 months of bilateral effusion with bilateral hearing deficit would most likely be managed therapeutically by:
    a. tonsillectomy.
    b. steroids.
    c. polyvalent pneumococcal polysaccharide vaccine.
    d. tympanostomy tubes.

32. Children with tympanostomy tubes should:
    a. swim only in fresh water lakes without earplugs.
    b. keep bath water out of the ear.
    c. notify the physician immediately if a grommet appears.
    d. never allow any water to enter their ears.

33. Which one of the following techniques would be *contraindicated* for the nurse to recommend to parents to prevent recurrent otitis externa?
    a. Place a combination of vinegar and alcohol in each ear after swimming.
    b. Allow the child to swim every day for 2 to 4 hours.
    c. Dry the ear canal after swimming with a cotton swab.
    d. Use a hair dryer on low heat at 1 to 2 feet for 30 seconds several times a day.

34. Most children with croup:
    a. require hospitalization.
    b. will need to be intubated.
    c. can be cared for at home.
    d. are over 6 years old.

35. Of the following croup syndromes, the one that is potentially life threatening is:
    a. spasmodic croup.
    b. laryngotracheobronchitis.
    c. acute spasmodic laryngitis.
    d. acute epiglottitis.

36. The nurse should suspect epiglottitis if the child has:
    a. cough, sore throat, and agitation.
    b. cough, drooling, and retractions.
    c. drooling, agitation, and absence of cough.
    d. hoarseness, retractions, and absence of cough.

37. In the child who is suspected of having epiglottitis, the nurse should:
    a. have intubation equipment available.
    b. prepare to immunize the child for *H. influenzae*.
    c. obtain a throat culture.
    d. do all of the above.

38. Since the advent of immunization for *H. influenza* type B, there has been a decrease in the incidence of:
    a. laryngotracheobronchitis.
    b. acute epiglottitis.
    c. bacterial tracheitis.
    d. bronchiolitis.

39. The primary therapeutic regimen for croup usually includes:
    a. vigilant assessment, cool mist, nebulized epinephrine, and corticosteroids.
    b. vigilant assessment, cool mist, racemic epinephrine, and antibiotics.
    c. intubation, cool mist, racemic epinephrine, and corticosteroids.
    d. intubation, nebulized epinephrine, and antibiotics.

40. Which of the following diagnostic adjuncts is often used to diagnose acute epiglottitis?
    a. A 2-view chest radiograph (anterior and lateral views)
    b. Throat inspection with tongue blade
    c. A lateral neck soft tissue radiograph
    d. Laryngoscopy with mild sedation

41. In the infant who is admitted with possible RSV, the nurse would expect the laboratory to perform:
    a. the ELISA or DFA antibody test on nasal secretions.
    b. a viral culture of the stool.
    c. a bacterial culture of nasal secretions.
    d. an anaerobic culture of the blood.

42. Which of the following is administered prophylactically to infants at high risk for the development of RSV?
    a. Ribavirin
    b. Palivizumab
    c. Pneumococcal vaccine
    d. Penicillin G

43. In an 8-month-old infant admitted with pertussis, the nurse should particularly assess the:
    a. living conditions of the infant.
    b. labor and delivery history of the mother.
    c. immunization status of the infant.
    d. alcohol and drug intake of the mother.

44. Infants under the age of 6 months who are diagnosed with pertussis are more likely to present with:
    a. severe cough.
    b. apnea.
    c. tachypnea.
    d. sore throat.

45. The best test to screen for tuberculosis in a child is the:
    a. chest x-ray.
    b. tuberculin skin test.
    c. sputum culture.
    d. multipuncture tests (MPT), such as the tine test.

46. The recommended treatment for the child who has clinically active tuberculosis includes a 6-month regimen of:
    i. isoniazid (INH).
    ii. rifampin.
    iii. pyrazinamide (PZA).
    iv. ethambutol.
    v. ocephin

    a. i, ii, and iv
    b. iv and v
    c. i, ii, iii, and iv
    d. i, ii, and iii

47. A congenital diaphragmatic hernia is suspected when the newborn has which of the following?
    a. Acute respiratory distress
    b. Scaphoid abdomen
    c. Signs of shock
    d. Unresponsive to bag and mask ventilation
    e. All of the above

218

48. Which of the following is not usually a cause of ARDS/ALI in children?
    a. Smoke inhalation
    b. Near-drowning
    c. Sepsis
    d. Gastroesophageal reflux

49. Strategies to prevent ventilator-associated pneumonia in infants and children include all of the following *except*:
    a. endotracheal suctioning every 2 hours.
    b. elevation of the head of the bed (30 degrees).
    c. oral care every 4 hours.
    d. closed suctioning system.

50. List the three primary goals of pharmacologic therapy for asthma.

51. The age-group with the highest asthma mortality risk includes:
    a. infants and toddlers.
    b. preschoolers.
    c. school age.
    d. adolescents.

52. List the overall goals of asthma management in children and adolescents.

53. The most common early manifestation of cystic fibrosis is:
    a. meconium aspiration.
    b. meconium ileus.
    c. growth failure.
    d. chronic cough.

54. Identify which of the following therapies is *not* usually included in the care of the child or adolescent with cystic fibrosis.
    a. Insulin administration
    b. Administration of pancreatic enzymes
    c. Airway clearance therapy
    d. Administration of fat-soluble vitamins
    e. Administration of water-soluble vitamins

CRITICAL THINKING—CASE STUDY

Six-month-old Jessica is seen in the emergency room with a history of not nursing or eating well for the last 2 days and breathing difficulty. She has an axillary temperature of 39.3° C (102.7° F), abundant nasal secretions, irritability and crying, a pulse oximetry reading of 89% on room air, tachypnea, wheezing, nonproductive cough, and a capillary refill of 3 seconds. The initial presumptive diagnosis is respiratory syncytial virus and acute otitis media.

55. List two possible nursing diagnoses for Jessica.

56. Identify a priority collaborative (nursing and medicine) intervention that should be performed for Jessica.

57. List five nursing interventions that would be appropriate for Jessica.

58. Given Jessica's history of poor fluid intake and the fact that she has only had one wet diaper in the last 24 hours, what would be the best method to hydrate Jessica?

59. Jessica improves following treatment with nebulized albuterol and parenteral fluids and is discharged home. List three measures the nurse should show the mother how to perform at home to help Jessica deal with the clinical manifestations of RSV.

60. Is Jessica a candidate for antibiotic therapy? Explain your rationale.

29 The Child with Cardiovascular Dysfunction

1. The following terms are related to the therapeutic management of heart failure. Match each term with its description.

   a. Digoxin
   b. Angiotensin-converting enzyme (ACE) inhibitor
   c. Lisinopril, captopril, enalapril
   d. Furosemide

   e. Chlorothiazide
   f. Spironolactone
   g. Carvedilol

   _____ A beta blocker; blocks α- and β-adrenergic receptors, causing decreased heart rate, decreased blood pressure, and vasodilation; used selectively in children; improves symptoms and left ventricular function

   _____ Blocks action of aldosterone to produce diuresis; allows retention of potassium

   _____ Acts directly on distal tubules and possibly proximal tubules to decrease sodium, water, potassium, chloride, and bicarbonate absorption; decreases urinary diluting capacity; may need to supplement potassium

   _____ Causes vasodilation that decreases pulmonary and systemic vascular resistance, decreased blood pressure, reduced afterload, and decreased right and left atrial pressures

   _____ Blocks reabsorption of sodium and water to produce diuresis

   _____ Used because of its rapid onset and decreased risk for toxicity; increases the force of contraction (positive inotropic effect), decreases the heart rate (negative chronotropic effect), slows the conduction of impulses through the AV node (negative dromotropic effect), and indirectly enhances diuresis

   _____ ACE inhibitors that are frequently used in pediatrics

2. The embryologic development of the heart results in a heartbeat by the:
   a. fourth week.
   b. fifth week.
   c. sixth week.
   d. eighth week.

3. During embryologic development of the lower heart, the muscular septum develops from:
   a. fusion of the chambers of the common ventricle.
   b. growth of endocardial cushions.
   c. growth of the conal cushions.
   d. fusion of the conotruncal septum.

4. The process of the formation of the heart's atrial septum results in a temporary flap called the:
   a. truncus arteriosus.
   b. foramen ovale.
   c. sinus venosus.
   d. ductus venosus.

5. In fetal circulation, the umbilical vein divides and sends blood directly to the inferior vena cava by way of the ductus venosus. This division occurs at the:
   a. heart.
   b. lungs.
   c. liver.
   d. placenta.

6. In fetal circulation the majority of the oxygenated blood is pumped through the:
   a. foramen ovale.
   b. lungs.
   c. liver.
   d. coronary sinus.

7. When obtaining a history from the parents of an infant suspected of having altered cardiac function, the nurse would expect:
   a. specific concerns related to palpitations the infant is having.
   b. feeding difficulty, sweating with activity, and poor weight gain.
   c. specific concerns about the infant's shortness of breath.
   d. concerns related to the infant's lack of crying.

8. A clue in the mother's history that is important in the diagnosis of congenital heart disease is:
   a. rheumatoid arthritis.
   b. rheumatic fever.
   c. streptococcal infection.
   d. rubella.

9. Coarctation of the aorta should be suspected when:
   a. the blood pressure in the arms is different from the blood pressure in the legs.
   b. the blood pressure in the right arm is different from the blood pressure in the left arm.
   c. apical pulse is stronger than the radial pulse.
   d. point of maximum impulse is shifted to the left.

10. Of the following descriptions, the heart sound that would be considered normal in a young child is:
    a. splitting of S_1.
    b. splitting of S_2.
    c. splitting of S_3.
    d. splitting of S_4.

11. The standard pediatric ECG has:
    a. 6 leads.
    b. 12 leads.
    c. 15 leads.
    d. 18 leads.

12. The diagnostic test that requires intravenous sedation and has been used increasingly in recent years to confirm the diagnosis of a congenital heart defect without a cardiac catheterization is the:
    a. ECG.
    b. echocardiogram.
    c. transesophageal echocardiogram.
    d. two-dimensional echocardiogram.

13. In children, the usual approach to the left ventricle of the heart in a cardiac catheterization is through the:
    a. left side of the heart.
    b. right side of the heart.

14. List at least five of the most significant signs of complications after a cardiac catheterization in an infant or young child.

15. If bleeding occurs at the insertion site after a cardiac catheterization, the nurse should apply:
    a. warmth to the unaffected extremity.
    b. pressure 1 inch below the insertion site.
    c. warmth to the affected extremity.
    d. pressure 1 inch above the insertion site.

16. When children develop heart failure from a congenital heart defect, the failure is usually:
    a. right-sided only.
    b. left-sided only.
    c. both right- and left-sided.

17. Which one of the following heart rates would be considered tachycardia in an infant?
    a. A resting heart rate of 120 beats/min
    b. A crying heart rate of 200 beats/min
    c. A resting heart rate of 170 beats/min
    d. A crying heart rate of 180 beats/min

18. Pulmonary congestion in an infant may be identified by:
    a. inability to feed.
    b. mild cyanosis.
    c. costal retractions.
    d. all of the above.

19. Evaluation of the infant for edema is different from that of the older child in that:
    a. weight is not reliable as an early sign.
    b. pedal edema is most pronounced in the newborn.
    c. edema is usually generalized and difficult to detect.
    d. distended neck veins are the most reliable sign.

20. In the child taking digoxin, ECG signs that the drug is having the intended effect are:
    a. prolonged P-R interval and slowed ventricular rate.
    b. shortened P-R interval and slowed ventricular rate.
    c. prolonged P-R interval and faster ventricular rate.
    d. shortened P-R interval and faster ventricular rate.

21. The electrolyte that is usually depleted with most diuretic therapy and is most likely to cause dysrhythmias is:
    a. sodium.
    b. chloride.
    c. potassium.
    d. magnesium.

22. The nutritional needs of the infant with heart failure are usually:
    a. the same as an adult's.
    b. less than a healthy infant's.
    c. the same as a healthy infant's.
    d. greater than a healthy infant's.

23. The calories are usually increased for an infant with heart failure by:
    a. increasing the number of feedings.
    b. introducing solids into the diet.
    c. increasing the caloric density of the formula.
    d. gastrostomy feeding.

24. Chronic hypoxemia is manifested clinically by which of the following signs?
    a. Fatigue
    b. Polycythemia
    c. Clubbing
    d. All of the above

25. List three interventions for the infant having a hypercyanotic spell.

26. Prostaglandin is administered to the newborn with a congenital heart defect to:
    a. close the ductus arteriosus.
    b. keep the ductus arteriosus open.
    c. keep the foramen ovale open.
    d. close the foramen ovale.

27. The presence of poor ventricular function and atrial arrhythmias increases the risk for:
    a. infection.
    b. CVA.
    c. fever.
    d. air embolism.

28. Air embolism may form in the venous system, traveling directly to the brain in the child with:
    a. a right-to-left shunt.
    b. a left-to-right shunt.
    c. dehydration and hypoxemia.
    d. hypernatremia and hypokalemia.

29. Match the type of defect with the specific disorder. (Defects may be used more than once.)

    a. Defects with decreased pulmonary blood flow
    b. Mixed defects
    c. Defects with increased pulmonary blood flow
    d. Obstructive defects

    ___C___ Patent ductus arteriosus → HTN

    ___D___ Coarctation of the aorta

    ___A___ Ventricular septal defect

    ___BB___ Subvalvular aortic stenosis

    _____ Hypoplastic left heart syndrome

    ___A___ AV canal defect

    ___B___ Pulmonic stenosis

    ___A___ Tetralogy of Fallot

    ___B___ Aortic stenosis

    ___A___ Tricuspid atresia

    ___B___ Valvular aortic stenosis

    _____ Truncus arteriosus

    ___A___ Atrial septal defect

    _____ Transposition of the great vessels

    _____ Total anomalous pulmonary venous connection

30. Which one of the following defects has the best prognosis?
    a. Tetralogy of Fallot
    b. Ventricular septal defect
    c. Atrial septal defect
    d. Hypoplastic left heart syndrome

31. Which of the following defects has the worst prognosis?
    a. Tetralogy of Fallot
    b. Atrial ventricular canal defect
    c. Transposition of the great vessels
    d. Hypoplastic left heart syndrome

32. Tetralogy of Fallot consists of these defects:
    - i. VSD
    - ii. ASD
    - iii. Right ventricular hypertrophy
    - iv. Pulmonic stenosis
    - v. Overriding aorta
    - vi. Patent ductus arteriosus

    a. ii, iii, iv, and vi
    b. i, iii, iv, and v
    c. ii, iv, v, and vi

33. The clinical manifestations of the main types of congenital heart disease fall into which of the following two categories?
    a. Decreased cardiac output and low blood pressure
    b. Heart failure and murmurs
    c. Increased blood pressure and pulse

34. Surgical intervention is usually necessary in the first few months of life when an infant is born with:
    a. atrial septal defect.
    b. ventricular septal defect.
    c. transposition of the great vessels.
    d. patent ductus arteriosus.

35. The best approach for the nurse to use in advising parents about how to discipline the child with a congenital defect is to:
    a. provide the parents with anticipatory guidance.
    b. teach the parents to overcompensate.
    c. help the parents focus on the child's defect.
    d. teach the parents to use benevolent overreaction.

36. For parents using the Internet to obtain information about their child's cardiac diagnosis, it is important for the nurse to remind them that:
    a. information is difficult to access.
    b. most information found will not be helpful.
    c. not all websites offer accurate information.
    d. information on the Internet is usually reliable.

37. Parents of the child with a congenital heart defect should know the signs of heart failure, which include:
    a. poor feeding.
    b. sudden weight gain.
    c. increased efforts to breathe.
    d. all of the above.

38. The most common cause of heart failure in infants and children is _____ _____.

39. An infant is receiving Lanoxin elixir 0.028 mg once daily. Lanoxin is available in an elixir concentration of 50 mcg/ml. The correct dose to draw up and administer is:
    a. 0.56 ml.
    b. 0.28 ml.
    c. 0.84 ml.
    d. 1.12 ml.

$$\frac{28}{50} \times 1 = 0.56$$

40. List at least three major topics that should be included in a discharge teaching plan for parents of a child with a congenital heart disorder.

41. A visit to the intensive care unit (ICU) before open-heart surgery for a young child should take place:
   a. one week before the surgery.
   b. at a busy time with a lot to see and hear.
   c. the day before surgery.
   d. several weeks before the surgery.

42. Children who will undergo cardiac surgery should be informed about:
   a. the location of the intravenous lines.
   b. the pain at the intravenous insertion sites.
   c. the need to lie still at all times after surgery.
   d. all of the above.

43. Which one of the following patterns is indicative of infection in the postoperative period following cardiac surgery?
   a. Temperature of 38.6° C (101.5° F) 72 hours after surgery
   b. Temperature of 37.7° C (100° F) 36 hours after surgery
   c. Hypothermia in the early postoperative period

44. After cardiac surgery in a child, the central venous pressure (CVP) line may be used to:
   a. administer fluids.
   b. obtain vital information.
   c. act as a central line outside the ICU.
   d. do all of the above.

45. When suctioning an infant after cardiac surgery, the nurse should:
   a. hyperoxygenate before suctioning.
   b. suction for no more than 5 seconds.
   c. provide supplemental oxygen.
   d. perform all of the above.

46. Which one of the following is *not* a common reason for chest tube drainage in the child after cardiac surgery?
   a. Removal of secretions
   b. Removal of air
   c. Prevention of pneumothorax
   d. Removal of an empyema

47. The most painful part of cardiac surgery for the child is usually the:
   a. thoracotomy incision site.
   b. graft site on the leg.
   c. sternotomy incision site.
   d. intravenous insertion site.

48. An infant who weighs 7 kg (15.4 lb) has just returned to the ICU after cardiac surgery. The chest tube has drained 30 ml in the past hour. In this situation, what is the first action for the nurse to take?
   a. Notify the surgeon.
   b. Identify any other signs of hemorrhage.
   c. Suction the patient.
   d. Identify any other signs of renal failure.

49. An infant who weighs 7 kg (15.4 lb) has just returned to the ICU after cardiac surgery. The urinary output has been 20 ml in the past hour. In this situation, what is the first action for the nurse to take?
   a. Notify the surgeon.
   b. Identify any other signs of hypervolemia.
   c. Suction the patient.
   d. Identify any other signs of renal failure.

50. The leading cause of death in the first 3 years after heart transplantation (the greatest risk in the first 6 months) in children is:
    a. heart failure.
    b. infection.
    c. rejection.
    d. renal dysfunction.

51. After cardiac surgery, fluid intake calculations for a child would include:
    a. intravenous fluids.
    b. arterial and CVP line flushes.
    c. fluid used to dilute medications.
    d. all of the above.

52. Fluids are especially important to monitor after cardiac surgery, because during surgery:
    a. the cardiopulmonary pump uses a large volume of extra fluid.
    b. the patient's blood is diluted by the use of the pump.
    c. there is total body edema.
    d. all of the above may occur.

53. One of the strategies the nurse can use to progressively increase a child's activity in the postoperative period after cardiac surgery is to:
    a. ambulate on the first day.
    b. keep the child on strict bedrest.
    c. ambulate after analgesic medication.

54. Which one of the following patients with bacterial endocarditis (BE) is at highest risk for death?
    a. A 15-year-old with BE caused by a bacterium that is susceptible to ampicillin
    b. A 2-month-old infant with BE caused by a fungus
    c. A 5-year-old child with BE following a mitral valve replacement
    d. A 9-year-old with BE and aortic stenosis

55. One of the most important factors in preventing BE in high-risk patients is:
    a. administration of prophylactic antibiotic therapy.
    b. surgical repair of the defect.
    c. administration of routine childhood immunizations.
    d. administration of antibiotics after dental work.

56. A common finding on physical examination of the child with acute rheumatic heart disease is:
    a. a systolic murmur.
    b. a pleural friction rub.
    c. an ejection click.
    d. a split S_2.

57. The test that provides the most reliable evidence of recent streptococcal infection is the:
    a. throat culture.
    b. Mantoux test.
    c. elevation of liver enzymes.
    d. ASLO titer test.

58. Which of the following is *not* a major manifestation of rheumatic fever?
    a. Carditis
    b. Chorea
    c. Erythema marginatum
    d. Uveitis
    e. Polyarthritis

59. Children who have been treated for rheumatic fever:
    a. do not need additional prophylaxis against BE.
    b. are immune to rheumatic fever for the rest of their lives.
    c. will have transitory manifestations of chorea for the rest of their lives.
    d. may need antibiotic therapy for years.

60. The peak age for the incidence of Kawasaki disease is in the:
    a. infant age-group.
    b. toddler age-group.
    c. school-age group.
    d. adolescent age-group.

61. The standard treatment for Kawasaki disease is:
    a. aspirin and immune globulin.
    b. aspirin and cryoprecipitate.
    c. meperidine hydrochloride and immune globulin.
    d. meperidine hydrochloride and cryoprecipitate.

62. Because of the medication used for long-term therapy, children with Kawasaki disease are at increased risk for:
    a. chickenpox.
    b. influenza.
    c. Reye syndrome.
    d. myocardial infarction.

63. Most cases of hypertension in children are a result of:
    a. systemic hypertension.
    b. secondary hypertension.
    c. primary hypertension.
    d. congenital heart defects.

64. The goal of pharmacologic therapy in systemic hypertension is to reduce the child's BP levels below the _____ percentile.

65. The nurse's role in relation to hypertension may include:
    a. routine accurate assessment of blood pressure in infants and children.
    b. providing information.
    c. follow-up of the child with hypertension.
    d. all of the above.

66. Elevated cholesterol in childhood:
    a. can predict the long-term risk for heart disease for the individual.
    b. can predict the risk for hypertension in adulthood.
    c. is a major predictor of the adult cholesterol level.
    d. is usually symptomatic.

67. Current recommendations for cholesterol screening in children include:
    a. all children over 2 years of age.
    b. children over 2 years of age with a family history of elevated cholesterol.
    c. children with congenital heart disease.
    d. all children.

68. The most common type of cardiomyopathy found in children is:
    a. dilated cardiomyopathy.
    b. hypertrophic cardiomyopathy.
    c. restrictive cardiomyopathy.
    d. secondary cardiomyopathy.

69. The heart transplant procedure in which the recipient's own heart is left in place is the:
    a. heterotopic heart transplantation.
    b. orthotopic heart transplantation.

70. The first-line pharmacologic agent of choice for supraventricular tachycardia in a child is:
    a. digoxin
    b. adenosine
    c. amiodarone
    d. lidocaine

CRITICAL THINKING—CASE STUDY

Pauline is a 3-year-old child admitted for repair of an atrial septal defect. Her parents have known about the defect since her birth. She has had numerous respiratory tract infections with occasional episodes of heart failure in the past year. Pauline has taken digoxin and furosemide in the past but currently takes only vitamins with iron. Her parents state that they are eager to have the surgery over with, so that they can treat Pauline like the other children. They have three other children who are older than Pauline.

71. On admission Pauline is afebrile and playful and has no signs of heart failure. As part of the admission process, the nurse wants to be sure to have a baseline assessment of:
    a. Pauline's sucking and swallowing abilities.
    b. Pauline's reading ability.
    c. Pauline's exercise tolerance level.
    d. Pauline's toileting habits.

72. When developing a nursing care plan for Pauline and her family, the nurse would most likely have chosen a nursing diagnosis of:
    a. Interrupted Family Processes.
    b. Impaired Skin Integrity.
    c. Parental Role Conflict.
    d. Risk for Decreased Cardiac Tissue Perfusion.

73. One of the best ways for the nurse to provide emotional support for Pauline and her family in the stressful post-operative period is to:
    a. facilitate a swift transfer out of ICU.
    b. expect courage and bravery from Pauline.
    c. limit Pauline's expression of anger toward her parents.
    d. praise Pauline for her efforts to cooperate.

30 The Child with Hematologic or Immunologic Dysfunction

1. Match the term with its description.

   a. Blood
   b. Plasma
   c. Macrophages
   d. Phagocytosis
   e. Erythropoiesis
   f. Polycythemia
   g. Polymorphonuclear leukocytes
   h. Neutrophilia
   i. Monocytosis
   j. Eosinophilia
   k. Basophilia
   l. Thrombocyte

   m. Petechiae
   n. Anemia
   o. Normochromic
   p. Hypochromic
   q. Hyperchromic
   r. Leukocytosis
   s. Mean corpuscular hemoglobin concentration (MCHC)
   t. Mean corpuscular volume (MCV)
   u. Fetal hemoglobin
   v. Mean corpuscular hemoglobin (MCH)
   w. Granulocytes
   x. Agranulocytes

   _____ About 90% water and 10% solutes with principal solutes being albumin, electrolytes, and proteins

   _____ Increased number of basophils

   _____ Active red blood cell (RBC) production

   _____ Reduction in RBC mass and or hemoglobin concentration compared with normal values for age

   _____ Cells with many-formed nuclei

   _____ Term means "clot" and "cell" and accurately describes the main function of platelets

   _____ Increased number of monocytes

   _____ Capable of ingestion and digestion of foreign substances, formation of immune bodies, and differentiation into other cells, such as hemocytoblasts

   _____ Increased number of eosinophils

   _____ Composed of a fluid portion called plasma and a cellular portion known as the formed elements

   _____ Small hemorrhagic areas formed under the skin

   _____ Increased numbers of neutrophils

   _____ Ingestion and digestion of foreign substances

   _____ Increase in the number of erythrocytes

   _____ Sufficient or normal hemoglobin concentration

   _____ Increased amount of hemoglobin concentration

   _____ Reduced amount of hemoglobin concentration

   _____ Indicates the average concentration of hemoglobin in the RBC

   _____ Increase in leukocytes

   _____ Indicates the average volume or size of a single RBC

   _____ Two α and two γ chains; has a greater affinity for oxygen

_____ Indicates the average weight of hemoglobin in each RBC

_____ Monocytes, lymphocytes

_____ Neutrophils, basophils, eosinophils

2. Identify the following statements as true or false.

_____ The major physiologic component of red blood cells (RBCs) is erythropoietin.

_____ A complete blood count with differential describes the components of blood known as platelets.

_____ A child with a suspected bacterial infection would have a differential count that shows a shift to the left with more mature cells present.

_____ Erythrocytes supply oxygen and remove carbon dioxide from cells.

_____ The mature RBC has no nucleus.

_____ Reticulocytes indicate active RBC production.

_____ The regulator of erythrocyte production is tissue oxygenation and renal production of erythropoietin.

_____ The regulatory mechanism for the production of erythrocytes is their circulating numbers.

_____ The absolute neutrophil count reflects the body's ability to handle bacterial infection.

_____ Monocytes and lymphocytes are granulocytes.

_____ In the child with increased numbers of eosinophils, the nurse should suspect allergies or parasitic infection.

_____ Monocytosis is more evident in acute inflammation.

_____ The hematocrit is approximately three times the hemoglobin content.

_____ Bands are immature neutrophils, and they increase in number during bacterial infections.

_____ The life span of the RBC is 120 days.

3. The nurse would expect laboratory results for the patient with chronic blood loss to include:
   a. high iron levels.
   b. macrocytic and hyperchromic erythrocytes.
   c. microcytic and hypochromic erythrocytes.
   d. normocytic and normochromic erythrocytes.

4. What are the main causes of anemia?

5. What is the basic physiologic defect caused by anemia?

6. Identify the causes of leukocytosis.

7. Routine screening of hemoglobin or hematocrit, as recommended by the American Academy of Pediatrics, includes which of the following?
   a. Screening should be performed once during infancy (9 to 12 months of age), childhood (1 to 5 years of age), late childhood (5 to 12 years of age), and adolescence (14 to 20 years of age).
   b. All children should be screened once during childhood.
   c. Screening should be performed on all children at high risk for iron deficiency anemia, preterm infants, infants born of a multiple pregnancy or to iron-deficient women, and children in low socioeconomic groups.
   d. Screening should not be performed unless history and physical examination suggest anemia.

8. When the hemoglobin level falls sufficiently to produce clinical manifestations of anemia, the patient experiences:
   a. cyanosis.
   b. tissue hypoxia.
   c. nausea and vomiting.
   d. feelings of anxiety.

9. Which of the following does the nurse expect to include in the care plan of a patient with anemia?
   i. Prepare the child for laboratory tests.
   ii. Observe for complications of therapy.
   iii. Decrease tissue oxygen needs.
   iv. Implement safety precautions.

   a. i and iv
   b. i, ii, iii, and iv
   c. ii and iii
   d. i and ii

10. The nurse is scheduled to administer 100 ml of packed RBCs to 3-year-old Amy. Which one of the following is *not* a correct guideline when administering the blood?
    a. Take vital signs before administration.
    b. Infuse the blood through an appropriate filter.
    c. Administer 50 ml of the blood within the first few minutes to detect for possible reactions before proceeding with the remainder of the infusion.
    d. Start the blood within 30 minutes of its arrival from the blood bank or return it to the blood bank.

11. Lucas, age 7 years, is receiving a transfusion of packed RBCs. After 45 minutes, he begins to have chills, fever, a sensation of tightness in his chest, and headache. The priority action of the nurse is to:
    a. stop the transfusion, maintain a patent intravenous (IV) line with normal saline and new tubing, and administer acetaminophen.
    b. stop the transfusion, maintain a patent IV line with normal saline and new tubing, and notify the practitioner.
    c. slow the transfusion rate until the symptoms subside.
    d. slow the transfusion and send a sample of the patient's blood and urine to the laboratory.

12. At birth, the normal full-term newborn has maternal stores of iron sufficient to last how long?
    a. The first 5 to 6 months of life
    b. The first 2 to 3 months of life
    c. The first 8 months of life
    d. Less than 1 month of life

13. Which one of the following laboratory values is diagnostic of anemia caused by inadequate intake or absorption of iron?
    a. Elevated total iron-binding capacity (TIBC) and reduced serum iron concentration (SIC)
    b. Reduced TIBC and SIC
    c. Elevated TIBC and SIC
    d. Reduced TIBC and elevated SIC

14. Angie, age 11 months, is brought into the clinic by her mother for a routine checkup. On physical examination, the nurse observes that Angie appears chubby; that her skin looks pale, almost porcelain-like; and that Angie has poor muscle development. Based on these observations, which one of the following questions is most important for the nurse to include when completing Angie's history?
    a. "Did you have any complications during pregnancy or delivery of Angie?"
    b. "Tell me about what you are currently feeding Angie."
    c. "Has Angie had any recent infections or high fevers?"
    d. "Have you noticed whether Angie is having difficulty with her movements or advancing in her growth and development abilities?"

15. The nurse is instructing a new mother in how to prevent iron-deficiency anemia in her new premature infant when she takes her home. The mother intends to breastfeed. Which one of the following statements reflects a need for further education of the new mother?
    a. "I will use only breast milk or formula as a source of milk for my baby until she is at least 12 months old."
    b. "My baby will need to have iron supplements introduced when she is 2 months old."
    c. "As my baby is able to tolerate other foods, such as cereal, I should limit her formula intake to about 1 liter per day to encourage intake of iron-rich cereals."
    d. "I will need to add iron supplements to my baby's diet when she is 6 months old."

16. When teaching the parents of 4-year-old Tony how to administer the iron supplement ordered for his iron deficiency, the nurse should include which one of the following in the teaching plan?
    a. Give the iron twice daily in divided doses with orange juice.
    b. Give the iron twice daily with milk.
    c. Administer the oral liquid iron preparation with the use of a syringe or medicine dropper directly into each side of the mouth in the cheek areas.
    d. Make certain the parents have at least a 3-month supply of the iron preparation on hand so that they will not run out.

17. On a return clinical visit after Tony has been taking the iron supplement, his mother tells the nurse she is concerned because Tony's stools are now greenish black. What would your response be?

18. Hereditary spherocytosis (HS) is:
    a. always transmitted as an autosomal recessive disease.
    b. a hemolytic disorder caused by a defect in the proteins that form the RBC membrane.
    c. rarely evident until the infant is 4 to 6 months of age.
    d. usually resolved when additional folic acid supplements are administered.

19. Splenectomy, a treatment for HS:
    a. is generally reserved for children younger than 5 years of age with symptomatic anemia.
    b. requires immunizations with the pneumoccocal, meningococcal, and *Haemophilus influenzae* type b vaccines before surgery.
    c. requires prophylactic penicillin administration for several months after surgery.
    d. has a goal of decreasing hemolysis while maintaining splenic phagocytic function.

20. Sally and David Brown are returning with Jason, their 6-week-old infant, for a routine newborn examination. Sally is a carrier for sickle cell anemia; David is not. What is the chance that Jason was born with sickle cell anemia?
    a. 25% chance
    b. 50% chance
    c. 75% chance
    d. 0% chance

21. Infants are often not diagnosed with sickle cell anemia until they are 1 year of age. Why?
    a. Usually there are no symptoms until after age 1 year.
    b. High intake of fluids from formula prevents sickle cell crises during this age.
    c. Fetal hemoglobin is present during the first year of life.
    d. Increased hemoglobin and hematocrit amounts compensate during this period.

22. Under what four conditions does the relatively insoluble HgbS, in sickle cell amenia, change its molecular structure to filamentous crystals to distort the cell membrane to a crescent- or sickle-shaped RBC?

23. Persons diagnosed with sickle cell trait:
    a. have 50% or more of the total hemoglobin in HgbS.
    b. cannot pass the trait to their children.
    c. can have painful gross hematuria as a major complication.
    d. never develop symptoms of anemia.

24. Bruce, age 12 years, is admitted to your unit with a diagnosis of sickle cell crisis. Which one of the following activities is most likely to have precipitated this episode?
    a. Attending the football game with his friends
    b. Going camping and hiking in the mountains with his friends
    c. Going to the beach and surfing with his friends
    d. Staying indoors and reading for several hours

25. Pat is a 5-year-old being admitted because of diminished RBC production triggered by a viral infection. What type of sickle cell crisis is she most likely experiencing?
    a. Vasoocclusive crisis
    b. Splenic sequestration crisis
    c. Aplastic crisis
    d. Hyperhemolytic crisis

26. Which of the following diagnostic tests can distinguish between those children with sickle cell trait and those with sickle cell disease?
    a. Complete blood count with differential
    b. Sickledex
    c. Bleeding time
    d. Hemoglobin electrophoresis

27. Therapeutic management of sickle cell crisis generally includes which one of the following?
    a. Long-term oxygen use to enable the oxygen to reach the sickled RBCs
    b. Decrease in fluids to increase hemoconcentration
    c. Diet high in iron to decrease anemia
    d. Bed rest to minimize energy expenditure

28. _____ is a useful noninvasive diagnostic test that screens for stroke risk in children with sickle cell disease. It is performed yearly on children ages 2 to 16 years and measures the vascular flow within the large cerebral arteries.
    a. CAT scan of the head
    b. Transcranial Doppler
    c. Ultrasound of the carotid arteries
    d. Magnetic resonance imaging of the head

29. To control pain related to vasoocclusive sickle cell crisis, which one of the following can the nurse expect to be included in the care plan?
    a. Administration of long-term oxygen
    b. Application of cold compresses to the area
    c. Administration of meperidine (Demerol) titrated to a therapeutic level
    d. Codeine added to acetaminophen or ibuprofen if neither one of these is effective in relieving the pain alone

30. In planning for a child's discharge after a sickle cell crisis, the nurse recognizes which one of the following as a critical factor to include in the teaching plan?
    a. Ingestion of large quantities of liquids to promote adequate hydration
    b. Rigorous exercise schedule to promote muscle strength
    c. A high-caloric diet to improve nutrition
    d. At least 12 hours of sleep per night to promote adequate rest

234

31. Which of the following is the homozygous form of β-thalassemia, which results in a severe anemia and is not compatible with life without transfusion support?
a. Thalassemia minor
b. Thalassemia intermedia
c. Thalassemia major
d. Thalassemia trait

32. Norma, age 2 years, is to begin therapy for β-thalassemia. Which one of the following would be appropriate for the nurse to include in the educational session held with the parents?
    i. Norma will need frequent blood transfusions to keep her hemoglobin level above 12 g/dl.
    ii. Large doses of vitamin C will be needed throughout the disease.
    iii. Chelation therapy is delayed until after 6 years of age to promote normal physical development.
    iv. To minimize the effect of iron overload, deferoxamine (Desferal), an iron-chelating agent, will be given intravenously or subcutaneously.
    v. Deferasirox is an oral iron-chelating agent available for patients 2 years and older with chronic iron overload secondary to recurrent blood transfusions.

a. i, ii, and iv
b. iii, iv, and v
c. i, ii, iii, iv, and v
d. iv and v

33. Which of the following does the nurse recognize as an appropriate nursing objective when caring for the child with β-thalassemia?
a. Promote compliance with transfusion and chelation therapy.
b. Foster the family's adjustment to the acute illness.
c. Teach the family to prevent tissue deoxygenation.
d. Promote physical therapy and range-of-motion techniques to prevent bone changes.

34. What are the two types of aplastic anemia?

35. a. How is a definite diagnosis of aplastic anemia determined?

    b. What are the three clinical manifestations for a patient with a diagnosis of aplastic anemia?

    c. Identify two main approaches aimed at restoring function to the marrow in aplastic anemia.

36. Danny is scheduled to receive antithymocyte globulin (ATG) for treatment of his aplastic anemia. Based on knowledge about this therapy, which one of the following does the nurse recognize as true?
a. ATG is administered intramuscularly every 3 to 4 weeks.
b. ATG is administered intravenously in a peripheral vein over a 3-hour period.
c. All reactions to ATG, including skin rash and fever, occur within the first hour of administration.
d. ATG suppresses T cell–dependent autoimmune responses but does not cause bone marrow suppression.

Chapter **30** **The Child with Hematologic or Immunologic Dysfunction**

37. Match each term with its description.

   a. Bleeding time
   b. Prothrombin time (PT)
   c. Partial thromboplastin time (PTT)
   d. Thromboplastin generation test (TGT)

   e. Fibrinogen level
   f. Hemostasis
   g. Fibrinolysis

   _____ Allows for determination of specific factor deficiencies, especially factors VIII and IX

   _____ Clot breakdown

   _____ Not dependent on phase I or II deficiencies

   _____ Function depends on platelet aggregation and vasoconstriction

   _____ Measures factors necessary for prothrombin conversion to thrombin and fibrinogen

   _____ Measures the activity of thromboplastin; specific for factor deficiencies except factor VII

   _____ Process that stops bleeding when a blood vessel is injured

38. When discussing hemophilia with the parents of a child recently diagnosed with this disease, the nurse tells the parents that:
   a. hemophilia is an X-linked disorder in which the mother is the carrier of the illness but is not affected by it.
   b. hemophilia is a recessive disorder carried by either the mother or the father.
   c. all daughters of the parents will be carriers.
   d. each of their sons has a 75% chance of being affected.

39. Which one of the following is the most frequent form of internal bleeding in the child with hemophilia?
   a. Hemarthrosis
   b. Epistaxis
   c. Intracranial hemorrhage
   d. Gastrointestinal tract hemorrhage

40. Which one of the following is no longer recommended for use in treating factor VIII deficiency because the risk for hepatitis or human immunodeficiency virus (HIV) cannot be safely eliminated?
   a. Factor VIII concentrate
   b. Cryoprecipitate
   c. DDAVP (1-deamino-8-D-arginine vasopressin)
   d. ε-Aminocaproic acid (Amicar, EACA)

41. Donald, age 5 years and previously diagnosed with hemophilia, is being admitted with bleeding into the joints. The nurse knows that which of the following is contraindicated in his care plan?
      i. Ice packs to the affected area
     ii. Application of a splint or sling to the area
    iii. Administration of corticosteroids
     iv. Administration of aspirin, indomethacin (Indocin), or phenylbutazone (Butazolidin)
      v. Passive range-of-motion exercises
     vi. Active range-of-motion exercises
    vii. Teach Donald how to administer antihemophilic factor (AHF) to himself

   a. i, iii, and vi
   b. ii, iii, iv, and vi
   c. i, v, and vii
   d. iv, v, and vii

42. Which one of the following statements about von Willebrand disease is true?
   a. The characteristic clinical feature is an increased tendency toward bleeding from mucous membranes.
   b. It affects females but not males.
   c. It will be unsafe for the female affected with the disease to have children because of hemorrhage.
   d. It is an inherited autosomal recessive disease.

43. Sammy, age 8 years and diagnosed with von Willebrand disease, is brought to the school nurse with a nosebleed. Which of the following is an appropriate action for the nurse to take?
    a. Call Sammy's parents immediately so that they can arrange for him to have a dose of DDAVP to control the bleeding.
    b. After Sammy is lying down, apply cold packs to the back of the neck and over the bridge of the nose.
    c. Have Sammy sit up, lean forward, and apply continuous pressure to his nose with the thumb and forefinger.
    d. Notify emergency services for transport of Sammy to the hospital emergency room, since all bleeding with von Willebrand disease is a medical emergency.

44. Which of the following is an acquired hemorrhagic disorder characterized by thrombocytopenia, absence of severe signs of bleeding, and normal bone marrow with a normal or increased number of immature megakaryocytes and eosinophils?
    a. Immune thrombocytopenia (ITP)
    b. Disseminated intravascular coagulation
    c. Acute-onset neutropenia
    d. Henoch-Schönlein purpura

45. Which one of the following does the nurse recognize as true when administering anti-D antibody for ITP?
    a. The platelet count will increase immediately after administration.
    b. Eligible patients include those with lupus.
    c. Bone marrow examination to first rule out leukemia is necessary before administration.
    d. The patient should be premedicated with acetaminophen before medication is infused.

46. In severe cases of disseminated intravascular coagulation, treatment may include the administration of heparin. What is the rationale for this therapy?
    a. Inhibit thrombin formation
    b. Decrease platelet count
    c. Increase RBCs
    d. Increase prothrombin

47. Disseminated intravascular coagulation is:
    a. a primary disease characterized by abnormal coagulation.
    b. a secondary disorder characterized by bleeding and clotting, which occur simultaneously.
    c. characterized by an increased tendency to form clots, along with diagnostic findings that include low prothrombin levels and increased fibrinogen levels.
    d. treated with blood transfusion of whole blood and factor VIII concentrate.

48. Which of the following statements about chronic benign neutropenia is true?
    a. Nursing care management includes educating the parents to keep their child away from crowded areas and individuals who are ill.
    b. Diagnosis is usually made when the child is seen with weight loss and fatigue.
    c. The absolute neutrophil count is usually 1500/mm^3 or less at the time of diagnosis.
    d. Children with chronic benign neutropenia do not receive routine childhood immunizations because of the abnormal cellular immunity and antineutrophil antibodies associated with this disorder.

49. What are the four characteristics of Henoch-Schönlein purpura?

50. a. What is the antibody produced on initial exposure to an antigen by the B-lymphocyte system?

Chapter **30** **The Child with Hematologic or Immunologic Dysfunction**

b. What is the antibody produced on subsequent exposure to the antigen? (It is a secondary antibody response as with repeat immunizations.)

51. In children, HIV can be transmitted by which of the following methods?
    a. Exposure in utero, intrapartum, or after delivery through breast milk from an infected mother
    b. Exposure to blood or bloody fluids containing visible blood
    c. Adolescent engagement in high-risk behaviors (sex or IV drugs)
    d. All of the above

52. What are the seven most common clinical manifestations of HIV infection in children?

53. Goals of therapy for HIV infection in children are:

54. Which of the following statements about HIV or AIDS is *incorrect*?
    a. Kaposi sarcoma is found equally in adults and children affected with AIDS.
    b. *Pneumocystis carinii* pneumonia (PCP) is a frequent cause of death in children with AIDS.
    c. Expressive language is more frequently impaired than receptive language in children with AIDS.
    d. The majority of infants with perinatally acquired HIV infection are clinically normal at birth.

55. Immunization needs of the child with HIV infection include which one of the following?
    a. Delay of all immunizations until the child has the HIV infection under control
    b. Withholding of pneumococcal and influenza vaccines
    c. Administration of varicella vaccine at the age of 12 months only if there is no evidence of severe immunocompromise
    d. Provision of MMR vaccine to children receiving IV gammaglobulin prophylaxis

56. Why are the ELISA and Western blot immunoassay tests *not* used to determine HIV infection in infants born to HIV-infected mothers?

57. Two-year-old Jennifer is HIV infected. Her mother is concerned about placing Jennifer in daycare and is discussing this with the nurse at a routine pediatric follow-up visit. Which of the following is the best information to provide Jennifer's mother?
    a. The risk for HIV transmission is significant in daycare centers. Jennifer should not go to daycare until she is older.
    b. It will be all right for Jennifer to attend the daycare, but Jennifer's mother must tell the daycare that Jennifer is infected.
    c. Jennifer can go to daycare but will not be allowed to participate in sports or physical activity that could lead to injury.
    d. Jennifer should be admitted to the daycare without restrictions and allowed to participate in all activities as her health permits.

58. Infants born to HIV-infected women should receive prophylaxis during the first year of life until HIV infection is excluded. Which of the following is the drug of choice?
    a. Amoxicillin
    b. Trimethoprim-sulfamethoxazole (TMP-SMZ)
    c. IV immune globulin
    d. Dapsone

59. In Wiskott-Aldrich syndrome, the most notable effect of the disease at birth is which one of the following?
    a. Bleeding
    b. Infection
    c. Eczema
    d. Malignancy

60. Which of the following would be the definitive therapeutic management for the infant diagnosed with severe combined immunodeficiency disease?
    a. Histocompatible hematopoietic stem cell transplantation from a sibling with human leukocyte antigen (HLA)–matched bone marrow
    b. Histocompatible hematopoietic stem cell transplantation from an identical twin with HLA-matched bone marrow
    c. IV immune globulin
    d. Fetal liver and thymus transplants

CRITICAL THINKING—CASE STUDY

Mary, age 9, has sickle cell anemia. She is admitted to the hospital with knee and back pain and is diagnosed as being in vasoocclusive crisis.

61. The nurse, in developing a care plan for Mary, formulates a diagnosis of pain. The nurse understands that Mary's pain is related to which one of the following?
    a. Pooling of large amounts of blood in the liver and spleen
    b. Shorter life span of the RBCs and the fact that the bone marrow cannot produce enough RBCs
    c. Tissue anoxia brought on by sickle cells occluding blood vessels
    d. RBC destruction related to a viral infection or transfusion reaction

62. Describe interventions that the nurse can include in the care plan to control pain during this vasoocclusive crisis to prevent undermedicating Mary.

63. The nurse is developing an educational plan about sickle cell anemia for Mary and her parents. To prevent recurrence of a crisis, which one of the following is most important to include in the educational session?
    a. Explaining the signs of dehydration
    b. Explaining that frequent rest periods are required when the child is in a low-oxygen atmosphere
    c. Explaining that the child should avoid injury to joints to decrease sickling of blood cells
    d. Explaining the importance of avoiding infection by routine immunization and protection from known sources of infection

64. Evaluation of Mary's progress is best based on which one of the following observations?
    a. Mary's verbalization that she no longer has pain or need for pain medication
    b. Mary's ability to perform active range-of-motion exercises
    c. Mary's desire to drink the required level of fluids for hydration
    d. Mary's verbalization of how to prevent future sickle cell crises

31 The Child with Cancer

1. Match each of following terms with its description:

   a. Germline mutations
   b. Oncogenes
   c. Leukemia
   d. Gram-negative bacteria

   e. Tumor suppressor genes
   f. Biologic response modifiers (BRMs)
   g. Bone marrow test

   _____ Genes that keep tumor growth in check

   _____ Used to determine the presence or absence of tumor or response to therapy in this specific location.

   _____ Chromosome abnormalities that are not confined to the tumor alone but are present elsewhere; may be present in all cells

   _____ Genes that activate tumor growth

   _____ A broad term given to a group of malignant diseases of the bone marrow and lymphatic system

   _____ Agents tht modify the relationship between tumor and host by therapeutically changing the host's reaction to tumor cells

   _____ Examples are *Pseudomonas aeruginosa, Escherichia coli,* and *Proteus* and *Klebsiella* organisms

2. The following terms are related to the signs and symptoms of cancer. Match each term with its description.

   a. Pain
   b. Fever
   c. Skin assessment
   d. Anemia

   e. Abdominal mass
   f. Swollen lymph glands
   g. Leukocoria

   _____ Classic sign of retinoblastoma; cat's eye reflex

   _____ Common finding in children; if enlarged and firm for more than a week, may indicate a serious disease

   _____ Typical finding in children with Wilms tumor and neuroblastoma

   _____ Caused by the replacement of normal cells with malignant cells in the bone marrow

   _____ May show signs of low platelet count, ecchymosis, petechiae

   _____ A frequent occurrence caused by numerous illnesses other than cancer; with cancer, usually caused by infection secondary to the malignant process

   _____ May be an early or late initial sign of cancer

3. The following terms are related to the nursing care of children with cancer. Match each term with its description.

   a. Absolute neutrophil count
   b. Colony-stimulating factors
   c. Granulocyte colony-stimulating factor

   d. Postirradiation somnolence
   e. Moon face
   f. Mood changes

   _____ Filgrastim; pegfilgrastim; directs granulocyte development and can decrease the duration of neutropenia following immunosuppressive therapy

   _____ One of the effects of long-term steroid treatment that can be extremely distressing to older children; child's face becomes rounded and puffy

   _____ May be experienced shortly after beginning steroid therapy; range from feelings of well-being and euphoria to depression and irritability

_____ If lower than 500/mm³, risk for infection and major complications

_____ A neurologic syndrome that may develop 5 to 8 weeks after central nervous system irradiation; characterized by somnolence with or without fever, anorexia, and nausea and vomiting; may be an early indicator of long-term neurologic sequelae after cranial irradiation

_____ A family of glycoprotein hormones that regulate the reproduction, maturation, and function of blood cells; used as a supportive measure to prevent the side effects caused by low blood counts

4. The cancer that occurs with the most frequency in children is:
   a. lymphoma.
   b. neuroblastoma.
   c. leukemia.
   d. melanoma.

5. Which one of the following carcinogenic agents has been implicated in the development of childhood cancer?
   a. Low doses of radiation
   b. Excessive sun exposure
   c. Exposure to cigarette smoke
   d. Vitamin K given at birth

6. Of the following assessment findings, the one that would most likely be seen in a child with leukemia is:
   a. weakness of the eye muscle.
   b. bruising, nosebleeds, pallor, and fatigue.
   c. wheezing and shortness of breath.
   d. abdominal swelling.

7. The severe cellular damage that is caused by chemotherapy drugs infiltrating into surrounding tissue occurs when the chemotherapeutic agent is a(n):
   a. hormone.
   b. steroid.
   c. vesiccant.
   d. antimetabolite.

8. Most chemotherapeutic drugs act to suppress cancer cells by interfering with the cell's function or production of _____ or _____.

9. The nurse is administering a dose of intravenous vincristine when the child suddenly starts complaining of difficulty breathing and is markedly flushed. The nurse's highest priority is to:
   a. administer an oral antihistamine.
   b. stop the infusion immediately.
   c. slow down the infusion rate.
   d. call the practitioner.

10. A 10-year-old child has received a dose of L-asparaginase to which he had an anaphylactic reaction a month ago. The boy's mother urges him to get his belongings together so they can leave the outpatient area. The nurse, however, insists that he stay for a period to be observed, because he had a previous reaction. The safe minimum time of observation for this child should be:
    a. 20 minutes.
    b. 30 minutes.
    c. 60 minutes.
    d. 90 minutes.

11. Name four types of early side effects of radiotherapy, and describe one nursing intervention for each type.

241

12. A candidate for bone marrow transplantation is the child who:
    a. is unlikely to be cured by other means.
    b. has acute leukemia.
    c. has chronic leukemia.
    d. has a compatible donor in his or her family.

13. A major benefit of using umbilical cord blood for stem cell transplantation is:
    a. stem cells are found in low frequency in newborns.
    b. umbilical cord blood is relatively immunodeficient.
    c. there is a lower risk for acute tumor lysis syndrome.
    d. umbilical cord blood has a greater number of neutrophils.

14. List five cardinal symptoms of cancer in children.

15. The family of glycoprotein hormones that regulate the function of blood cells is called _____-
    _____ _____.

16. A 9-year-old with leukemia presents with a fever for 2 days; lab shows an absolute neutrophil count (ANC) of 190/mm^3. Nursing care for this child should include:
    a. placing the child in isolation to prevent contamination of other patients.
    b. wearing a face mask and practicing meticulous hand washing.
    c. avoiding needlesticks and skin punctures such as IM injections.
    d. immediately placing the child on 100% oxygen by face mask.

17. Calculate the absolute neutrophil count for a child with the following: WBC 2600; neutrophils 9%; unsegmented neutrophils (bands) 5%.

    The ANC is _____.

18. Children who have profound anemia during induction therapy should:
    a. strictly limit their activities.
    b. regulate their own activity with adult supervision.
    c. receive blood transfusions until the hemoglobin level approaches 10 g/dl.
    d. receive chemotherapy until the hemoglobin level reaches 10 g/dl.

19. The nursing intervention that would be most helpful for the child who has stomatitis from cancer chemotherapy would be:
    a. an anesthetic preparation without alcohol.
    b. viscous lidocaine (Xylocaine).
    c. lemon glycerin swabs.
    d. a mild sedative.

20. Describe three strategies the nurse can use to prevent sterile hemorrhagic cystitis.

21. An 8-year-old is to receive a chemotherapeutic drug in the outpatient clinic; his mother comments that he is not eating well because he gets so nauseous with the chemo. One way to minimize these effects is to:
    a. administer an antiemetic when the child complains of nausea.
    b. avoid foods in the room that make him nauseous.
    c. administer an antiemetic 30 minutes to an hour before the chemo infusion.
    d. omit the chemo therapeutic drug from his regimen.

22. Parents sometimes view the child's moon face from steroids as an appearance of:
    a. an anorexic, undernourished child.
    b. a malnourished child with a swollen abdomen.
    c. an overweight but undernourished child.
    d. a well-nourished, healthy child.

23. The child who receives a bone marrow transplant will require:
    a. meticulous personal hygiene.
    b. multiple peripheral sites for intravenous therapy.
    c. less chemotherapy before the transplant.
    d. a room with laminar air flow.

24. After bone marrow aspiration is performed on a child, the nurse should:
    a. apply an adhesive bandage.
    b. place the child in the Trendelenburg position.
    c. ask the child to remain in the supine position.
    d. apply a pressure bandage.

25. Dental care for a child whose platelet count is 32,000/mm^3 and granulocyte count is 450/mm^3 should include daily:
    a. toothbrushing with flossing.
    b. toothbrushing without flossing.
    c. flossing without toothbrushing.
    d. wiping with moistened sponges.

26. Delaying vaccinations is usually recommended in the immunosuppressed child because the immune response is likely to be suboptimal; however, it is considered safe to administer:
    a. any vaccines.
    b. any live attenuated vaccines.
    c. any inactivated vaccines.
    d. the varicella vaccine.

27. Leukemia is characterized by:
    a. a high leukocyte count.
    b. destruction of normal cells by abnormal cells.
    c. low numbers of blast cells.
    d. overproduction of blast cells.

28. Identify the three main consequences of bone marrow dysfunction, along with their causes.

29. Important prognostic factors in determining long-term survival for children with acute lymphoblastic leukemia include:
    a. leukocyte count and leukemia cell burden.
    b. age and gender.
    c. immunologic subtype, FAB morphology, and cytogenetics.
    d. all of the above.

30. Children who receive reinduction therapy for a relapse of their acute lymphocytic leukemia are likely to:
    a. recover rapidly.
    b. receive vincristine and prednisone.
    c. receive a bone marrow transplant.
    d. relapse 5 years after a complete remission.

31. Which one of the following children with acute lymphoid leukemia has the best prognosis?
    a. A 1-year-old girl with a leukocyte count of 30,000/mm³
    b. A 6-year-old boy with a leukocyte count of 120,000/mm³
    c. A 6-year-old boy with a leukocyte count of 30,000/mm³
    d. A 1-year-old girl with a leukocyte count of 120,000/mm³

32. In an attempt to prevent central nervous system invasion of malignant cells, children with leukemia usually receive prophylactic:
    a. cranial-spinal irradiation.
    b. intravenous steroid therapy.
    c. intrathecal chemotherapy.
    d. intravenous methotrexate and cytarabine.

33. A complete remission of leukemia is determined by:
    i.   absence of clinical signs or symptoms.
    ii. presence of more than 9% blast cells in the bone marrow.
    iii. WBC count of 10/mm³ to 12/mm³.
    iv. presence of less than 5% blast cells in the bone marrow.

    a. i and iii
    b. i, ii, and iv
    c. i and iv

34. The nurse counsels the family of a 4-year-old child that in the period immediately following remission he must:
    a. consume a large amount of food items containing potassium to maintain adequate potassium levels.
    b. consume a large amount of foods containing iron to replenish deleted iron stores.
    c. wear a surgical mask and practice meticulous hand washing when going out of his house.
    d. All of the above are important in this time period.

35. Hodgkin disease increases in incidence in children between the ages of:
    a. 1 and 5 years.
    b. 5 and 10 years.
    c. 11 and 14 years.
    d. 15 and 19 years.

36. Using present treatment protocols, prognosis for Hodgkin disease may be estimated with:
    a. the Ann Arbor Staging Classification.
    b. histologic staging.
    c. degree of tumor burden.
    d. initial leukocyte count.

37. A child with Hodgkin disease who has lesions in both the left and right supraclavicular area, the mediastinum, and the lungs would be classified as:
    a. stage I.
    b. stage II.
    c. stage III.
    d. stage IV.

38. The Reed-Sternberg cell is a significant finding, because it:
    a. is absent in all diseases other than Hodgkin disease.
    b. is absent in all diseases other than the lymphomas.
    c. eliminates the need for laparotomy to determine the stage of the disease.
    d. is absent in all lymphomas other than Hodgkin disease.

39. A particular area of concern for the adolescent receiving radiotherapy is:
    a. frequent vomiting.
    b. altered sexual function.
    c. high risk for sterility.
    d. precocious puberty.

40. Burkitt lymphoma is a type of:
    a. Hodgkin disease.
    b. non-Hodgkin lymphoma.
    c. acute myelocytic leukemia.
    d. neuroblastoma.

41. The early signs and symptoms of brain tumor in the infant:
    a. are similar to those of a young child's.
    b. may be undetectable while the sutures are open.
    c. will be demonstrated as vomiting after feedings.
    d. will be demonstrated as headache and vomiting.

42. Match each major brain tumor of childhood with its corresponding characteristics.

    a. Medulloblastoma   d. Ependymoma
    b. Astrocytoma   e. Brainstem glioma
    c. Craniopharyngioma

    _____ Arises from pons or medulla; 10% of childhood brain tumors; slow growing

    _____ Considered to have benign properties but is life threatening because of its location near vital structures
              (pituitary gland)

    _____ Arises from lining tissue of the ventricle; supratentorial and infratentorial tumors comprise 13% of all
              brain tumors in children

    _____ Invades surrounding tissue, but a slow-growing tumor

    _____ Fast growing; arises from the cerebellum; can invade fourth ventricle and subarachnoid space and
              cerbrospinal fluid; 18% of all brain tumors in children

43. The surgical technique that uses computed tomography and magnetic resonance imaging is called:
    a. sclerotherapy.
    b. microsurgery.
    c. laser surgery.
    d. stereotactic surgery.

44. An assessment finding that is consistent with the presence of a brain tumor is increased:
    a. temporal headaches.
    b. appetite.
    c. pulse rate.
    d. blood pressure.

45. Describe three strategies the nurse can use to help prepare the child for shaving the hair before surgery to remove a
    brain tumor.

46. If a child vomits in the postoperative period following surgery for a brain tumor, it may predispose the child to:
    a. incisional rupture.
    b. increased intracranial pressure.
    c. aspiration.
    d. all of the above.

47. Of the following assessment findings in the postoperative care of a child who had surgery to remove a brain tumor, the one with the most serious implications is:
    a. a comatose child.
    b. serosanguineous drainage on the dressing.
    c. colorless drainage on the dressing.
    d. decreased muscle strength.

48. Neuroblastoma is often classified as a silent tumor because:
    a. diagnosis is not usually made until after metastasis.
    b. the primary site is intracranial.
    c. the primary site is the bone marrow.
    d. diagnosis is made based on the location of the primary site.

49. The most common bone cancer is most likely to occur in a child age:
    a. birth to 4 years.
    b. 4 years to 8 years.
    c. 8 years to 10 years.
    d. 11 years or older.

50. The most common bone cancer in children is:
    a. Ewing sarcoma.
    b. Osteosarcoma.

51. A limb salvage procedure is the treatment of choice with which bone cancer?
    a. Ewing sarcoma
    b. Osteosarcoma

52. Treatment for Ewing sarcoma usually involves:
    a. radiation alone.
    b. radiation and chemotherapy.
    c. amputation and chemotherapy.
    d. chemotherapy alone.

53. Treatment for Wilms tumor is based on clinical stage and histologic pattern and includes:
    a. chemotherapy and radiation.
    b. radiation alone.
    c. surgery, chemotherapy, and radiation.
    d. surgery alone.

54. The most common clinical manifestation of Wilms tumor is:
    a. painless, firm abdominal mass that does not cross the midline.
    b. painful abdominal mass that crosses the midline.
    c. nausea and vomiting.
    d. anorexia.

55. Preoperative palpation and manipulation of a Wilms tumor should be avoided because it might cause

    _____ _____.

56. Rhabdomyosarcoma is a:
    a. malignant bone neoplasm.
    b. nonmalignant soft tissue tumor.
    c. nonmalignant solid tumor.
    d. malignant solid tumor of the soft tissue.

57. Hereditary retinoblastomas are almost always considered to be transmitted as:
    a. an autosomal dominant trait.
    b. a somatic mutation.
    c. a chromosomal aberration.
    d. an autosomal recessive trait.

58. Which of the following assessment findings would be expected in an infant with retinoblastoma?
    a. Visible red reflex
    b. Leukocoria
    c. Nystagmus
    d. Strabismus

59. Preoperative instructions to prepare parents of a child who is scheduled for eye enucleation should include:
    a. there will be a cavity in the skull where the eye was.
    b. the child's face may be edematous and ecchymotic.
    c. the eyelids will be open and the surgical site will be sunken.

CRITICAL THINKING—CASE STUDY

Cory is a 6-year-old child who has been diagnosed with acute lymphoid leukemia. She receives chemotherapy on an outpatient basis regularly. Her parents are divorced, and she is an only child. She lives with her mother and rarely sees her father. Cory attends first grade when she can. She had little difficulty with school before her diagnosis, but lately she has had trouble keeping up with the activities because she is so tired.

60. Today Cory arrives at the chemotherapy clinic for her regular chemo infusion regimen. A complete blood count shows that her ANC is 350/mm^3. The most appropriate nursing diagnosis for Cory today based on the above information would be:
    a. Altered Family Process related to the therapy.
    b. Risk for Hemorrhagic Cystitis related to effects of chemotherapy drug.
    c. Risk for Infection related to depressed body defenses.
    d. Altered Mucous Membranes related to administration of chemotherapy.

61. Cory's mother tells the nurse that she has noticed that after the chemotherapy, Cory's appetite is usually poor. The mother knows that nutrition is essential, so she is trying everything to get Cory to eat even when she is nauseated after the chemotherapy. Strategies the nurse might suggest include:
    a. gargling with viscous lidocaine to relieve pain.
    b. permitting only nutritious snacks.
    c. starting Cory on a regimen of total parenteral nutrition.
    d. administering an antiemetic drug such as Zofran.

62. Since Cory has missed school, her mother is concerned she will have to repeat the first grade. What could the nurse suggest for dealing with this concern?

32 The Child with Cerebral Dysfunction

1. Match each term with its description.

   a. Central nervous system
   b. Peripheral nervous system
   c. Autonomic nervous system
   d. Meninges
   e. Dura mater
   f. Epidural space
   g. Falx cerebri
   h. Falx cerebelli
   i. Tentorium
   j. Tentorial hiatus

   k. Arachnoid membrane
   l. Subdural area
   m. Pia mater
   n. Subarachnoid space
   o. Arachnoid trabeculae
   p. Longitudinal fissure
   q. Corpus callosum
   r. Basal ganglia
   s. Brainstem
   t. Autoregulation

   _____ Cerebral nuclei; situated deep within each hemisphere and on each side of the midline; serve as vital sorting areas for messages passing to and from the hemispheres

   _____ The large gap through which the brainstem passes; the site of herniation in untreated increased intracranial pressure

   _____ The part of the nervous system that is composed of the sympathetic and parasympathetic systems, which provide automatic control of vital functions

   _____ A potential space that normally contains only enough fluid to prevent adhesion between the arachnoid and the dura mater

   _____ A double-layered membrane that serves as the outer meningeal layer and the inner periosteum of the cranial bones

   _____ Located between the pia mater and the arachnoid membrane; filled with cerebrospinal fluid (CSF), which acts as a protective cushion for the brain tissue

   _____ A segment of the sheet of dura that separates the cerebral hemispheres

   _____ Connected to the hemispheres by thick bunches of nerve fibers; all nerve fibers traverse through this structure as they pass from the hemispheres to the cerebellum and the spinal cord; extends from the base of the hemispheres through the foramen magnum, where it is continuous with the spinal cord

   _____ A segment of the sheet of dura that separates the cerebellar hemispheres

   _____ The part of the nervous system that is composed of the cranial nerves that arise from or travel to the brainstem and the spinal nerves that travel to or from the spinal cord and which may be motor (efferent) or sensory (afferent)

   _____ A segment of dura that separates the cerebellum from the occipital lobe of the cerebrum; a tentlike structure

   _____ Separates the outer meningeal layer and the inner periosteum of the cranial bones

   _____ The middle meningeal layer; a delicate, avascular, weblike structure that loosely surrounds the brain

   _____ The innermost covering layer of the brain; a delicate, transparent membrane that, unlike other coverings, adheres closely to the outer surface of the brain, conforming to the folds (gyri) and furrows (sulci)

   _____ The unique ability of the cerebral arterial vessels to change their diameter in response to fluctuating cerebral perfusion pressure

_____ Fibrous filaments that provide protection by helping to anchor the brain

_____ The membranes that cover and protect the brain; the dura mater, arachnoid membranes, and pia mater

_____ Separates the upper part of the two large cerebral hemispheres that occupy the anterior and medial fossae of the skull

_____ The part of the nervous system that is composed of two cerebral hemispheres, the brainstem, the cerebellum, and the spinal cord

_____ The largest fiber bundle in the brain; joins the central part of the cerebral hemispheres; interconnects cortical areas of the right and left hemispheres

2. The following terms are related to the evaluation of neurologic status. Match each term with its description.

a. Neurologic physical examination
b. Choreiform movements
c. Level of development
d. Alertness
e. Cognitive power
f. Unconsciousness
g. Coma
h. Comatose state
i. Glasgow Coma Scale
j. Brain death

k. Descriptive and detailed documentation
l. Pulse, respiration, blood pressure
m. Autonomic activity
n. Body temperature
o. Corneal reflex
p. Doll's head maneuver
q. Caloric test
r. Papilledema
s. Flexion posturing
t. Extension posturing

_____ Quick, jerky, grossly uncoordinated movements that may disappear on relaxation

_____ An arousal-waking state that includes the ability to respond to stimuli; an aspect of consciousness

_____ Includes observation of the size and shape of the head, spontaneous activity, postural reflex activity, sensory responses, symmetry of movement

_____ Depressed cerebral function; the inability to respond to sensory stimuli and have subjective experiences

_____ Provide information regarding the adequacy of circulation and the possible underlying cause of altered consciousness

_____ The aspect of consciousness that includes the ability to process stimuli and produce verbal and motor responses

_____ The continuum of diminished alertness as a result of pathologic conditions

_____ Provides essential information about neurologic function; developmental tests used to determine this element of the neurologic assessment

_____ Often elevated in head injury; sometimes extreme and unresponsive to therapeutic measures

_____ Consists of a three-part assessment; created to meet a clinical need of experienced nurses for objective criteria for the consciousness level; the most popular tool that attempts to standardize the description and interpretation of depressed consciousness

_____ A sign of increased intracranial pressure observed in the eyes

_____ The total cessation of brainstem and cortical brain function

_____ A sign of dysfunction at the level of the midbrain; characterized by rigid extension and pronation of the arms and legs

_____ Most intensively disturbed in deep coma and in brainstem lesions

_____ Blinking of the eyelids when the cornea is touched with a wisp of cotton; used to test the integrity of the ophthalmic division of the cranial nerve

_____ The fashion in which neurologic examination should be documented; enables detection of subtle changes in neurologic status over time

_____ Child's head rotated quickly to one side and then the other; normally, eyes will move in the direction opposite the head rotation

_____ A state of unconsciousness from which the patient cannot be aroused, even with powerful stimuli

_____ Oculovestibular response; elicited by irrigating the external auditory canal with ice water; causes movement of the eyes toward the side of the stimulation

_____ Seen with severe dysfunction of the cerebral cortex; includes adduction of the arms and shoulders; arms flexed on the chest; wrists flexed; hands fisted; lower extremities extended and adducted

3. The following terms are related to head injury. Match each term with its description.

a. Acceleration/deceleration
b. Deformation
c. Coup
d. Contrecoup
e. Shearing stresses
f. Cytotoxic edema
g. Vasogenic edema
h. Concussion
i. Contusion, laceration
j. Linear fractures

k. Depressed fractures
l. Compound fractures
m. Basilar fracture
n. Growing fracture
o. Epidural hematoma
p. Subdural hematoma
q. Postconcussion syndrome
r. Posttraumatic seizures
s. Structural complications

_____ A fracture in which the bone is locally broken, usually into several irregular fragments that are pushed inward, causing pressure on the brain

_____ Bruising at the point of impact

_____ Physical forces that act on the head when the stationary head receives a blow; the circumstances responsible for most head injuries; when the head receives a blow

_____ A common sequela to brain injury with or without loss of consciousness; symptoms typically develop within days of the injury and typically resolve within 3 months; involves headaches, dizziness, fatigue, irritability, anxiety, insomnia, loss of concentration, and memory impairment

_____ Caused by hemorrhage into the space between the dura and the skull

_____ Involves the basilar portion of the frontal, ethmoid, sphenoid, temporal, or occipital bones

_____ Actual bruising and tearing of cerebral tissue

_____ An effect of brain movement that is caused by unequal movement or different rates of acceleration at various levels of the brain; may tear small arteries; the area of the brainstem often most seriously affected

_____ Distortion and cavitation that occur as the brain changes shape in response to the force transmitted from impact to the brain

_____ Occur in a number of children who survive a head injury; more common in children than in adults; more likely to occur with severe head injury; usually occur within the first few days after injury

_____ Results from fracture with and underlying tear in the dura that fails to heal properly; parietal bone is the most common location

_____ A result of direct cell injury and caused by intracellular swelling

_____ Bruising at a distance from the point of impact

_____ Nerve cells not primarily injured; caused by increased permeability of capillary endothelial cells, which results in increased intracellular fluid

_____ Occur as a result of head injuries; include hydrocephalus and motor deficits

_____ The most common head injury; a transient and reversible neuronal dysfunction with instantaneous loss of awareness and responsiveness from trauma to the head

_____ Consists of a skin laceration that extends to the site of the bony fracture

_____ Uncommon before age 2 or 3, but constitute the majority of childhood skull fractures; often asymptomatic in older children

_____ Caused by hemorrhage between the dura and the arachnoid membrane.

4. The following terms are related to intracranial infections. Match each term with its description.

a. Meningitis
b. Encephalitis
c. Human diploid cell rabies vaccine
d. Bacterial meningitis
e. Viral meningitis

f. Tuberculous meningitis
g. *Streptococcus pneumoniae* meningitis
h. Meningococcal sepsis
i. Waterhouse-Friderichsen syndrome
j. Hydrophobia

_____ The sudden, severe, and fulminating onset of meningococcemia

_____ Inflammatory process that affects the brain

_____ The term used to describe the symptoms of rabies; severe spasm of respiratory muscles resulting in apnea, cyanosis, and anoxia

_____ An acute inflammation of the meninges and CSF; antimicrobial therapy has a marked effect on course and prognosis; dramatic decrease in incidence with increased use of *Haemophilus influenzae* type B and *S. pneumoniae* vaccines

_____ Vaccine administered to confer active immunity after a rabid animal bite; administered with immune globulin and followed with injections at 3, 7, 14, and 28 days after the first dose

_____ Aseptic meningitis

_____ Has decreased in incidence since the use of vaccine in 2000; remains the most common cause of bacterial meningitis in children between 3 months and 11 years of age

_____ Inflammatory process that affects the meninges

_____ Meningococcemia; one of the most dramatic and serious complications associated with meningococcal infection

_____ Meningitis that is more likely to disseminate in very young or immunosuppressed children; more children predisposed to this form of meningitis with the increase in drug-resistant tuberculosis

5. Match each neurologic diagnostic procedure with its description.

a. Lumbar puncture (LP)
b. Subdural tap
c. Ventricular puncture
d. Electroencephalography (EEG)
e. Nuclear brain scan
f. Endocephalography
g. Real-time ultrasonography (RTUS)

h. Radiography
i. Computed tomography (CT) scan
j. Magnetic resonance imaging (MRI)
k. Positron emission tomography (PET)
l. Digital subtraction angiography (DSA)
m. Single-photon emission computed tomography (SPECT)

_____ Needle inserted into anterior fontanel or coronal suture

_____ Identifies shifts in midline structures from their normal positions as a result of intracranial lesions; simple, safe, and rapid procedure; fontanel must be patent

_____ After contrast dye injected intravenously, computer "subtracts" all tissues without contrast medium, leaving clear image of contrast medium in vessels; safe alternative to angiography

_____ Similar to CT but uses ultrasound instead of ionizing radiation; especially useful in neonatal central nervous system problems

_____ Detects and measures blood volume and flow in brain, metabolic activity, biochemical changes within tissue; requires lengthy period of immobility; minimum exposure to radiation occurs; patient often needs sedation

_____ Needle inserted into lateral ventricle via coronal suture

_____ Pinpoint x-ray beam directed on horizontal or vertical plane to provide series of images that are fed into a computer and assembled in image displayed on video screen; uses ionizing radiation; rapid

_____ Radioisotope injected intravenously, then counted and recorded after fixed time intervals; radioisotope accumulates in areas where blood-brain barrier is defective; visualizes CSF pathways

_____ Provides information regarding blood flow to tissues/organs

_____ Records changes in electrical potential of brain; used to determine brain death and to indicate the potential for seizures

_____ Skull films taken from different views—lateral, posterolateral, axial; shows fractures

_____ Radiofrequency images produced from elements and converted to visual images by computer; no exposure to radiation; may require sedation

_____ Spinal needle inserted between L3 and L4 or L4 and L5 vertebral spaces into subarachnoid space; measures spinal fluid pressure; can obtain CSF for laboratory analysis

6. Cerebral blood flow, oxygen consumption, and brain growth are all:
   a. less in adults than in children.
   b. greater in adults than in children.
   c. greater in adults than in infants.
   d. less in infants than in children.

7. Match each seizure term with its description.

   a. Cryptogenic seizures
   b. Symptomatic seizures
   c. Epileptogenic focus
   d. Ictal state
   e. Postictal state
   f. Simple partial seizures with motor signs
   g. Atonic seizures
   h. Idiopathic seizures
   i. Absence seizures
   j. Simple partial seizures with sensory signs
   k. Simple partial seizures

   l. Generalized seizures
   m. Complex partial seizures
   n. Aura
   o. Automatism
   p. Status epilepticus
   q. Tonic-clonic seizures
   r. Lennox-Gastaut syndrome
   s. West syndrome
   t. Refractory seizures
   u. Corpuscallosotomy
   v. Multiple subpial transection

   _____ Seizures are associated with an acquired cause; associated with pathologic abnormalities

   _____ Formerly called *petit mal;* characterized by brief loss of consciousness

   _____ Seizures with no clear cause

   _____ Occurs in one part of the brain and causes no alteration of consciousness but may experience sudden feeling of joy, sadness

   _____ Complex symptoms that results in a change or loss of consciousness

   _____ Arise from the area of the brain that controls muscle movement

   _____ Seizures are genetic in origin

   _____ Horizontal fibers of the motor cortex divided to reduce seizures; vertical fibers spared to allow for function

   _____ A group of hyperexcitable cells that initiate the spontaneous electric discharge that produces a seizure

_____ The period during the time the seizure is occurring

_____ The period following a seizure

_____ Characterized by various sensations, including numbness, tingling, prickling, paresthesia, or pain that originates in one area and spreads to other parts of the body

_____ Seizures that involve both hemispheres of the brain

_____ Sensation or sensory phenomenon that precedes the seizure

_____ A characteristic of the complex partial seizure; repeated activities without purpose and carried out in a dreamy state such as smacking, chewing, drooling, or swallowing

_____ Sudden momentary loss of muscle tone

_____ Separation of the connections between the two hemispheres of the brain; used to treat some generalized seizures

_____ A seizure that lasts 30 minutes or longer or a series of seizures at intervals too brief to allow the child to regain consciousness between each seizure; requires emergency intervention

_____ Onset occurs between 1 and 8 years of age; multiple tonic seizures daily are typical

_____ Disorder also known as massive spasms, salaam seizures, flexion spasms, jackknife seizures, massive myoclonic jerks, or infantile myoclonic spasms; more common in males than in females

_____ Formerly know as grand mal seizures

_____ Persistence of seizures despite adequate trials of three antiepileptic medications.

8. The blood-brain barrier in a newborn is:
   a. less permeable than in the adult.
   b. impermeable to protein.
   c. impermeable to glucose.
   d. permeable to large molecules.

9. Which one of the following signs is used to evaluate increased intracranial pressure in the infant but not in the older child?
   a. Projectile vomiting
   b. Headache
   c. Tense or bulging fontanel
   d. Fatigue

10. Which of the following indicators is best to use to determine the depth of the comatose state?
    a. Motor activity
    b. Level of consciousness
    c. Reflexes
    d. Vital signs

11. Define the term *persistent vegetative state.*

12. The guidelines for establishing brain death in children:
    a. differ from age to age.
    b. are the same as in the adult.
    c. require an observation period of at least 7 days.
    d. require an observation period of at least 48 hours.

13. The drug mannitol is often administered to treat ICP resulting from cerebral edema. The nurse knows which of the following statements to be correct?
    a. Mannitol is always given by slow IV infusion.
    b. Mannitol is given with adrenocorticosteroids for cerebral edema secondary to head trauma.
    c. Mannitol is always given by rapid IV infusion.
    d. An indwelling catheter is inserted to ensure bladder emptying because of the profound diuretic effect of the drug.

14. A child in a very deep comatose state would exhibit:
    a. hyperkinetic activity.
    b. purposeless plucking movements.
    c. few spontaneous movements.
    d. combative behavior.

15. After a seizure in a child over 3 years of age, the Babinski reflex often:
    a. remains positive.
    b. remains negative.
    c. fluctuates.
    d. is unable to be tested correctly.

16. A cerebral dysfunction gait that is described as narrow-based gait with a tendency to walk on toes, along with flexion at knees and hips and shuffling, is:
    a. ataxia.
    b. spastic paraplegic gait.
    c. extrapyramidal gait.
    d. spastic hemiplegic gait.

17. If the patient has an increase in intracranial pressure, one test that is contraindicated is the:
    a. LP.
    b. subdural tap.
    c. CT.
    d. DSA.

18. The diagnostic procedure that is usually noninvasive and permits visualization of the neurologic structures using radiofrequency emissions from elements is called:
    a. DSA.
    b. PET.
    c. MRI.
    d. CT.

19. The factor that is likely to have the greatest impact on the outcome and recovery of the unconscious child is the:
    a. gradual reduction in intracranial pressure.
    b. level of nursing care and observation skills.
    c. emotional response of the parents.
    d. level of discomfort the child experiences.

20. The nurse should suspect pain in the comatose child if the child exhibits:
    a. increased flaccidity.
    b. increased oxygen saturation.
    c. decreased blood pressure.
    d. increased agitation.

21. Intracranial pressure monitoring has been found to be useful in pediatric critical care to:
    a. provide quick and effective relief of increased pressure.
    b. evaluate children with Glasgow Coma Scale scores less than 8.
    c. maintain $Paco_2$ at 25 to 30 mm Hg.
    d. prevent herniation.

22. Of the following activities, the one that has been shown to increase intracranial pressure is:
    a. using earplugs to eliminate noise.
    b. range-of-motion exercises.
    c. suctioning.
    d. osmotherapy.

23. The medications that are controversial in the management of increased intracranial pressure are:
    a. barbiturates.
    b. paralyzing agents.
    c. sedatives.
    d. antiepileptics.

24. If a child is permanently unconscious, it would be inappropriate for the nurse to:
    a. permit the parents to bring a child's favorite toy.
    b. provide guidance and clarify information that the physician has already given.
    c. suggest the parents plan for periodic relief from the continual care of their child.
    d. use reflexive muscle contractions as a sign of hope for recovery.

25. Because of the ability of the cranium to expand, very young children may tolerate which one of the following neurologic conditions better than an adult?
    a. Cerebral edema
    b. Hypoxic brain damage
    c. Epilepsy
    d. Subdural hemorrhage

26. Head injury that causes the brain to be forced though the tentorial opening is usually referred to as:
    a. tentorial contrecoup.
    b. concussion.
    c. tentorial herniation.
    d. deformation.

27. Of the following symptoms, the one that would not be considered a hallmark of concussion in a child is:
    a. alteration of mental status.
    b. amnesia.
    c. loss of consciousness.
    d. confusion.

28. Epidural hemorrhage is less common in children under 2 years of age than in adults because:
    a. the middle meningeal artery is embedded in the bone surface of the skull until approximately 2 years of age.
    b. fractures are less likely to lacerate the middle meningeal artery in children under 2 years of age.
    c. separation of the dura from bleeding is more likely to occur in children than in adults.
    d. there is an increased tendency for the skull to fracture in children under 2 years of age.

29. Which one of the following features is usually associated with acute subdural hematoma?
    a. Arterial hemorrhage is usually present.
    b. Skull fracture is almost always present.
    c. It is more common than epidural hematoma.
    d. It occurs in patients older than 2 years.

30. Which of the following diagnostic tests, for the child presenting with head injury, is *least* helpful in providing a more definitive diagnosis of the type and extent of the trauma?
    a. CT scan
    b. MRI
    c. History and physical
    d. Skull x-ray

31. Emergency treatment of a child with a head injury would generally *not* include:
    a. administering analgesics.
    b. checking pupils' reaction to light. ✓
    c. stabilizing the neck and spine. ✓
    d. checking level of consciousness. ✓

32. The clinical manifestation that indicates a progression from minor head injury to severe head injury is:
    a. confusion.
    b. mounting agitation.
    c. an episode of vomiting.
    d. pallor.

33. Compared with adults who have suffered craniocerebral trauma, children usually have a:
    a. lower incidence of psychologic disturbances.
    b. higher mortality rate.
    c. less favorable prognosis.
    d. higher incidence of psychologic disturbances.

34. Family support for the child who has suffered head injury includes all of the following (except) encouraging the parents to:
    a. hold and cuddle the child.
    b. bring familiar belongings into the child's room.
    c. make a tape recording of familiar voices or sounds.
    d. search for clues that the child is recovering.

35. What should the nurse emphasize when providing anticipatory guidance for parents in regard to children spending time near the water?

36. The major pulmonary changes that occur in submersion injury are directly related to:
    a. duration of submersion and severity of the hypoxia.
    b. amount of fluid aspirated and the type of fluid aspirated.
    c. the amount of blood shunted away from the lungs and the amount of water swallowed.
    d. the victim's physiologic response and amount of fluid aspirated.

37. Of the following factors, the best predictor of outcome in near-drowning victims is:
    a. respiratory rate.
    b. degree of acidosis on admission.
    c. level of consciousness.
    d. length of time the child was submerged.

38. The etiology of bacterial meningitis has changed in recent years because of the:
    a. increased surveillance of tuberculosis.
    b. increased awareness of rubella and polio vaccines.
    c. routine use of *H. influenzae* type B and *Streptococcus pneumoniae* vaccines.
    d. routine use of hepatitis B and hepatitis A vaccines.

39. The most common mode of transmission for bacterial meningitis is:
    a. vascular dissemination of a respiratory tract infection.
    b. direct implantation from an invasive procedure.
    c. direct extension from an infection in the mastoid sinuses.
    d. direct extension from an infection in the nasal sinuses.

40. A child who is ill and develops a purpuric or petechial rash may possibly have developed:
    a. aseptic meningitis.
    b. Waterhouse-Friderichsen syndrome.
    c. *Citrobacter diversus* meningitis.
    d. herpes simplex encephalitis.

41. Secondary problems from bacterial meningitis are most likely to occur in the:
    a. child with meningococcal meningitis.
    b. infant under 2 months of age.
    c. infant over 2 months of age.
    d. child with *H. influenzae* type B meningitis.

42. Which one of the following types of meningitis is self-limiting and least serious?
    a. Meningococcal meningitis
    b. Tuberculous meningitis
    c. *H. influenzae* meningitis
    d. Nonbacterial (aseptic) meningitis

43. Although an uncommon disease, the type of encephalitis that is responsible for 30% of cases in children is caused by:
    a. herpes simplex.
    b. measles.
    c. mumps.
    d. rubella.

44. The main focus of nursing care management for the patient with encephalitis is:
    a. isolation.
    b. control of rising ICP.
    c. support for the parents.
    d. control of nutritional deficiencies.

45. In the United States, most human fatalities associated with rabies occur in people who:
    a. are unaware of their exposure.
    b. have not been immunized.
    c. live near raccoons and bats.
    d. provoke an unvaccinated dog.

46. The recommended postexposure treatment for rabies includes:
    a. mass immunization using human rabies immune globulin.
    b. administration of human diploid cell rabies vaccine according to schedule.
    c. mass immunization using human diploid cell rabies vaccine.
    d. administration of human rabies immune globulin 90 days after the exposure.

47. Reye syndrome is widely believed to be linked to:
    a. administration of nonsteroidal medications for fever during an acute viral infection.
    b. encephalitis.
    c. administration of aspirin for fever in children with varicella or influenza.
    d. bacterial infections.

48. Symptoms that are similar to those of Reye syndrome have occurred during viral illnesses when the child was given an:
    a. antiemetic drug.
    b. analgesic drug.
    c. antiepileptic drug.
    d. antiarrhythmic drug.

49. The drug that reduces the chance that the human immunodeficiency virus (HIV)-infected pregnant mother will infect her infant is called:
    a. valproate.
    b. zidovudine.
    c. nitrazepam.
    d. felbamate.

50. An example of a nonrecurrent acute seizure is:
    a. febrile episodes.
    b. idiopathic epilepsy.
    c. epilepsy secondary to hemorrhage.
    d. hypoglycemic status hypopituitarism.

51. A child having a complex partial seizure rather than a simple partial seizure is more likely to exhibit:
    a. impaired consciousness.
    b. clonic movements.
    c. a seizure duration of less than 1 minute.
    d. all of the above.

52. One strategy that may provide a clue to the origin of a seizure is:
    a. to attempt to place an airway in the mouth.
    b. to gently open the eyes to observe their movement.
    c. to provide a clear description of events before the seizure.
    d. to provide a clear description of events after the seizure.

53. Which one of the following types of seizures is most common in children between the ages of 5 and 12 years?
    a. Salaam seizures
    b. Absence seizures
    c. Atonic seizures
    d. Jackknife seizures

54. The therapy for infantile spasms is likely to include:
    a. adrenocorticotropic hormone or vigabatrin.
    b. valproic acid and vigabatrin.
    c. ethosuximide only.
    d. felbamate only.

55. The drug approved for first-line therapy in the treatment of Lennox-Gastaut syndrome is:
    a. nitrazepam.
    b. clonazepam.
    c. gabapentin.
    d. valproate.

56. Therapy for epilepsy should begin with:
    a. short-term drug therapy.
    b. combination drug therapy.
    c. only one drug.
    d. drugs that correct the brain wave pattern.

57. The intravenous medication that is used to treat seizures and may be given in either saline or glucose is:
    a. fosphenytoin.
    b. phenytoin.
    c. valproic acid.
    d. felbamate.

A fat ↓ carb — prtn

58. Which of the following statements about the ketogenic diet is true?
    a. It is a high-carbohydrate, high-fat diet with adequate protein.
    b. It has shown effectiveness for treatment of epilepsy.
    c. Consumption of the diet forces the body to shift from using fat as the primary source to using glucose, thus developing a state of ketosis.
    d. Vitamin supplements are rarely necessary with the diet.

59. A simple, effective, and safe treatment for home or prehospital management of status epilepticus is:
    a. intranasal midazolam.
    b. intravenous diazepam.
    c. intravenous lorazepam.
    d. rectal fosphenytoin.

60. Which of the following statements related to prognosis of seizures in children is *incorrect?*
    a. A history of two unprovoked seizures is sufficient to diagnose epilepsy.
    b. The etiology and specific epilepsy syndromes are the most important factors affecting prognosis.
    c. Mortality is increased twofold in children with epilepsy.
    d. Children who have cognitive impairments, as compared to children who have no cognitive impairments, are at no higher risk for developing epilepsy.

61. Nursing intervention for a child during a tonic-clonic seizure should include attempts to:
    a. halt the seizure as soon as it begins.
    b. restrain the child.
    c. remain calm and prevent the child from sustaining any harm.
    d. place an oral airway in the child's mouth.

62. Emergency care of the child during a seizure includes:
    a. giving ice chips slowly.
    b. restraining the child.
    c. putting a tongue blade in the child's mouth.
    d. loosening restrictive clothing.

63. To prevent submersion injuries in children with epilepsy, the child should be instructed to:
    a. never go swimming.
    b. take showers.
    c. wear a bicycle helmet.
    d. do all of the above.

64. In most children who have a febrile seizure, the factor that triggers the seizure tends to be:
    a. rapidity of the temperature elevation.
    b. duration of the temperature elevation.
    c. height of the temperature elevation.
    d. any of the above.

65. When a child has a febrile seizure, it is important for the parents to know that the child will:
    a. probably not develop epilepsy.
    b. most likely develop epilepsy.
    c. most likely develop neurologic damage.
    d. usually need tepid sponge baths to control fever.

66. Migraine headaches in children:
    a. have typical symptoms of abdominal pain and episodic pallor in the older child.
    b. occur most often in the morning, awakening the child from sleep.
    c. are more common in boys after the onset of puberty.
    d. have typical symptoms of nausea, vomiting, and abdominal pain that are relieved by sleep.

67. Treatment for migraine headaches in adolescents over 12 years of age may include:
    a. ergots.
    b. opioids.
    c. almotriptan.
    d. all of the above.

68. The primary diagnostic tool for detecting hydrocephalus in older infants and children is:
    a. computed tomography or magnetic resonance imaging.
    b. measuring head circumference.
    c. echoencephalography.
    d. ultrasonography.

69. Most cases of hydrocephalus are a result of:
    a. developmental malformations.
    b. neoplasm.
    c. infection.
    d. trauma.

70. The infant with hydrocephalus has which of the following clinical manifestations?
    a. Upward eye slanting
    b. Strabismus
    c. Setting-sun sign
    d. Decreased head circumference

71. Surgical shunts are often required to provide drainage in the treatment of hydrocephalus. What is the preferred shunt for infants?
    a. Ventriculoperitoneal shunt
    b. Ventriculoatrial shunt
    c. Ventricular bypass
    d. Ventriculopleural shunt

72. The nurse recognizes that which one of the following should be included in the postoperative care of a patient with a shunt?
    a. Positioning the patient in a head-up position
    b. Continuous pumping of the shunt to assess function
    c. Monitoring for abdominal or peritoneal distention
    d. Positioning the child on the side of the operative site to facilitate drainage

CRITICAL THINKING—CASE STUDY

Jackson was riding his bike in the street by his house when he was hit by a car. He is 9 years old. He was not wearing a helmet at the time. He has been unconscious since the accident 8 hours ago. His mother and father both work full-time, and there are five other siblings at home ranging in ages from 7 to 19 years old.

73. Based on the preceding information, which of the following nursing diagnoses would have the highest priority?
    a. Risk for Impaired Skin Integrity related to immobility
    b. Self-Care Deficit related to physical immobility
    c. Interrupted Family Process related to potential permanent disability
    d. Risk for Aspiration: Ineffective Airway Clearance related to depressed sensorium

74. To effectively deal with the interrupted family process related to the hospitalization, the nurse should:
    a. provide information about bicycle safety helmets.
    b. encourage expression of feelings.
    c. encourage the family to take care of Jackson's hygiene needs.
    d. provide auditory stimulation for Jackson.

75. To help Jackson receive appropriate sensory stimulation, the nurse should:
    a. hang a black-and-white mobile above his bed.
    b. hang a calendar at the foot of his bed.
    c. encourage the family to bring a tape of his favorite music.
    d. administer pain medications as needed.

76. Jackson's parents visit him every day, but they never come together. The nurse should be concerned about:
    a. marital problems that usually occur during stressful times like this.
    b. whether Jackson's parents are able to receive adequate support from each other with this arrangement.
    c. whether Jackson's siblings are being adequately cared for.
    d. all of the above.

33 The Child with Endocrine Dysfunction

1. Overproduction of the anterior pituitary hormones can result in:
   a. hyperthyroidism.
   b. hypogonadism (functional).
   c. precocious puberty.
   d. all of the above.

2. The most common organic cause of pituitary undersecretion is:
   a. tumor in the adrenocortical region.
   b. autoimmune hypophysitis.
   c. tumor in the pituitary or hypothalamic region.
   d. perinatal trauma.

3. A child with growth hormone deficiency will exhibit the signs of:
   a. restricted height and weight.
   b. abnormal skeletal proportions.
   c. malnutrition.
   d. short stature but proportional height and weight.

4. In a child with hypopituitarism, the growth hormone levels would usually be:
   a. elevated after 20 minutes of strenuous exercise.
   b. elevated 45 to 90 minutes after the onset of sleep.
   c. lower than normal or not measurable at all.
   d. increased in response to insulin.

5. Treatment of choice for the child with idiopathic hypopituitarism may include:
   a. biosynthetic growth hormone.
   b. human growth hormone.
   c. chemotherapy.
   d. administration of clonidine.

6. In the child with idiopathic hypopituitarism, growth hormone replacement therapy:
   a. will continue for life.
   b. will not result in achievement of a normal familial height.
   c. requires subcutaneous injection.
   d. requires intramuscular injection.

7. Tests that use neuromodulators to stimulate the release of growth hormone:
   a. are the best method to diagnose growth hormone deficiency.
   b. suppress the release of growth hormone.
   c. may be less sensitive indicators than growth hormone assays.
   d. are recommended whenever growth delays occur.

8. Explain the difference between acromegaly and the pituitary hyperfunction that is not considered to be acromegaly.

9. Parents of the child with precocious puberty need to know that:
   a. dress and activities should be aligned with the child's sexual development.
   b. heterosexual interest will usually be advanced.
   c. the child's mental age is congruent with the chronologic age.
   d. overt manifestations of affection represent sexual advances.

10. Desmopressin acetate (DDAVP) may be administered:
    a. by mouth.
    b. intranasally.
    c. topically.
    d. by all of the above routes.

11. Diabetes insipidus (DI) may manifest in a child by sudden episodes of _____ and _____ _____.

12. Compare and contrast clinical manifestations of DI and diabetes mellitus (DM) in the table below.

Diabetes Insipidus	Diabetes Mellitus

13. Which one of the following is *not* considered a secondary cause of DI?
    a. Head trauma
    b. Phenytoin
    c. Meningitis
    d. Obesity

14. The immediate management of syndrome of inappropriate antidiuretic hormone (SIADH) consists of:
    a. increasing fluids.
    b. administering antibiotics.
    c. restricting fluids.
    d. administering vasopressin.

15. One of the most common causes of thyroid disease in children and adolescents is:
    a. Hashimoto disease.
    b. Graves disease.
    c. goiter.
    d. thyrotoxicosis.

16. The initial treatment for the child with hyperthyroidism is:
    a. subtotal thyroidectomy.
    b. total thyroidectomy.
    c. ablation with radioactive iodide.
    d. administration of antithyroid medication.

17. When a thyroidectomy is planned, the nurse should explain to the child that:
    a. iodine preparations will be mixed with flavored foods and then eaten.
    b. he or she will need to hyperextend the neck postoperatively.
    c. the skin, not the throat, will be cut.
    d. laryngospasm can be a life-threatening complication.

18. The child with longstanding hypoparathyroidism will usually exhibit:
    a. short, stubby fingers.
    b. dimpling of the skin over the knuckles.
    c. skeletal growth restriction.
    d. a short, thick neck.

19. A common cause of secondary hyperparathyroidism is:
    a. maternal hyperparathyroidism.
    b. chronic renal disease.
    c. maternal diabetes mellitus.
    d. adenoma of the parathyroid gland.

20. Hyperfunction of the adrenal medulla results in:
    a. release of epinephrine and norepinephrine from the sympathetic nervous system.
    b. pheochromocytoma.
    c. adrenal crisis.
    d. myxedema.

21. Diagnosis of acute adrenocortical insufficiency is based on:
    a. elevated plasma cortisol levels.
    b. the clinical presentation.
    c. depressed plasma cortisol levels.
    d. depressed aldosterone levels.

22. Parents of a child who has Addison disease should be instructed to:
    a. use extra hydrocortisone only when signs of crisis are present.
    b. discontinue the child's cortisone if side effects develop.
    c. decrease the cortisone dose during times of stress.
    d. administer hydrocortisone intramuscularly.

23. Which one of the following diagnostic tests is particularly useful in diagnosing congenital adrenal hyperplasia?
    a. Chromosomal typing
    b. Pelvic ultrasound
    c. Pelvic x-ray
    d. Testosterone levels

24. The temporary treatment for hyperaldosteronism before surgery usually involves administration of:
    a. spironolactone and potassium.
    b. phentolamine and sodium.
    c. furosemide and phosphorus.
    d. phenoxybenzamine.

25. Definitive treatment for pheochromocytoma consists of:
    a. surgical removal of the thyroid.
    b. administration of potassium.
    c. surgical removal of the tumor.
    d. administration of beta blockers.

26. Most children with diabetes mellitus tend to exhibit characteristics of:
    a. maturity-onset diabetes of youth.
    b. gestational-onset diabetes.
    c. type 2 diabetes.
    d. type 1 diabetes.

27. The currently accepted etiology of type 1 diabetes mellitus takes into account:
    a. genetic factors.
    b. autoimmune mechanisms.
    c. environmental factors.
    d. all of the above.

264

28. An early sign of type 2 diabetes mellitus in the adolescent is:
    a. acanthosis nigricans.
    b. obesity.
    c. Kussmaul respirations.
    d. increased hunger.

29. Of the following blood glucose levels, the value that most certainly indicates a diagnosis of type 1 diabetes mellitus is a:
    a. fasting blood glucose of 120 mg/dl.
    b. random blood glucose of 160 mg/dl.
    c. fasting blood glucose of 160 mg/dl.
    d. glucose tolerance test (oral) value of 160 mg/dl for the 2-hour sample.

30. State the goal of insulin replacement therapy.

31. Glycosylated hemoglobin is an acceptable method used to:
    a. assess for ketoacidosis.
    b. assess the control of diabetes.
    c. assess oxygen saturation of the hemoglobin.
    d. accurately determine blood glucose levels.

32. Even with optimal glucose control, a child with type 1 diabetes mellitus may frequently suffer the acute complication of:
    a. retinopathy.
    b. ketoacidosis.
    c. hypoglycemia.
    d. hyperosmolar nonketotic coma.

33. Describe the treatment for a mild hypoglycemic episode in a young child with diabetes mellitus.

34. Which of the following is *not* one of the principles of managing diabetes during illness?
    a. Blood glucose should be monitored every 3 hours.
    b. Insulin dosage requirements may increase, decrease, or remain the same.
    c. Insulin should always be omitted when excessive vomiting occurs.
    d. Oral fluids should be encouraged to avoid dehydration.

35. Diabetic ketoacidosis in children with type 1 diabetes mellitus:
    a. is the most common chronic complication.
    b. is a result of too much insulin.
    c. is a life-threatening complication.
    d. rarely requires hospitalization.

36. Which one of the following cardiac wave patterns is indicative of hypokalemia?
    a. Widening of the Q-T interval with a flattened T wave
    b. Shortening of the Q-T interval with an elevated T wave
    c. Shortening of the Q-T interval with a flattened T wave
    d. Widening of the Q-T interval with an elevated T wave

37. The best approach to effectively teach a child and his or her family the complex concepts of the home management of type 1 diabetes mellitus is to:
    a. provide intensive training a day or so after diagnosis.
    b. provide intensive training the first 3 or 4 days after diagnosis.
    c. teach nothing until 2 weeks after diagnosis.
    d. teach essentials at diagnosis, followed by intense information later.

38. Children with DKA require fluid volume replacement with what type of IV fluid initially?
    a. Dextrose 5% in water (D_5W)
    b. Dextrose 5% in 0.9% normal saline with 20 mEq/KCl per liter
    c. 0.9% normal saline
    d. 10% dextrose with 10 mEq sodium bicarbonate per liter

39. The child with type 1 diabetes mellitus is taught to weigh and measure food to:
    a. receive the nutrients prescribed.
    b. prevent hypoglycemia.
    c. learn to estimate food portions.
    d. prevent hyperglycemia.

40. In regard to meal planning for the child with type 1 diabetes mellitus, parents should be aware that:
    a. fast foods must be eliminated.
    b. foods must be always be weighed and measured.
    c. the exchange list is limited to one type of food.
    d. foods with sorbitol are metabolized into glucose.

41. The most efficient rotation pattern for insulin injections involves giving injections in:
    a. one area of the body 1 inch apart.
    b. different areas of the body each day.

42. In regard to insulin administration:
    a. insulin should never be premixed.
    b. insulin syringes should never be reused.
    c. insulin doses under 2 units may be diluted.
    d. an air bubble in the syringe is insignificant.

43. The child with type 1 diabetes mellitus needs to test his or her urine:
    a. for ketones every day.
    b. for ketones at times of illness.
    c. for glucose every day.
    d. for glucose at times of illness.

44. Exercise for the child with type 1 diabetes mellitus may:
    a. be restricted to noncontact sports.
    b. require a decreased intake of food.
    c. necessitate an increased insulin dose.
    d. require an increased intake of food.

45. Problems with the child adjusting to the self-management of type 1 diabetes are most likely to occur when the condition is diagnosed in:
    a. infancy.
    b. adolescence.
    c. the toddler years.
    d. the school-age years.

CRITICAL THINKING—CASE STUDY

Rebecca Bennett is an 8-year-old who was recently diagnosed with type 1 diabetes mellitus. She is hospitalized with diabetic ketoacidosis, and she is beginning to learn about the disease process. Her parents are with her continually. She has an identical twin sister who is staying with her maternal grandparents.

46. Mrs. Bennett is concerned that Rebecca's sister will also develop diabetes. Based on the preceding information, an acceptable response for the nurse to make would be to:
    a. reassure the parents that the disease is not contagious.
    b. discuss the hereditary and viral factors of type 1 diabetes mellitus.
    c. discuss the hereditary factors of type 1 diabetes mellitus.
    d. discuss the viral factors of type 1 diabetes mellitus.

47. Which one of the following nursing diagnoses is most appropriate for Rebecca once the acute phase of DKA has been resolved?
    a. Fluid Volume Deficit related to uncontrolled diabetes
    b. Fluid Volume Excess related to hormonal disturbances
    c. Deficient Knowledge related to newly diagnosed type 1 diabetes mellitus
    d. Impaired Respiratory Function related to fluid imbalance

48. In preparing the Bennett family for discharge, the nurse should plan to teach:
    a. only Rebecca how to inject insulin.
    b. only Rebecca's parents how to inject insulin.
    c. both Rebecca and her parents how to inject insulin.
    d. the family how to administer oral hypoglycemics.

49. To evaluate Rebecca's progress in relation to her diabetes self-management, the best outcome measure would be Rebecca's:
    a. parents' verbalizations about the disease process.
    b. blood glucose levels.
    c. glycosylated hemoglobin values.
    d. demonstration of her insulin injection technique.

34 The Child with Musculoskeletal or Articular Dysfunction

1. a. What topics does the community nurse include in the educational plan to promote injury prevention among children?

   b. Besides conducting educational programs, what methods can the nurse use to promote injury prevention in children?

2. The nurse is suspicious of child abuse (nonaccidental injury) when:
    i. there is a delay in seeking medical assistance for the injury.
    ii. the parent's history of the injury is not congruent with the actual injury.
    iii. x-ray studies demonstrate previous fractures in different stages of healing.
    iv. the child is crying and fearful of separation from the parent.

   a. i, ii, iii, and iv
   b. i, ii, and iii
   c. ii and iii
   d. ii, iii, and iv

3. A nurse discovers 5-year-old Jimmy, a neighbor, lying in the street next to his bicycle. The nurse sends another witness to activate the emergency medical services (EMS) while the nurse begins a primary assessment of Jimmy. Which one of the following *best* describes the primary assessment and its correct sequence?
   a. Body inspection, head-to-toe survey, and airway patency
   b. Airway patency, respiratory effectiveness, circulatory status
   c. Open airway, head-to-toe assessment for injuries, and chest compressions
   d. Weight estimation, symptom analysis, blood pressure measurement

4. The nurse suspects that Jimmy (from question 3) has a spinal cord injury. Describe the safest immobilization technique.

5. Major consequences of immobility in the pediatric patient include which one of the following?
   a. Bone demineralization leading to osteoporosis
   b. Orthostatic hypertension
   c. Dependent edema in the lower extremities
   d. Decrease in the metabolic rate

6. What are the three major cardiovascular consequences of immobility?

7. List four symptoms of neurologic impairment that should be immediately evaluated in an immobilized child.

8. Nursing interventions aimed at preventing problems associated with immobility include which one of the following?
   a. Encouraging self-care
   b. Restricting fluids with strict intake and output
   c. Limiting active range-of-motion exercises to once per day
   d. Decreasing sensory stimulation to allow adequate rest

9. Match each term with its description.

   a. Orthotics
   b. Prosthetics
   c. Trough crutches
   d. Ankle-foot orthosis (AFO)
   e. Knee-ankle-foot orthosis (KAFO)
   f. Hip-knee-ankle-foot orthosis (HKAFO)

   g. Reciprocal gait orthosis (RGO)
   h. Thoracolumbosacral orthosis (TLSO)
   i. Boston brace
   j. Jewett-Taylor brace
   k. Axillary swing-through crutches
   l. Forearm crutches

   _____ The fabrication and fitting of braces

   _____ Provides support for the knee, ankle, and hip; used for flail lower limb and paralysis

   _____ The fabrication and fitting of artificial limbs

   _____ Sometimes used to support the spine and trunk during ambulation to prevent compression after fracture of the spinal column

   _____ Used to prevent buckling of the knee, to support the extremity when there is paralysis or marked weakness of the knee extension or quadriceps muscle

   _____ Custom molded and fits snugly around the truck of the body to exert pressure on the ribs and back to support the spine in a straight position

   _____ An underarm orthosis customized from prefabricated plastic shells, with corrective forces for each patient supplied by lateral pads; prevent progression of curves in the spine

   _____ Allows children with paraplegia to walk on a flat surface; used in children with spinal cord injury, sacral agenesis, and spina bifida

   _____ Used to prevent footdrop due to bed rest, trauma to the foot, or paralysis of muscles that flex the foot

   _____ Usual selection for children who anticipate permanent use; used for paraplegic children who are unable to use braces

   _____ Used most frequently for temporary assistance

   _____ Allows the weight to be assumed by the elbow

10. Which one of the following is a complication of immobility that is easily prevented with appropriate nursing intervention?
    a. Disuse atrophy and loss of muscle mass
    b. Constipation
    c. Hypocalcemia
    d. Pain

11. Which one of the following is not included in the teaching plan of a child with a brace or prosthesis?
    a. Frequent assessment of all areas in contact with the brace for signs of skin irritation
    b. Assessment of the stump area before application of the prosthesis
    c. Removal of the prosthesis limited to bedtime unless skin breakage occurs
    d. Use of protective clothing under the brace

12. List five effects that prolonged immobilization or disability of the child may have on the family.

13. Continuous pressure on the radial nerve may result in:
    a. footdrop
    b. wristdrop

14. List five interventions aimed at preventig circulatory stasis and development of DVT in an immobilized child.

15. All children who are immobilized for a prolonged period are at risk for skin breakdown. Identify three intrinsic risk factors that place immobilized children at increased risk for skin breakdown.

16. Bone healing is characteristically more rapid in children than in adults because:
    a. children have less constant muscle contraction associated with the fracture.
    b. children's fractures are less severe than adults'.
    c. children have an active growth plate that helps speed repair with less likelihood of deformity.
    d. children have thickened periosteum and a more generous blood supply.

17. The method of fracture reduction is *not* determined by:
    a. The child's age
    b. The manner in which the fracture occurred
    c. The degree of displacement
    d. The amount of edema

18. What are the "five *P*s" of ischemia that are considered when assessing fractures to rule out vascular injury?

19. Emergency treatment for the child with a fracture includes:
    a. moving the child to allow removal of clothing from the area of injury.
    b. immobilization of the limb, usually including joints above and below the injury site.
    c. pushing the protruding bone under the skin.
    d. keeping the area of injury in a dependent position.

20. What are the four goals of fracture management?

21. An appropriate nursing intervention for the care of a child with an extremity in a new cast is to:
    a. keep the cast covered with a sheet.
    b. use the fingertips when handling the cast to prevent pressure areas.
    c. use heated fans or dryers to circulate air and speed the cast-drying process.
    d. turn the child at least every 2 hours to help dry the cast evenly.

22. A 10-year-old presents to the ED with a suspected radial fracture incurred in a fall from a treehouse. List three nursing interventions for the initial care of this child.

23. A 9-year-old with a new long arm cast is discharged home with a prescription for pain medication. What main points should the nurse include in the home care of the child in a cast?

24. Match each term with its description.

a. Spiral
b. Open, or compound fracture
c. Buckle, or torus, fracture
d. Complete fracture
e. Incomplete fracture
f. Transverse fracture

g. Simple, or closed fracture
h. Plastic deformation
i. Complicated fracture
j. Comminuted fracture
k. Greenstick fracture

_____ Fracture with an open wound from which the bone has protruded

_____ Fracture in which fracture fragments are separated

_____ Fracture in which fracture fragments remain attached

_____ Fracture that is crosswise, at right angles to the long axis of the bone

_____ Fracture in which small fragments of bone are broken from the fractured shaft and lie in surrounding tissue

_____ Fracture in which bone fragments cause damage to surrounding organs or tissue

_____ Fracture that is slanting and circular, twisting around the bone shaft

_____ Appears as a raising or bulging at the site of the fracture

_____ Occurs when a bone is angulated beyond the limits of bending

_____ Fracture that has not produced a break in the skin

_____ Occurs when bone is bent but not broken

25. To reduce anxiety in the child undergoing cast removal, which of the following nursing interventions would the nurse expect to be *least* effective?
   a. Demonstrate how the cast cutter works before beginning the procedure.
   b. Use the analogy of having fingernails or hair cut.
   c. Explain that it will take only a few minutes.
   d. Continue to reassure that all is going well and that the child's behavior is accepted during the removal process.

26. Julie, age 10, has just returned from surgery for repair of an open fracture; she has a dressing and elastic bandage wrap on her leg from upper thigh to mid-calf. The nurse immediately notifies the physician if assessment findings include which of the following?
   a. Appearance of blood-stained area the size of a dime on the dressing
   b. 2+ pedal pulse
   c. Inability to move the toes
   d. Report of pain level of 4/10 on Wong-Baker Faces Pain Rating Scale

27. List five possible clinical manifestations of compartment syndrome.

28. The nurse is caring for 7-year-old Charles after application of skeletal traction. Which of the following is contraindicated?
    a. Gently massage over pressure areas to stimulate circulation.
    b. Release the traction when repositioning Charles in bed.
    c. Inspect pin sites for bleeding or infection.
    d. Assess for alterations in neurovascular status.

29. The nurse is assessing Carol, age 8, for complications related to her recent fracture and the application of a fiberglass cast to her forearm and elbow. Carol is crying with pain, the nurse is unable to locate pulses in the affected extremity, and there is lack of sensitivity to the area as well as some edema. Which of the following would the nurse suspect as most likely to be occurring?
    a. Normal occurrence for the first few hours after application of traction
    b. Volkmann contracture
    c. Nerve compression syndrome
    d. Epiphyseal damage

30. Johnny, a 12-year-old with fracture of the femur, has developed sudden chest pain and shortness of breath. The astute nurse suspects:
    a. pulmonary embolism.
    b. compartment syndrome.
    c. myocardial infarction.
    d. pneumonia.

31. The priority nursing action for Johnny (in item 30) is to:
    a. elevate the affected extremity.
    b. administer oxygen.
    c. administer pain medication.
    d. start an intravenous (IV) infusion of heparin.

32. Match the term with its description.

    a. Contusion   f. Myositis ossificans
    b. Ecchymosis   g. Stress fracture
    c. Dislocation   h. Overuse injury
    d. Strain   i. Nursemaid's elbow
    e. Sprain

    _____ Occurs when the force of stress on the ligament is so great that it displaces the normal position of the opposing bone ends or the bone end in relation to its socket

    _____ Partial dislocation of the radial head in the elbow

    _____ Occurs as a result of repeated muscle contraction from repetitive weight-bearing sports

    _____ Damage to the soft tissue, subcutaneous structures, and muscle

    _____ Occurs when trauma to a joint is so severe that a ligament is either stretched or partially or completely torn by the force created as a joint is twisted or wrenched

    _____ Repetitive microtrauma that occurs to a particular anatomic structure

    _____ Occurs from deep contusions to the biceps or quadriceps muscles, resulting in a restriction of the flexibility of the affected limb

    _____ Escape of blood into the tissues

    _____ Microscopic tear to the musculotendinous unit

33. Which of the following statements about "nursemaid's elbow" is correct?
    a. This most common partial dislocation of the radial head of the elbow is usually found in children ages 1 to 3 years.
    b. This condition is caused by a sudden pull at the wrist while the arm is fully extended and the forearm is pronated.
    c. The longer the dislocation is present, the longer it takes the child to recover mobility after treatment.
    d. All of the above statements are correct.

34. Immediate treatment of sprains and strains includes:
    a. rest and cold application.
    b. disregarding the pain and "working out" the sprain or strain.
    c. rest, elevation, and pain medication.
    d. compression of the area and heat application.

35. Major sprains or tears to the ligamentous tissues rarely occur in growing children because the _____ are stronger than bone. The _____ or _____ _____ is the weakest part of the bone and the usual site of injury.

36. Ben, a 15-year-old high school student, is at a track event. He has been running multiple events. He was feeling unwell before the event and had been vomiting. Now he is complaining of thirst, headache, fatigue, dizziness, and nausea. He seems to be somewhat disoriented and is sweating. Ben's temperature is normal. Which of the following is the most likely to describe Ben's condition?
    a. Heat cramps
    b. Dehydration
    c. Heat exhaustion
    d. Heatstroke

37. Which of the following statements made to the athlete by the nurse is correct?
    a. It is more important to replace sodium and chloride than water.
    b. Recommended dietary energy intake for adolescents involved in sports is 50% of caloric intake from carbohydrates.
    c. Iron replacement is necessary only for the female athlete.
    d. Energy for prolonged exercise is best obtained from high-carbohydrate foods eaten 2 hours before the event.

38. Sixteen-year-old Ben has been brought to the school nurse's office for heatstroke. He has a temperature of 40° C (104° F) and is awake but disoriented. Which of the following is contraindicated?
    a. Immediate removal of clothing and application of cool water to the skin
    b. Administration of antipyretics
    c. Use of fans directed at Ben
    d. Activation of EMS for transport to hospital

39. Zac, a 16-year-old football star at the local high school, is at the school nurse practitioner's office for acne that is not clearing with the over-the-counter medications. During the physical examination, the nurse notes that Zac has achieved a marked increase in muscle and strength in a very short time. Which of the following would the nurse suspect caused these changes?
    a. Use of an ergogenic aid, anabolic steroids
    b. More frequent and more strenuous workouts in the gym
    c. Increased protein and vitamins in the diet
    d. Use of methylphenidate (Ritalin) or phenmetrazine (Preludin)

40. Commotio cordis:
    a. occurs after a blunt, nonpenetrating blow to the chest, which produces ventricular fibrillation.
    b. rarely causes death.
    c. occurs almost exclusively in athletes with hypertrophic cardiomyopathy.
    d. occurs in athletes who have a history of sudden death in a relative under the age of 50 years.

41. List the three characteristics of the female athlete triad.

42. The condition recognized in the infant with limited neck motion, in which the neck is flexed and turned to the affected side as a result of shortening of the sternocleidomastoid muscle, is:
    a. torticollis.
    b. brachial plexus palsy.
    c. lordosis.
    d. kyphosis.

43. Bob, age 7, is diagnosed with Legg-Calvé-Perthes disease. Which of the following manifestations is *not* consistent with this diagnosis?
    a. Intermittent appearance of a limp on the affected side
    b. Hip soreness, ache, or stiffness that can be constant or intermittent
    c. Pain and limp most evident on arising and at the end of a long day of activities
    d. Specific history of injury to the area

44. Slipped capital femoral epiphysis is suspected when:
    a. an adolescent or preadolescent begins to limp and complains of continuous or intermittent pain in the hip.
    b. an examination reveals no restriction on internal rotation or adduction but restriction on external rotation.
    c. referred pain goes into the sacral and lumbar areas.
    d. all of the above occur.

45. The primary diagnostic tool used in developmental dysplasia of the hip (DDH) in a newborn is:
    a. a radiograph
    b. an ultrasound
    c. magnetic resonance imaging
    d. the Barlow and Ortolani maneuvers

46. The recommended treatment for DDH in an infant 2 months old is:
    a. surgical fixation.
    b. hip spica cast.
    c. Pavlik harness.
    d. hip abduction orthosis.

47. Osteomyelitis resulting from a blood-borne bacterium that could have developed from an infected lesion is termed:
    a. acute hematogenous osteomyelitis.
    b. exogenous osteomyelitis.
    c. subacute osteomyelitis.
    d. chronic osteomyelitis.

48. The care plan for the child during the acute phase of osteomyelitis always includes:
    a. performing wound irrigations.
    b. ensuring administration of antibiotics.
    c. isolating the child.
    d. incorporating passive range-of-motion exercises for the affected area.

49. Which of the following statements about septic arthritis is true?
    a. The most common causative agent in children under 2 years of age is *Haemophilus influenzae*.
    b. Knees, hips, ankles, hands, and feet are the joints most commonly affected.
    c. Early radiographic findings show soft tissue swelling and erosions of the bone.
    d. IV antibiotic use is based on Gram stain and clinical presentation.

50. Nursing considerations for the patient diagnosed with osteogenesis imperfecta include:
    a. preventing fractures by holding onto the child's ankles when changing diapers.
    b. providing nonjudgmental support while parents may be dealing with accusations of child abuse.
    c. providing guidelines to the parents in avoiding all exercise and sports for the child.
    d. educating parents that the use of braces and splints can increase the rate of fracture.

51. In addition to the prevention of fractures, the nursing care of a child with osteogenesis imperfecta should include:
    a. oral and dental care.
    b. meticulous skin care.
    c. care related to the effects of drug treatment.
    d. all of the above.

52. Diagnostic evaluation is important for early recognition of scoliosis. Which of the following is the correct procedure for the school nurse conducting this examination?
    a. View the child, who is standing and walking fully clothed, to look for uneven hanging of clothing.
    b. View all children from the left and right side to look mainly for asymmetry of the hip height.
    c. Completely undress all children before the examination.
    d. View the child, who is wearing underpants, from behind when the child bends forward at the hips.

53. The surgical technique for the correction of scoliosis (arthrodesis) consists of:

54. Marilyn, age 12, has been diagnosed with scoliosis and placed in a thoracolumbosacral orthotic (TLSO) brace. Which of the following information provided by the nurse to Marilyn is correct?
    a. "The brace will cure your curvature."
    b. "The brace is an underarm brace made of plastic that will be molded and shaped to your body to correct the curvature."
    c. "The brace includes a neck ring to extend the neck."
    d. "The brace will only be worn in bed, since it prevents walking because of the severity of the trunk bend."

55. Nursing care directed toward nonsurgical management in a teenager with scoliosis primarily includes:
    a. promoting self-esteem and positive body image.
    b. preventing immobility.
    c. promoting adequate nutrition.
    d. preventing infection.

56. Which of the following nursing goals is most appropriate for the child with juvenile idiopathic arthritis?
    a. Child will exhibit signs of reduced joint inflammation and adequate joint function.
    b. Child will exhibit no signs of impaired skin integrity due to rash.
    c. Child will exhibit normal weight and nutritional status.
    d. Child will exhibit no alteration in respiratory patterns or respiratory tract infection.

57. What should the nurse teach the patient and family of the child diagnosed with systemic lupus erythematosus (SLE) regarding each of the following topics?
    a. Diet

    b. Sun exposure

    c. Birth control medication

Chapter **34 The Child with Musculoskeletal or Articular Dysfunction**

58. What are the two goals of therapeutic management for SLE?

59. The principal drugs used in SLE to control inflammation are the _____.

60. What is the primary nursing goal for the child with SLE?

CRITICAL THINKING—CASE STUDY

Sandy age 10, has developed joint and leg pain, some joint swelling, fever, malaise, and pleuritis. The physician has ordered laboratory testing to include sedimentation rate, rheumatoid factor, and a complete blood count. Tentative diagnosis has been established as juvenile idiopathic arthritis (JIA).

61. If the diagnosis is correct, which of the following would represent the expected laboratory results?
    a. Leukocytosis
    b. Elevated sedimentation rate
    c. Negative rheumatoid factor
    d. All of the above may be present.

62. A group of drugs prescribed for JIA are nonsteroidal antiinflammatory drugs. Education regarding the use of these drugs should include which of the following?
    a. They produce excellent analgesic and antiinflammatory effects but little antipyretic effect.
    b. They are administered in the lowest effective dose and given on alternate days rather than daily.
    c. Antiinflammatory effect occurs 3 to 4 weeks after therapy is begun.
    d. Because there is a narrow margin between effective and toxic dosage, levels need to be monitored regularly until therapeutic dosage is established.

63. Which of the following is the most appropriate nursing intervention to promote adequate joint function in the child with JIA?
    a. Incorporate therapeutic exercises in play activities.
    b. Provide heat to affected joints by use of tub baths.
    c. Provide written information for all treatments ordered.
    d. Explore and develop activities in which the child can succeed.

64. An expected outcome for the nursing diagnosis of Disturbed Body Image related to the disease process of JIA is:
    a. the patient and family members are able to explain the disease process.
    b. the patient is accepted by peers.
    c. the patient will express feelings and concerns about how the condition affects her life.
    d. the child will understand and use effective communication techniques.

35 The Child with Neuromuscular or Muscular Dysfunction

1. The nurse knows that the etiology of CP is most commonly related to which of the following?
   a. Existing prenatal brain abnormalities
   b. Maternal asphyxia
   c. Childhood meningitis
   d. Preeclampsia

2. The nurse is preparing the long-term care plan for a child with CP. Which of the following is included in the plan?
   a. No delay in gross motor development is expected.
   b. The illness is not progressively degenerative. ✓
   c. There will be no persistence of primitive infantile reflexes.
   d. All children will need genetic counseling as they get older before planning for a family.

3. Match each term with its description.

   a. Dyskinetic CP   e. Dystonic
   b. Mixed-type CP   f. Diplegia
   c. Spastic CP   g. Hemiplegia
   d. Ataxic CP

   _____ Slow, twisting movement of the trunk or extremities; abnormal posture

   _____ Most common form of spastic CP; motor deficit greater in upper extremity; one side of the body affected

   _____ Characterized by abnormal involuntary movement, such as athetosis—slow, wormlike, writhing movements that usually involve the extremities, trunk, neck, facial muscles, and tongue

   _____ Characterized by wide-based gait; rapid, repetitive movements performed poorly; disintegration of movements of the upper extremities when the child reaches for objects

   _____ Combination of spastic CP and dyskinetic CP

   ___C___ The most common clinical type of CP; physical signs of increased stretch reflexes, hypertonicity, poor control of posture, balance, and coordinated motion; impairment of fine and gross motor skills

   _____ Type of spastic CP; all extremities affected—lower more than upper

4. Children with CP often have manifestations that include alterations of muscle tone. Which of the following is an example of a finding in a child with altered muscle tone?
   a. Demonstrates increased or decreased resistance to passive movements
   b. Develops hand dominance by the age of 5 months
   c. Has an asymmetric crawl
   d. When placed in prone position, maintains hips higher than trunk, with legs and arms flexed or drawn under the body

5. Associated disabilities and problems related to the child with CP include which of the following?
   a. All children with CP have intelligence testing in the abnormal range.
   b. A large number of eye cataracts are associated with CP and require surgical correction.
   c. Seizures are a common occurrence among children with athetosis and diplegia.
   d. Coughing and choking, especially while eating, predispose children with CP to aspiration. ✓

6. The nurse is completing a physical examination on 6-month-old Brian. Which of the following would be an abnormal finding suggestive of CP?
   a. Brian is able to hold onto the nurse's hands while being pulled to a sitting position.
   b. Brian has no Moro reflex.
   c. Brian has no tonic neck reflex.
   d. Brian has an obligatory tonic neck reflex.

7. Recommended diagnostic evaluation for infants at risk for CP includes:
   a. magnetic resonance imaging of the brain.
   b. computed tomographic scan of the brain.
   c. laboratory testing.
   d. metabolic and genetic testing when structural abnormality is identified.

8. The goal of therapeutic management for the child with CP is:
   a. assisting with motor control of voluntary muscle.
   b. promoting an optimal developmental course to enable children to achieve their maximal potential.
   c. delaying the development of sensory deprivation.
   d. surgically correcting deformities.

9. Identify the five broad areas of therapeutic management for the child with CP.

10. Identify the following statements as true or false.

   _____ Ankle-foot orthoses are molded to fit the feet and worn inside shoes to reduce deformity.

   _____ Surgical intervention is used in the child with CP to correct contractures or spastic deformities and provide stability.

   _____ Baclofen and diazepam are effective in improving muscle coordination in children with CP and in decreasing overall spasticity.

   _____ Prime candidates for botulinum toxin type A (Botox) injections are children with spasticity confined to the lower extremities.

   _____ CP patients are screened before Baclofen pump placement by the infusion of a test dose of intrathecal baclofen delivered via a lumbar puncture.

   _____ The application of technical aids makes it possible for older persons with CP to eventually function in their own apartments and can be extended into the workplace.

   _____ Children receiving phenytoin are at risk for developing gum hyperplasia.

   _____ Physical therapy consisting of stretching, passive, active, and resistive movements applied to specific muscle groups is able to achieve spectacular changes in the ultimate outcome of the CP child.

   _____ Children who have CP and sucking and swallowing difficulty should be held in a semireclining posture during feeding to make use of gravity flow.

   _____ Feeding techniques such as forcing the child to use the lips and tongue in eating can facilitate speech.

   _____ Education requirements of all children with CP are determined by the child's needs and potential.

11. List the most common side effects of medications (baclofen, dantrolene sodium, and diazepam) administered to children with CP to decrease overall spasticity.

12. Give three reasons why children with CP have difficulty meeting their nutritional needs.

13. Which of the following would be expected in the infant with hypotonia?
    a. When held in horizontal suspension, the infant responds by slightly raising the head.
    b. When pulled to a sitting position, the infant demonstrates head lag that is quickly corrected to a normal position.
    c. When placed in horizontal suspension position, the infant's head droops over the examiner's supporting hand and the infant's extremities hang loosely.
    d. The infant has a slower weight gain but a good sucking reflex.

14. Infantile spinal muscular atrophy (SMA type 1):
    a. may be diagnosed prenatally by genetic analysis of circulating fetal cells in maternal blood or amniotic fluid.
    b. can be cured with surgery performed in utero.
    c. is associated with nutritional failure to thrive, the most serious complication, often leading to the infant's early death.
    d. is associated with children who are intellectually delayed.

15. The disease inherited only as an autosomal recessive trait and characterized by progressive weakness and wasting of skeletal muscles caused by degeneration of anterior horn cells is:
    a. cerebral palsy.
    b. Kugelberg-Welander disease.
    c. infantile SMA type 1 (Werdnig-Hoffmann disease).
    d. Guillain-Barré syndrome (GBS).

16. Nursing considerations for the infant with SMA type 1 should include which of the following to promote developmental care?
    a. Feeding by nasogastric tube
    b. Using an infant walker to develop muscle strength
    c. Incorporating verbal, tactile, and auditory stimulation
    d. Encouraging the parents to seek genetic counseling

17. a. What are the most serious orthopedic problems associated with SMA type 1?

    b. Describe the goal of treatment for nursing care for the child with SMA type 1.

18. Which of the following is a true statement about Guillain-Barré syndrome (GBS)?
    a. GBS is an autosomal recessive inherited disease.
    b. GBS is more likely to affect children than adults, with children under the age of 4 years having the higher susceptibility.
    c. GBS is an acute demyelinating polyneuropathy with a progressive, usually ascending, flaccid paralysis.
    d. GBS is an autoimmune disorder associated with the attack of circulating antibodies on the acetylcholine receptors.

19. Diagnostic evaluation for the patient with GBS would include which of the following results?
    a. Complete blood count elevated
    b. Cerebrospinal fluid high in protein
    c. Creatinine phosphokinase elevated
    d. Sensory nerve conduction time increased

20. The priority nursing consideration for the child in the acute phase of GBS is:
    a. careful observation for difficulty in swallowing and respiratory involvement.
    b. prevention of contractures.
    c. prevention of bowel and bladder complications.
    d. prevention of sensory impairment.

21. Which one of the following is *not* considered a standard treatment for GBS?
    a. Plasmapheresis
    b. Corticosteroids
    c. Administration of IVIG
    d. Administration of neostigmine

22. What are the characteristic symptoms of generalized tetanus?

23. Terry, age 11 years, comes to the urgent care clinic with a major laceration sustained while working on a cattle fence. The laceration requires extensive cleaning and suturing. Terry last received a tetanus booster on entry to school at age 7 years. Ideally, Terry should receive which of the following for protection against tetanus?
    a. Tetanus antitoxin and tetanus toxoid
    b. Tetanus immunoglobulin (TIG) and tetanus toxoid
    c. Tetanus immunoglobulin (TIG) and tetanus antitoxin

24. Primary nursing implementations for the child with tetanus include:
    i. controlling or eliminating stimulation from sound, light, and touch.
    ii. placing the child in isolation.
    iii. arranging for the child not to be left alone, since these children are mentally alert.
    iv. realizing that vecuronium does not cause total paralysis.
    v. encouraging high intake of fluid.
    vi. decreasing the environmental stimuli.

    a. i, ii, iii, and vi
    b. ii, iv, and v
    c. iii, v, and vi
    d. i, iii, and vi

25. A common risk factor for infant botulism includes:
    a. contamination of the umbilical stump after birth.
    b. ingestion of an uncooked meat product.
    c. ingestion of uncooked and unwashed vegetables.
    d. ingestion of honey.

26. Infant botulism usually manifests with symptoms of:
    a. diarrhea and vomiting.
    b. constipation and generalized weakness.
    c. high fever and decrease in spontaneous movement.
    d. failure to thrive.

27. What is the treatment for infant botulism?

28. Nursing considerations aimed at parental support for the infant with botulism include:
    a. teaching the parents the importance of administering enemas and cathartics for bowel function after discharge.
    b. preparing the parents for the fact that the child will have muscular disability after the illness.
    c. teaching the parents the proper administration of antibiotics to continue treatment after discharge.
    d. teaching parents that the child will fatigue easily when muscular action is sustained and that timing of feedings after discharge is important.

29. Tammy, age 13, is diagnosed with myasthenia gravis. The nurse, in preparing a teaching plan for the family, includes which of the following as a priority?
    a. Observing for signs of overmedication of anticholinesterase drugs, which include respiratory distress, choking, and aspiration
    b. Encouraging Tammy to be involved in strenuous activity and sports
    c. Suggesting to Tammy and her parents that they limit Tammy's scholastic activities in school to allow for adequate rest
    d. Reducing Tammy's weight to reduce symptom occurrence

30. Neonatal myasthenia gravis:
    a. occurs in approximately 30% to 50% of infants born to mothers with myasthenia gravis.
    b. produces exaggerated Moro reflex and shrill cry in the infant.
    c. may require administration of cholinesterase inhibitors to improve feeding ability.
    d. produces strength changes in the infant even after the maternal acetylcholine receptor antibodies have cleared the infant's system.

31. Upon the delivery of an infant with myelomeningocele, which one of the following nursing actions is contraindicated?
    a. Examination of the membranous cyst for intactness
    b. Diapering the infant
    c. Keeping moist, sterile normal saline dressings on the defect
    d. Keeping the infant in the prone position

32. Therapeutic management that provides the most favorable morbidity and mortality outcomes for the child born with myelomeningocele is:
    a. early physical therapy.
    b. surgical closure of the defect within the first 24 to 72 hours.
    c. vigorous antibiotic therapy.
    d. splint application to lower extremities.

33. The major anomaly most frequently associated with myelomeningocele is:
    a. Chiari malformation.
    b. hydrocephalus.
    c. clubfoot.
    d. developmental dysplasia of the hips.

34. a. What is the optimal management goal for genitourinary function in the infant born with myelomeningocele?

    b. What is the optimal goal for the older child born with the same condition?

35. Management of the genitourinary function in the patient with myelomeningocele includes clean intermittent catheterization (CIC) and anticholinergic medication. Which of the following statements about their use is correct?

    i. CIC is used to prevent spontaneous voiding.
    ii. Parents are taught to catheterize the infant every 4 hours during the day and once at night.
    iii. Anticholinergic medications enhance sphincter competence.
    iv. Anticholinergic medications reduce detrusor muscle tone and reduce bladder pressure.

    a. i and iii
    b. i and iv
    c. ii and iii
    d. ii and iv

36. Research has shown that maternal supplementation of folic acid can reduce the recurrence rates of spina bifida, anencephaly, or encephalocele. How should this supplement be administered?
    a. Daily folic acid dose of 4 mg beginning 1 month before conception and during the first trimester
    b. Daily folic acid dose of 0.4 mg as soon as pregnancy is confirmed
    c. Daily folic acid dose of 4 mg given through the use of multivitamin preparations beginning 1 month before conception and throughout the first trimester
    d. Daily folic acid dose of 4 mg beginning with the confirmation of pregnancy and continuing throughout pregnancy

37. Children with spina bifida who are confined to a wheelchair are at increased risk for:
    a. tethered cord syndrome.
    b. Chiari malformation.
    c. skin breakdown.
    d. orthopedic deformities.

38. Spinal cord injuries are classified as either complete or incomplete. In a complete spinal cord injury:
    a. there is loss of sensation, pain, and proprioception with normal cord function, including motor function.
    b. there is transient loss of neural function below the level of the acute spinal cord lesion, resulting in flaccid paralysis and loss of tendon autonomic and cutaneous reflex activity.
    c. there is no motor or sensory function more than three segments below the neurologic level of the injury.
    d. there is tetraplegia, commonly with sacral sparing, with patients gaining some motor recovery.

39. Diagnostic evaluation of the child who is seen with a spinal cord injury includes a complete neurologic examination. Motor system evaluation is done by:
    a. stimulating peripheral receptors by eliciting reflex such as the patellar.
    b. observing gait if the child is able to walk; noting balance maintenance; and assessing the ability to lift, flex, and extend extremities.
    c. testing all 12 cranial nerves.
    d. using the blunt end of a safety pin and the sharp point to test each dermatome.

40. What is the general guideline used when determining whether a paraplegic person has the capacity for self-help in learning to walk?

41. Discuss the benefits of functional electrical stimulation (FES) for the child with spinal cord injury.

42. The nurse caring for the child with spinal cord injury and neurogenic bladder knows:
   a. to keep the patient's urine alkaline.
   b. that administration of dicyclomine (Bentyl) will relax the bladder musculature but will not promote increased bladder capacity or more adequate emptying.
   c. that the bladder that empties periodically by reflex action will not need intermittent catheterization.
   d. that pyelonephritis and renal failure are the most significant causes of death in longstanding paraplegic patients.

43. In discussing sexuality with the teenager who has a spinal injury, the nurse correctly includes which of the following in the discussion?
   a. Development of secondary sexual characteristics will be delayed.
   b. Well-motivated young people can look forward to successful participation in marital and family activities.
   c. If injury occurs before onset of menstruation, ovulation and conception are not possible.
   d. Females can easily experience vaginal or clitoral orgasms.

44. Clinical manifestations of juvenile dermatomyositis include:
   i. proximal limb and trunk muscle weakness.
   ii. stiff and sore muscles.
   iii. decreased ductal muscle strength and reflex response.
   iv. red rash over the malar areas and nose and violet discoloration of the eyelids.
   v. erythematous, scaly, atopic skin over extensor muscle surfaces.

   a. i, ii, iii, and iv
   b. i, ii, iv, and v
   c. iii, iv, and v
   d. ii, iii, and iv

45. Corticosteroid administration in muscular dystrophy has been shown to do all of the following *except*:
   a. increase muscle bulk and muscle power.
   b. improve pulmonary function.
   c. prolong ambulation.
   d. increase incidence of scoliosis.

46. What are the major complications of muscular dystrophy?

47. Major goals in the therapeutic management of children with muscular dystrophy include which of the following?
   a. Promoting strenuous activity and exercise
   b. Promoting large caloric intake
   c. Promoting optimum function in all muscles for as long as possible
   d. Preventing cognitive impairment

48. Characteristic features of Duchenne muscular dystrophy include all of the following *except*:
   a. waddling gait.
   b. lordosis.
   c. calf muscle hypertrophy.
   d. neurogenic bladder.

Kevin, age 4, has a history of premature delivery, with CP being diagnosed around age 2 years. Assessment findings include tetraplegia and deficient verbal communication skills but apparently normal level of intelligence. Kevin has been hospitalized several times in the past because of respiratory tract infection and gastric reflux. During Kevin's regular follow-up visit, his mother tells the nurse it is becoming harder to care for Kevin because of his needs. Because of Kevin's recent admission to the hospital for pneumonia, she worries that she is not giving Kevin the care he needs.

49. Which of the following assessment findings could most help explain why Kevin is having respiratory problems?
    a. Constant drooling, which contributes to wet clothing and chilling
    b. Dietary imbalance with poor nutritional intake
    c. Nystagmus and amblyopia
    d. Coughing and choking, especially while eating, and history of gastric reflux

50. Kevin's mother asks the nurse how she can improve Kevin's communication skills, and a nursing diagnosis of Impaired Verbal Communication is developed. Which of the following plans would be most appropriate for Kevin at this time to improve his communication skills?
    a. Purchase an electric typewriter or computer to facilitate communication skills.
    b. Facilitate a consult with a speech language pathologist.
    c. Teach Kevin the use of nonverbal communication skills like sign language.
    d. Use audiotapes with Kevin to improve his speech abilities.

51. The nurse recognizes that an additional diagnosis is Altered Family Processes related to a child with a lifelong disability. Which of the following interventions should the nurse recognize as being important to include in Kevin's care plan?
    a. Explore potential for additional caregiving support.
    b. Refer the family to a support group of other parents of children with CP.
    c. Refer the parents to social services for additional suggestions.
    d. All of the above are important.

52. Based on the information given about Kevin, identify the nursing goals that would assist him and his family.

53. While Kevin is in the hospital, the nurse should plan appropriate play activities that include:
    a. minimized speaking, since Kevin has difficulty with his speech.
    b. solitary play to allow Kevin's parents to be away from Kevin so that they can rest.
    c. helping Kevin relax muscles that are tense.
    d. those that require little intellectual functioning.

Answer Key

CHAPTER 1

1. b (p. 2)
2. d (p. 3)
3. c (p. 6)
4. c (p. 6)
5. a (p. 6)
6. d (p. 7, Table 1-2)
7. c (p. 7)
8. c (p. 7)
9. c (p. 7)
10. a (p. 8)
11. c (p. 7, Table 1-3)
12. d (p. 8)
13. Possible answers: Respiratory illnesses, infection, acute illness (p. 8)
14. Possible answers: Homelessness, poverty, low birth weight, chronic illnesses, adoption, daycare attendance (p. 8)
15. a (p. 2)
16. b (p. 4)
17. Car restraints, bicycle helmets, and smoke detectors (p. 4)
18. b (p. 3, Table 1-1)
19. d (p. 11)
20. Anticipatory guidance (p. 10)
21. Atraumatic care is the provision of care that minimizes or eliminates psychologic and physical distress experienced by children and their families. The three principles are: prevent or minimize child's separation from family; promote a sense of control in the child and family; and prevent or minimize bodily injury or pain (pp. 8-9)
22. a (p. 8)
23. c (p. 8)
24. c (p. 9)
25. Evidence-based practice (p. 11)
26. c (p. 12)
27. e, b, g, f, i, d, c, h, a (pp. 9-11)
28. c (pp. 12-14)
29. a (pp. 12-14)
30. d (pp. 12-14)
31. c (pp. 12-14)
32. b (pp. 12-14)
33. a (pp. 12-14)
34. Possible answers include: Falls prevalence; Failure to rescue; Central line catheter infection. (p. 14; Box 1-5)

CHAPTER 2

1. f (p. 24), r (p. 17), j (p. 22), m (p. 17), a (p. 17), c (p. 17), e (p. 24), h (p. 30), d (p. 20), n (p. 17), b (p. 20), g (p. 26), o (p. 19), i (p. 30), p (p. 19), s (p. 32), k (p. 26), l (p. 20), q (p. 25)
2. c (p. 17)
3. b, a, a, b, c, c (pp. 18-20; Table 2-1)
4. b (p. 20)
5. c (pp. 20, 21)
6. In guiding the nurse throughout the nursing process to help predict ways that families can cope and respond to stressful events, in providing individualized support that builds on family strengths and functioning style and in assisting family members in obtaining resources (p. 22)
7. T, F, T, T, F, T (pp. 22, 23)
8. c (p. 23)
9. b (p. 24)
10. b, a, c (p. 24)
11. a (p. 25; Family-Centered Care box)
12. a (p. 24)
13. a (p. 26)
14. b (pp. 25, 26)
15. a (p. 27)
16. d (p. 27)
17. c (pp. 26, 27)
18. F, T, F, T, T, T, T, F (pp. 29, 30; Box 2-5)
19. c (p. 30)
20. c (p. 30)
21. a, c, b (p. 31)
22. j (p. 35), c (p. 34), a (p. 33), d (p. 32), g (p. 33), f (p. 35), k (p. 35), i (p. 34), b (p. 34), h (p. 34), l (p. 35), m (p. 35), e (p. 35)
23. d (p. 33)
24. a. Support, Empowerment, Boundaries and expectations; Constructive use of time
    b. Commitment to learning, Positive values, Social competencies, Positive identity (p. 34)
25. b (pp. 32, 39, 40)
26. a (p. 36)
27. d (p. 37, Box 2-6)
28. d. (p. 37)
29. b, d, c, a (p. 37)
30. c (p. 38)
31. d (p. 38)
32. a (p. 40)
33. c (p. 40)
34. a (p. 35)
35. e, c, b, d, a (p. 41, Box 2-9)
36. d (pp. 18, 19; Box 2-1, Table 2-1)
37. a (pp. 18-20; Box 2-1, Box 2-2, Table 2-1)
38. b (pp. 18-20; Box 2-1, Box 2-2, Table 2-1)
39. d (p. 19)
40. Establish a healthy family unit. Seek support from extended family; seek parenting instruction. Attend support group for parents with twins. Identify community

resources available for the family (pp. 18-20; Box 2-2; Table 2-1).

41. a. Occurs without any intervention; effective only when the consequences are meaningful; for example, forgetting ballet slippers results in the child's having to dance in stocking feet.

 b. Directly related to the rule; for example, child is not permitted to visit a friend's house for 1 day after coming home late from that friend's house.

 c. Those that are imposed deliberately; for example, no watching TV until homework is finished (p. 26).

42. Corporal punishment usually takes the form of spanking and causes a dramatic short-term decrease in the behavior. However, the flaws include the following:

 a. It teaches children that violence is acceptable.

 b. It may physically harm the child if it is the result of parental rage.

 c. Children become "accustomed" to spanking, requiring more severe corporal punishment over time.

 d. It can result in severe physical and psychological injury.

 e. It interferes with the parent-child interaction.

 f. When the parents are not around, the child is likely to misbehave, since the child has not learned to behave well for his or her own sake or what behavior is acceptable.

 g. It interferes with the child's development of moral reasoning (p. 26).

CHAPTER 3

1. c (p. 49), e (p. 48), a (p. 46), f (p. 46), g (p. 49), i (p. 54), k (p. 50), h (p. 45), p (p. 50), r (p. 50), b (p. 46), m (p. 48), t (p. 54), l (p. 47), n (p. 47), q (p. 47), v (p. 55), s (p. 48), o (p. 47), u (p. 47), d (p. 48), j (p. 49).
2. d (p. 53), f (p. 55), c (pp. 52, 66), a (pp. 48, 70), e (p. 53), b (p. 66)
3. d (p. 51)
4. c (pp. 54-55; Table 3-2; Figure 3-6)
5. a (p. 48; Box 3-1)
6. b, b, a, a, c, b, c, c, b, a, b, b, b, a, a, a, b, b (pp. 58-62; Table 3-4)
7. d (p. 47; Box 3-1; p. 68)
8. c (p. 68)
9. a (p. 75)
10. a (pp. 71-72, 79)
11. d (pp. 82-83; Box 3-8)
12. b (pp. 78-79)
13. c (pp. 78-79)
14. c, b, d, a (pp. 79, 80; Boxes 3-1 and 3-3)
15. d (p. 80)
16. a (pp. 82, 86-87)
17. d (p. 81)
18. a (p. 81)
19. b (p. 82)
20. c (p. 84)

21. d (p. 82; Box 3-7)
22. b (p. 84)
23. d (p. 86)
24. a (pp. 78-79, 82-83)
25. a (pp. 80-82)
26. a (pp. 80-82)
27. c (pp. 80-82)
28. d (p. 71)
29. d (pp. 71-72)
30. a (p. 74)

CHAPTER 4

1. d (p. 96), i (p. 116), g (p. 93), m (p. 116), o (p. 94), c (p. 93), b (p. 93), e (p. 103), k (p. 116), a (p. 91), h (p. 110), n (p. 99), l (p. 116), f (p. 92), j (p. 123)
2. c (pp. 91, 92)
3. b (p. 91)
4. b (p. 93)
5. d (pp. 92-94; Box 4-2)
6. d (p. 92; Box 4-1)
7. b (p. 93)
8. d (pp. 94, 95; Nursing Care Guidelines box)
9. F, T, T, T, F (p. 95; Figure 4-2; Nursing Care Guidelines box)
10. d (p. 94)
11. b, a, b, c, c, d (pp. 95, 96)
12. d (p. 97)
13. a. Storytelling
 b. "I" messages
 c. Bibliotherapy
 d. Drawing
 e. Directed play (pp. 98, 99; Box 4-3)
14. Identifying information, chief complaint, present illness, past history, review of systems, family medical history, psychosocial history, sexual history, family history, nutritional assessment (pp. 99, 100; Box 4-4)
15. b (pp. 99, 100)
16. c (p. 100)
17. a (pp. 100, 101; Box 4-4)
18. Approximate weight at 6 months, 1 year, 2 years, and 5 years of age; approximate length at 1 and 4 years; dentition, including age of onset, number of teeth, and symptoms during teething (p. 102)
19. Age of holding up head steadily; age of sitting alone without support; age of walking without assistance; age of saying first words with meaning; present grade in school; scholastic performance; whether the child has a best friend, and interaction with other children, peers, and adults (p. 102)
20. d (pp. 102, 103; Box 4-6)
21. Type, location, severity, duration, and influencing factors (pp. 100, 101; Nursing Care Guidelines box)
22. a (p. 104; Nursing Care Guidelines Box)
23. b (pp. 103, 104; Box 4-7)
24. Family composition, home and community environment, occupation and education of family members, cultural and religious traditions (p. 103)

25. c (pp. 106, 107; Box 4-8)
26. b (p. 110)
27. a (pp. 110-112; Nursing Care Guidelines box, Table 4-2)
28. d (p. 111, Nursing Care Guidelines box)
29. a (p. 112)
30. With the child in a supine position, fully extend the body by holding the head in midline position, grasping the knees together gently, and pushing down on the knees until the legs are fully extended and flat against the table. Using a length board, place the head firmly at the top of the board and the heels of the feet firmly against the footboard. (p. 113)
31. b (p. 108; Table 4-1)
32. b (pp. 116, 117)
33. Apical; 1 full minute; abdominal; 1 full minute (p. 118)
34. b (pp. 118-120, Table 4-3, Translating Evidence Into Practice box)
35. c (p. 117)
36. c (pp. 118, 121, 123; Table 4-4)
37. d (p. 123)
38. a (p. 124; Table 4-6), d (p. 124; Table 4-6), b (p. 124; Table 4-6), w (p. 145), c (p. 124; Table 4-6), d (p. 124; Table 4-6), e (p. 124; Table 4-6), f (p. 124; Table 4-6), k (p. 139), v (p. 145), l (p. 126), m (p. 126), i (p. 135), j (p. 135), g (p. 125), h (p. 124), p (p. 136), o (p. 145), n (p. 145), q (p. 138), r (p. 138), s (p. 139), u (p. 139), t (p. 139)
39. d (p. 124)
40. c (p. 125)
41. a (pp. 125, 126)
42. Pupils equal, round, react to light, and accommodation (p. 126)
43. d (p. 126), g (p. 127), c (p. 126), e (p. 127), b (p. 126), f (p. 127), i (p. 129), a (p. 126), h (p. 129)
44. b (pp. 126, 127, 128; Table 4-7)
45. a, b, c (pp. 128, 129; Table 4-7)
46. d (pp. 128, 129; Table 4-7)
47. d (pp. 130, 131)
48. d (pp. 131, 132)
49. a (pp. 134, 135)
50. a (pp. 135, 136)
51. b (p. 118; Box 4-9)
52. a (p. 138)
53. a (p. 140, Table 4-9)
54. b (p. 140)
55. d (p. 142)
56. c (p. 144)
57. Normal, abnormal, normal, normal, normal (p. 145)
58. Behavior, sensory testing, motor functioning, cerebellar functioning, reflexes, and cranial nerves (p. 146)
59. d (p. 149)
60. d (pp. 91, 93-96; Box 4-2)
61. a (pp. 99, 100)
62. c (pp. 105, 107; Box 4-9)
63. a (pp. 108, 109, 124, 134; Table 4-1)
64. d (pp. 104, 110; Box 4-7)
65. b (pp. 95, 96, 97, 112; Nursing Care Guidelines box; Table 4-2)

66. d (pp. 140-142)
67. d (p. 140)
68. c (pp. 91, 93, 94, 95)
69. b (p. 140)
70. S1, apex; S2, base (p. 139)
71. d (p. 139)

CHAPTER 5

1. Pain assessment, administration of analgesics at subtherapeutic levels, prolonged intervals in between medications, and lack of systematic monitoring and evaluation of relief (p. 152)
2. b (p. 152)
3. d (p. 152)
4. b (pp. 152, 153; Box 5-1)
5. c (p. 153; Box 5-1)
6. a (pp. 153, 154; Table 5-1)
7. b (pp. 153, 154; Table 5-1)
8. d (pp. 154, 155; Table 5-2)
9. b (pp. 154, 155; Table 5-2)
10. a (pp. 154, 156; Table 5-2)
11. b (pp. 156, 157; Figure 5-3)
12. b (p. 157)
13. c (pp. 157, 158)
14. C: crying; R: requiring increased oxygen; I: increased vital signs: E: expression; S: sleeplessness (p. 159)
15. c (pp. 160, 161, 162: Figure 5-4)
16. a (p. 163)
17. d (p. 163)
18. Possible answers: Distraction, relaxation, guided imagery, positive self-talk, thought stopping, cutaneous stimulation, behavioral contracting (pp. 164, 165; Applying Evidence to Practice)
19. c (pp. 164, 165; Figure 5-5; Research Focus)
20. b (p. 158; Box 5-2)
21. b (p. 169; Applying Evidence to Practice)
22. biologically based, manipulation treatments, energy based, mind-body techniques, alterative medical systems (p. 170)
23. c (p. 171)
24. d (p. 171)
25. d (p. 171)
26. b (p. 175)
27. a (p. 175)
28. (1) Patient-administered boluses—can be infused according to the preset amount and lockout interval; (2) nurse-administered boluses—usually give an initial loading dose; (3) continuous basal infusion—delivers a constant amount of analgesic and is used when patient cannot control the infusion (pp. 176, 177; Box 5-3)
29. d (p. 176)
30. c (pp. 178, 179)
31. b (p. 179)
32. c (p. 177; Box 5-3)
33. a (pp. 177, 179; Box 5-3)
34. d (p. 180; Applying Evidence to Practice)

35. b (p. 176)
36. d (pp. 179, 180; Box 5-4)
37. c (p. 181)
38. b (p, 180; Community and Home Health Considerations box)
39. The effects of pain on the neonate and the lack of knowledge of immediate and long-term consequences of untreated pain (p. 183)
40. b (p. 184; Box 5-6)
41. d (p. 185)
42. a (p. 186)
43. Possible answers: Teaching patients self-control skills such as biofeedback and relaxation; modifying behavior patterns or techniques (p. 186)
44. c (pp. 186, 187)
45. c (p. 187)
46. T, F, T, T, F, T, T (pp. 187-189)
47. Need to acquire an understanding of the antecedents and consequences of headache pain. Explore with Beverly the fact that the headaches always occur in her first-period math class. Ask her to keep a headache diary in which she records the time of onset, activities before the onset, any worries or concerns as far back as 24 hours before the onset, severity and duration of the pain, pain medication taken and its effect, and activity pattern during headache episodes (p. 186).
48. Teach Beverly biofeedback techniques, relaxation training, and how to activate positive thoughts and engage in adaptive behavior appropriate to the situation (p. 186).
   Teach parents to focus attention on adaptive coping and maintenance of normal activity patterns (p. 186).
49. a (p. 189)
50. b (p. 189)

CHAPTER 6

1. f (p. 193), c (p. 193), a (p. 193), d (p. 194), e (p. 194), b (p. 193), h (p. 193), g (p. 193), i (p. 194), j (p. 194)
2. d (p. 193)
3. a (p. 195)
4. d (p. 193)
5. d (p. 195)
6. n, l, k, m, j, a, b, c, d, f, e, g, i, h (p. 196; Box 6-2)
7. c (p. 196)
8. b (p. 201)
9. b (p. 201)
10. d (pp. 198, 201; Figure 6-2)
11. a (pp. 201, 202)
12. b (pp. 201, 202)
13. c (p. 202)
14. d (p. 202)
15. b (p. 203)
16. a (p. 203)
17. a (pp. 197, 203; Figure 6-2)
18. c (p. 211)
19. b (p. 211)
20. d (pp. 211, 212)
21. a (p. 212)
22. a (p. 212)
23. c (p. 213)
24. a (p. 214; Atraumatic Care)
25. contraindication; precaution (p. 214)
26. d (pp. 215, 216)
27. Day, month, and year of administration of the vaccine; name of the vaccine given and the manufacturer of the vaccine with lot number of each vaccine; name and title of the person administering the vaccine and the location (address) where the vaccine was given; site and route of administration for each vaccine; evidence that the parent or legal guardian gave informed consent before the immunization was administered; VIS (vaccine information sheet) was given for each vaccine before it was administered and the publication date of the VIS. (p. 216)
28. c, a, b, d, g, f, e, h, j, i (p. 205; all taken from Table 6-2)
29. a (pp. 218, 219)
30. d (p. 218)
31. d (p. 219)
32. Varicella (chickenpox) and zoster (herpes zoster or shingles) (p. 219)
33. b (p. 220)
34. b (p. 220)
35. a (p. 220)
36. c (p. 220)
37. c (pp. 204, 220; Table 6-2)
38. a (p. 221)
39. d (p. 221)
40. T, T, T, T, F, F, F, T, F (p. 222)
41. c (p. 225; Box 6-4)
42. a (p. 223)
43. d (p. 226)
44. a (pp. 225, 226; Box 6-5)
45. c (p. 228)
46. a (pp. 228, 230; Table 6-6)
47. c (p. 231)
48. d (pp. 232, 233)
49. a. Observation of the white eggs (nits) firmly attached to the hair shafts that do not dislodge easily when removal is attempted; scratch marks and/or inflammatory papules caused by secondary infection may be found on the scalp (p. 234)
   b. Children with head lice are allowed to return to school after proper treatment. School "no nit" policy is discouraged.
   c. Permethrin 1% cream rinse (Nix)
50. a (pp. 234, 235)
51. b (p. 256)
52. e (p. 238; Table 6-8), d (p. 238; Table 6-8), f (p. 238; Table 6-8), a (p. 232; Table 6-7), c (p. 238; Table 6-8), b (p. 232; Table 6-7)
53. a (pp. 237, 238)
54. d (p. 239)
55. b (p. 239)
56. a (p. 239)

57. Possible answers include: explanation that MRSA is easily spread by self-inoculation and direct contact with the sores; the need to avoid touching the sores, scratching the sores or picking at the sores; the need for frequent hand washing especially after contact with the sores; the need to keep from reusing articles—clothes, towel, facecloths, etc—that have been exposed to MRSA until they are washed in hot water; the need to dispose of razors used for shaving; also could recommend using mupirocin in the nares for 1-2 weeks to prevent reinfection and could suggest bathing in a chlorine bath 1-2 times weekly (2.5 ml of bleach diluted with 13 gallons of water, and a 5-minute soak) (p. 226)
58. a (p. 221; Box 6-3)
59. b (pp. 218, 221)
60. b (pp. 218, 219, 221)
61. a (p. 221)
62. b (p. 221)
63. a (p. 221)

CHAPTER 7

1. Low oxygen, high carbon dioxide, low pH (p. 243)
2. The sudden chilling of the infant on entering a cooler environment from the warmer environment (p. 243)
3. c (p. 243)
4. b (p. 243)
5. a (p. 244)
6. T, F, T, F, T, F, F, T, F, F, T (pp. 244, 245, 246)
7. Rate of fluid exchange is seven times greater in infant; infant's rate of metabolism is twice as great in relation to body weight; infant's immature kidneys cannot sufficiently concentrate urine to conserve body water (p. 244).
8. b, a, c (p. 245; Box 7-1)
9. Maternal circulation; breast milk (p. 246)
10. d (p. 246)
11. a. 8 inches
    b. Yellow, green, pink, geometric shapes, checkerboards
    c. Low, high
    d. 20/100 and 20/400 (p. 246)
12. c (p. 247)
13. a, b, c (pp. 247, 248)
14. b (p. 248; Box 7-2)
15. a (p. 251)
16. c (pp. 253, 254; Table 7-3)
17. b (pp. 258, 259)
18. m (p. 255; Table 7-3), g (p. 255; Table 7-3), a (p. 254; Table 7-3), c (p. 254; Table 7-3), i (p. 255; Table 7-3), b (p. 254; Table 7-3), d (p. 255; Table 7-3), j (p. 255; Table 7-3), e (p. 254; Table 7-3), h (p. 255), f (p. 254; Table 7-3), l (p. 261), k (p. 261)
19. b (p. 253)
20. a (p. 259)
21. d (pp. 261, 262; Figure 7-8)
22. a (pp. 247, 248, 250, 253)
23. d (pp. 255, 266; Table 7-3)

24. a. Making a sharp, loud noise close to the infant's head should produce a startle reflex or other reaction, such as twitching of the eyelids (p. 262).
    b. Conduct auditory brainstem response or evoked otoacoustic emissions testing before discharge from the hospital (p. 270).
25. Obligatory nose breathers and are unable to breathe orally (p. 262)
26. c (pp. 255, 263; Table 7-3)
27. h (p. 263), c (p. 263; Table 7-4), d (p. 263; Table 7-4), e (p. 263; Table 7-4), a (pp. 257, 266), g (p. 263; Table 7-4), b (p. 263), f (p. 263)
28. c (p. 268)
29. a. Radiation
    b. Conduction
    c. Convection
    d. Evaporation (pp. 267, 268)
30. d (p. 267)
31. a. Silver nitrate, erythromycin, or tetracycline ophthalmic drops or ointment (p. 268)
    b. Vitamin K (p. 269)
    c. Hepatitis B vaccine (p. 269)
32. a (p. 269)
33. a (pp. 271, 272)
34. That current evidence indicates the health benefits of newborn male circumcision outweigh the risks, and that the procedure should be made available to families who choose it. Despite encouraging outcome data, the medical benefits of male newborn circumcision are not sufficient to recommend it as a routine procedure. The policy stresses the need for parents to determine what is best for their child after they have been given accurate and unbiased information about the risks and benefits and alternatives to this elective procedure. It also advised that procedural analgesic be given to the infant during circumcision. (p. 272).
35. d (pp. 275, 276; Box 7-5)
36. a (p. 275)
37. c (p. 277)
38. All statements are true (pp. 277, 279, 280; Nursing Alert on p. 279).
39. d (p. 281; Table 7-6)
40. d (pp. 283-285)
41. Prefeeding behavior such as crying; Approach behavior such as sucking movements; Attachment behavior such as activities that occur from the time the infant receives the nipple and sucks; Consummatory behavior such as coordinated sucking and swallowing; Satiety behavior lets the parent know that they are satisfied, usually falling asleep (p. 282)
42. c (p. 247; Table 7-1)
43. Posture—full flexion of the arms and legs; square window—full flexion, hand lies flat on ventral surface of forearm; arm recoil—quick return to full flexion after arms released from full extension; popliteal angle—less angle/degree behind knee, less than 90 degrees; scarf sign—elbow does not reach midline with infant's

arm pulled across the shoulder so that infant's hand touches shoulder; heel to ear—knees flexed with a popliteal angle of less than 10 degrees when the infant's foot is pulled as far as possible up toward ear (pp. 250, 251; Figure 7-1)

44. a (pp. 247, 248)
45. Infant will maintain a patent airway. Infant will maintain a stable body temperature. Infant will experience no infection or injury. Infant will receive optimum nutrition (pp. 267, 268, 274).
46. c (p. 279)
47. c (pp. 277-279, 282; Box 7-5)
48. a. Wet diapers: minimum of one for each day of life (day 2 = 2 wets; day 3 = 3 wets) until fifth or sixth day, at which time 5 or 6 per day to 14 days, then 6 to 10 per day
    b. Stools: at least two or three per day with breastfeeding
    c. Activity: has four or five wakeful periods per day; alerts to environmental sounds and voices
    d. Cord: keep above diaper line, nonodorous, drying
    e. Position for sleep: on back
    f. Safe transport home from hospital: use a federally approved infant care safety seat restraint, which should be a rear-facing safety seat with infant placed in the back seat; rolled blankets and towels may be needed between the crotch and legs to prevent slouching and can be placed along the sides to minimize lateral movement but should never be placed underneath or behind the infant (p. 288; Community and Home Health Consideration box)
49. d (p. 262)
50. Adherent patches on the tongue and/or palate that cannot be wiped off may indicate an abnormal condition called thrush (candidiasis). If the patches can be wiped off, it is a normal finding, probably from the milk (pp. 256, 263; Table 7-3).
51. a. Wash hands before working with each infant and between infants (p. 268).
    b. Use Standard Precautions of wearing gloves when handling infant until the blood and amniotic fluid are removed by bathing (p. 271).

CHAPTER 8

1. d (p. 311), m (p. 295; Box 8-2), g (p. 318), o (p. 331), a (p. 294), h (p. 322), l (p. 311), c (p. 312), p (p. 302), i (p. 307), b (p. 297), k (p. 312), j (p. 322), f (p. 323), n (p. 300), e (p. 313)
2. c (p. 294)
3. c (pp. 294, 295; Box 8-2)
4. d (p. 294)
5. c, b, a (pp. 295, 296; Figure 18-1)
6. a (p. 297)
7. b, a, a, c, b, a, c, a (pp. 297-299)
8. 2 months, 18 months, 12 years or older (p. 299)
9. F, T, T, F, T, T (p. 299)
10. c (p. 301)
11. a (p. 301)

12. d (pp. 301, 302)
13. c (p. 303)
14. Additional surgeries can be necessary; speech impairments that require speech therapy; improper drainage from the middle ear, resulting in recurrent otitis media, which can lead to hearing impairment and insertion of pressure equalizer tubes for prevention; extensive malposition of teeth and maxillary arches, requiring extensive orthodontics and dental prosthesis (pp. 304, 305)
15. c (pp. 305, 306)
16. d (pp. 306-308; Nursing Care Plan)
17. b (p. 307)
18. c (pp. 306, 309; Nursing Care Plan)
19. c (p. 307)
20. T, T, F, T, T, F, F, F, F (p. 310)
21. c (pp. 310, 311)
22. d (p. 311)
23. a. Port-wine stains (p. 312)
    b. Infantile hemangiomas (p. 312)
    c. Café-au-lait spots (p. 311)
    d. Cavernous venous hemangiomas (p. 312)
24. d (pp. 312, 313)
25. Hyperbilirubinemia, jaundice (p. 313)
26. Heme, globin, unconjugated bilirubin, conjugated bilirubin (p. 313)
27. c (p. 314)
28. a (p. 315
29. a (pp. 314, 315; Table 8-2)
30. c (pp. 315, 316)
31. a (p. 316)
32. b (pp. 315, 316)
33. a (pp. 316, 317)
34. Appearance of clinical jaundice within 24 hours of birth; Bilirubin level in the high-risk zone; Gestational age 35 to 36 weeks; Exclusive breastfeeding; Maternal race (e.g., Asian or Asian American), Significant bruising or cephalhematoma; Blood group incompatibility with a positive direct Coombs test; Hereditary hemolytic disease; Sibling with prior case of jaundice (p. 316)
35. d (pp. 318, 319)
36. b (pp. 319, 320)
37. a (pp. 318, 319)
38. a. Rh incompatibility (p. 333)
    b. Rh negative, Rh positive, O, A, B (p. 333)
    c. Indirect Coombs, direct Coombs (p. 325)
    d. 72 hours, 26 to 28, intramuscular (p. 325)
    e. Isoimmunization (p. 323)
39. Keeps the infant NPO during the procedure with a peripheral infusion of dextrose and electrolytes being established; Keeps documentation of blood volumes exchanged, the amount of blood withdrawn and infused, the time of each procedure, and the cumulative record of the total volume exchanged; vital signs monitored (usually electronically during the procedure) and evaluated frequently and correlated with the removal and infusion of blood; observation for signs of transfusion reaction, maintenance of adequate neonatal

thermoregulation, blood glucose levels, and fluid balance (p. 326)
40. a (p. 327)
41. c (p. 328)
42. b (pp. 328, 329)
43. a (pp. 327, 328)
44. c (p. 329)
45. 125 mg/dl, 150 mg/dl (p. 329)
46. d (p. 329)
47. b (p. 330)
48. d (pp. 330, 331)
49. Administer 0.5 to 1 mg into the vastus lateralis muscle or ventrogluteal muscle during the first 24 hours of life (p. 331).
50. d (p. 331)
51. c (pp. 313, 314, 315, 316; Table 8-2)
52. a (pp. 313, 314, 319; Table 8-2)
53. c (pp. 319, 320, 321; Nursing Care Plan)
54. d (p. 320)
55. d (pp. 320, 321)
56. Time phototherapy was started and stopped, proper shielding of eyes, type of fluorescent lamp by manufacturer, number of lamps, distance between lamp and infant (no less than 18 inches), used in combination with incubator or open bassinet, photometer measurement of light intensity, and occurrence of side effects (p. 320)
57. There is often an increase in the serum bilirubin level called "rebound effect"; this often resolves without resuming therapy (p. 322).
58. Teach to evaluate the number of voids and evidence of adequate breastfeeding; teach to bring infant to health care practitioner if indications of hyperbilirubinemia occur and for follow-up visit in 2 or 3 days for evaluation of feeding and elimination patterns (p. 322).

CHAPTER 9

1. a. Low-birth-weight infant (p. 338; Box 9-1)
   b. Extremely low-birth-weight infant (p. 338; Box 9-1)
   c. Small-for-gestational-age infant (p. 338; Box 9-1)
   d. Large-for-gestational-age infant (p. 338; Box 9-1)
   e. Preterm (premature) infant (p. 338; Box 9-1)
   f. Full-term infant (p. 338; Box 9-1)
   g. Postterm (postmature) infant (p. 338; Box 9-1)
   h. Fetal death (p. 338; Box 9-1)
   i. Neonatal death (p. 338; Box 9-1)
   j. Perinatal mortality (p. 338; Box 9-1)
   k. Late-preterm infant (p. 338; Box 9-1)
2. d (pp. 336, 338; Box 9-1)
3. c (pp. 337, 338)
4. c (p. 339)
5. Feeding behavior, activity, color, oxygen saturation (SpO_2), vital signs (p. 339)
6. a (p. 339)
7. T (p. 339), F (p. 339), F (p. 339), T (p. 340), T (p. 340), F (p. 341), F (p. 341)
8. Infant will exhibit adequate oxygenation; infant will maintain stable body temperature (p. 341).

9. Nonshivering thermogenesis (p. 341)
10. a (p. 341)
11. Hypoxia, metabolic acidosis, hypoglycemia (p. 342)
12. a (p. 342), b (p. 342), d (p. 343), c (p. 342), f (p. 343), e (p. 343)
13. b (p. 343)
14. Describe shape of chest (barrel, concave), symmetry, presence of incisions, chest tubes, or other deviation. Describe use of accessory muscles: nasal flaring or substernal, intercostal, or subclavicular retractions. Determine respiratory rate and regularity. Auscultate and describe breath sounds: stridor, crackles, wheezing, diminished sounds, areas of absence of sound, grunting, diminished air entry, equality of breath sounds. Determine whether suctioning is needed. Describe ambient oxygen and method of delivery; if intubated, describe size of tube, type of ventilator and settings, and method of securing tube. Determine oxygen saturation by pulse oximetry (p. 340; Nursing Care Guidelines box).
15. a (p. 322)
16. a. Peripheral veins on the dorsal surfaces of the hands or feet (p. 343)
    b. Redness, edema, or color change at site; blanching at site (p. 344)
17. b (p. 344)
18. c (p. 324)
19. T (p. 345), F (p. 346), F (p. 347), T (p. 346), F (p. 346), T (p. 346), T (p. 346), T (p. 346), F (p. 346), F (p. 346), F (p. 345), T (p. 345), T (p. 346)
20. a (pp. 347, 348)
21. b (p. 349; Box 9-3)
22. d (p. 347)
23. c (p. 347)
24. Nonnutritive sucking (p. 347)
25. d (p. 351)
26. d (pp. 351, 352; Applying Evidence to Practice box)
27. a. Benzyl alcohol (p. 352), b. Hyperosmolar (p. 352)
28. T (p. 353), T (p. 354), F (p. 355), T (p. 355), F (p. 355), T (p. 356), F (p. 356), T (p. 356), T (p. 358), T (p. 357), F (p. 358), T (p. 358)
29. Supine (p. 357)
30. a (pp. 359, 360)
31. a. Vulnerable child syndrome (p. 363), b. Anticipatory grief (p. 359)
32. a (p. 362)
33. c (pp. 363, 364)
34. b (p. 365)
35. d (pp. 366, 367)
36. d (p. 367)
37. c (p. 368)
38. b (p. 367)
39. a (p. 371)
40. Deficient surfactant production causes unequal inflation of alveoli on inspiration and the collapse of alveoli on end expiration; infants are unable to keep their lungs inflated and therefore exert a great deal of effort to reexpand the alveoli with each breath (pp. 369, 370).

41. c (p. 374, Table 9-7), j (p. 372), d (p. 374, Table 9-7), a (p. 370), e (p. 374, Table 9-7), b (p. 370), g (p. 371, Figure 9-14), f (p. 371, Figure 9-14), h (p. 374, Table 9-7), i (p, 375)
42. c (pp. 372, 373)
43. a (p. 376)
44. b (pp. 376, 377)
45. d (pp. 378, 379)
46. c (p. 380)
47. a (p. 382)
48. Because of the infant's poor response to pathogenic agents, there is often no local inflammatory response at the portal of entry to indicate an infection (p. 383).
49. d (p. 385)
50. d (p. 386)
51. c (p. 387)
52. b (p. 388)
53. a (p. 388)
54. Hematocrit of 65% or greater; the small-for-gestational-age infant (p. 388)
55. a (p. 389)
56. Infant may be stuporous or comatose; seizures may begin after 6 to 12 hours and become more frequent and severe. Between 24 and 72 hours, deterioration in the level of consciousness may occur. After 72 hours, stupor and disturbances of sucking and swallowing are seen. Muscular weakness of the hips and shoulders in the full-term infant and lower limb weakness in the preterm infant occur. Apneic episodes may occur (p. 390).
57. d (p. 392)
58. c (p. 392)
59. c (pp. 392, 393)
60. c (p. 393)
61. b (p. 395)
62. c (p. 396)
63. d (p. 397)
64. F (p. 398), T (p. 398), F (p. 398), T (p. 398), T (p. 398), F (p. 398), T (p. 399), T (p. 399), T (p. 400), F (p. 400), T (p. 400), T (p. 400), T (p. 400)
65. d (p. 400; Box 10-13)
66. d (pp. 401, 402)
67. Toxoplasmosis; Other agents such as hepatitis B, parvovirus, human immunodeficiency virus; Rubella; Cytomegalovirus infection; Herpes simplex; Syphilis (p. 402)
68. Transplacental, during vaginal delivery, or in breast milk (p. 403, Table 9-10)
69. c (p. 338; Box 9-1)
70. b (pp. 338, 339, 341)
71. b (pp. 373, 375, 376)
72. c (pp. 359-361)
73. a (pp. 341, 373, 377)
74. Number of apneic spells; the appearance of the infant during and after attacks, whether the infant self-recovers or whether tactile stimulation is needed to restore breathing (p. 368)
75. Strong, vigorous suck; coordination of sucking and swallowing; a gag reflex; sucking on the gavage tube, hands, or pacifier; rooting and wakefulness before and sleeping after feedings (p. 348)
76. The nurse should use therapeutic positioning to reduce the potential for acquired positional deformities and to accommodate necessary medical equipment and medical needs (p. 357).

CHAPTER 10

1. l (p. 423), a (p. 420), s (p. 441), c (p. 421), b (p. 420), e (p. 422), i (p. 422), d (p. 421), g (p. 422), f (p. 422), k (p. 423), h (p. 422), j (p. 423), p (p. 422), m (p. 423), r (p. 427), n (p. 427), o (p. 23), q (p. 425)
2. c (p. 413)
3. b (p. 413)
4. a (p. 413)
5. b (p. 426)
6. c (p. 414)
7. b (p. 415)
8. a (p. 426)
9. a (p. 416)
10. d (p. 416)
11. c (p. 416)
12. a (p. 416)
13. a (p. 416)
14. b (p. 416)
15. a (p. 417)
16. d (p. 417)
17. 4, 8 months (p. 425)
18. c (p. 417)
19. b (p. 417)
20. a (p. 419)
21. a (p. 420)
22. b (p. 422)
23. c (p. 424)
24. b (p. 431)
25. c (p. 425)
26. c (pp. 427-428)
27. c (p. 434)
28. c (p. 435)
29. c (p. 437)
30. a (p. 441)
31. d (p. 438)
32. d (p. 439)
33. c (p. 441)
34. d (p. 440)
35. b (p. 440)
36. a (p. 446)
37. b (p. 434)
38. Suffocation, motor vehicle–related deaths, and drowning (p. 442)
39. Bottle propping, giving milk bottle in bed, and giving juice in a bottle (p. 442).
40. a. True (p. 440)
    b. False (p. 439)
    c. False (p. 442)
    d. True (p. 440)
41. The following should be checked: Nutrition, sleep and activity, number and condition of teeth, immunization

status, and safety precautions used in the home. (p. 449)

42. c (p. 447-449)
43. b (p. 447-449)

CHAPTER 11

1. a (p. 468), g (p. 458), f (p. 454), i (p. 457), h (p. 462), j (p. 458), b (p. 462), k (p. 458), d (p. 458), c (p. 462), e (p. 462)
2. a. Children who are exclusively breastfed by mothers with an inadequate intake of vitamin D or are exclusively breastfed longer than 6 months without adequate maternal vitamin D intake or supplementation
   b. Children with dark skin pigmentation who are exposed to minimal sunlight because of socioeconomic, religious, or cultural beliefs or housing in urban areas with high levels of pollution, or who live above or below a latitude of 33 degrees north and south where sunlight does not produce vitamin A
   c. Children with diets that are low in sources of vitamin D and calcium
   d. Individuals who use milk products not supplemented with vitamin D (e.g., yogurt, raw cow's milk) as the primary source of milk
3. b (p. 453)
4. c (p. 453)
5. b (p. 454)
6. Cow's milk (whole) (p. 454)
7. c (p. 453)
8. World Health Organization (p. 454)
9. a (p. 454)
10. b (p. 455)
11. d (p. 455)
12. c (p. 456)
13. c (p. 456)
14. d (p. 458)
15. d (p. 460)
16. c (p. 461)
17. c (p. 461)
18. b (p. 461)
19. a (p. 462)
20. c (p. 462)
21. b (p. 462)
22. a (p. 471)
23. e (p. 471)
24. a (p. 463)
25. Possible responses: multifactorial and involves a combination of possible infant organic disease, dysfunctional parenting behaviors, subtle neurologic or behavioral problems, disturbed parent-child interactions, inadequate caloric intake, poverty (p. 463)
26. d (p. 463)
27. a (p. 463)
28. c (p. 464)
29. c (p. 465)

30. Moisture (wetness); increased pH; and fecal irritants (p. 466)
31. d (p. 467)
32. a (p. 468)
33. Hydrate the skin; relieve pruritus; prevent secondary infections; prevent or minimize flare-ups or inflammation (p. 469)
34. False (p. 476)
    True (p. 475)
    False (p. 475)
    False (p. 475)
    True (p. 476)
35. d (p. 479)
36. Maternal smoking during pregnancy; maternal alcohol use during pregnancy; cosleeping with an adult or child; soft bedding; prone or side sleeping position; blankets or other items in infant's sleeping bed (pp. 476-477)
37. Low Apgar scores at birth; low birthweight or preterm (<37 weeks' gestation); African American or Native American ethnicity (p. 477); recent viral illness; sibling of >2 SIDS sibs; male infant (pp. 475-476)
38. e (p. 481)
39. b (p. 479)
40. Reassure parents they are not doing anything wrong and that the infant is not experiencing any physical harm (provided that medical problems have been ruled out); help the parents understand the nature of infant crying and finding an appropriate for parents to deal with crying; encourage support from other community and family resources during crying times (p. 472).
41. a (pp. 472-474)
42. d (pp. 454-482)
43. a (pp. 457-461)
44. c (pp. 459-460)
45. b

CHAPTER 12

1. j (p. 492), g (p. 491), f (p. 490), d (p. 491), b (p. 491), m (p. 492), i (p. 493), n (p. 493), l (p. 493), k (p. 495), h (p. 495), e (p. 497), c (p. 502), o (p. 493), a (p. 504), p (p. 493)
2. 12-36 (p. 488)
3. b (p. 490)
4. a (p. 489)
5. b (p. 489)
6. c (p. 490)
7. c (p. 490)
8. a (p. 493)
9. a (p. 493)
10. d (p. 494)
11. c (p. 495)
12. b (p. 495)
13. c (p. 496)
14. a (p. 497)
15. a (p. 497)
16. Physical characteristics—Voluntary control of anal and urethral sphincters; ability to stay dry for 2 hours;

regular bowel movements; gross motor skills of sitting, walking, and squatting; fine motor skills to remove clothing

Mental characteristics—Recognizes urge to defecate or urinate; communicative skills to indicate needs; cognitive skills to imitate behavior and follow directions

Psychologic characteristics—Expresses willingness to please parent; able to sit for 5 to 10 minutes; demonstrates curiosity about toilet habits; impatient with soiled or wet diapers (pp. 500-501)

17. a (p. 502)
18. a (p. 500)
19. c (p. 502)
20. consistency (p. 503)
21. d (p. 503)
22. c (p. 504)
23. d (p. 504)
24. d (p. 504)
25. b (p. 504)
26. c (p. 504)
27. d (p. 505)
28. b (p. 505)
29. c (p. 505)
30. c (p. 506)
31. physiologic anorexia (p. 505)
32. Toddlers like to have the same plate, spoon or fork, cup, and food to eat at almost every meal. If some of these change the toddler may refuse to eat. Some believe it is a part of gaining autonomy or control (p. 505)
33. 3 tbsp. (p. 506)
34. milk; 24-28 oz. (p. 506)
35. a (p. 507)
36. b (p. 508)
37. a (p. 508)
38. a (p. 508)
39. d (p. 510)
40. c (p. 511)
41. b (p. 511)
42. d (p. 512)
43. Motor vehicle (p. 512)
44. b (p. 513)
45. 65 (p. 515)
46. b (p. 515)
47. b (p. 516)
48. b (p. 517)
49. Foods: Hot dogs, nuts, dried beans, pits from fruit, bones, gum
Play objects: Anything with small parts
Household objects: Drawstring jackets or hoods, thumbtacks, nails, screws, coins, jewelry, old refrigerators, storage chests
Electric: Outlets, garage doors, car windows (pp. 582-583)
50. Possible answers: Psychosocial development, achievement of major fine and gross motor skills, language, nutrition, sleep and activity, dental health, injury prevention (pp. 490, 509, 510, 512-519)

51. d (pp. 495-498)
52. Discuss the signs that signal Dora's readiness to toilet train. Also explore Ms. Jackson's ideas about when it is appropriate to toilet train a child (determines the method used). Discuss the common methods and explain that Dora may become toilet trained before the new baby arrives but may regress with the arrival of the new baby. (pp. 500-503)
53. Discuss toddler's eating habits, including picky eating and the need for fewer calories during this period. Obtain a weight and plot Dora's growth on an appropriate reference chart and discuss results with Ms. Jackson. Identify Ms. Jackson's knowledge about child nutrition and discuss some points on providing nutritious snacks for Dora to eat. (pp. 504-506)

CHAPTER 13

1. 3, 5 (p. 523)
2. 2-3 kg or 4.5 to 6.5 lb (p. 523)
3. b (p. 523)
4. 5 (p. 523)
5. initiative, guilt (pp. 524-525)
6. d (p. 524)
7. a (p. 525)
8. b (p. 525)
9. c (p. 526)
10. d (p. 526)
11. c (p. 527)
12. c (p. 527)
13. 2100 (p. 527)
14. a (p. 527)
15. c (p. 527)
16. d (pp. 527-528)
17. b (p. 531)
18. Present ideas as exciting; talk to the child about activities he or she will be involved with; behave confidently on the first day (p. 532)
19. Become friends in time of loneliness; they accomplish what the child is still attempting; they experience what the child wants to forget or remember; can be blamed for any wrongdoings (p. 531)
20. b (p. 532)
21. a (pp. 533-534)
22. c (p. 534)
23. d (p. 535)
24. b (p. 536)
25. c (p. 537)
26. Child ascribes lifelike qualities to inanimate objects (pp. 536-537)
27. Fear of loss of body parts, fear of the dark, fear of being left alone, ghosts, castration, painful interventions (p. 537)
28. b (p. 537)
29. d (pp. 539-540)
30. b (p. 538)
31. c (p. 539)
32. a (pp. 532-533)
33. c (pp. 532-533)

34. b (pp. 532-533)
35. d (pp. 532-533)

CHAPTER 14

1. c (p. 543)
2. daytime tiredness; behavior changes; hyperactivity; difficulty concentrating; impaired learning ability; poor control of emotions and impulses; strain on family relationships (p. 543)
3. d (pp. 543, 544)
4. a, b, b, a, a, b, b (p. 544; Table 14-1)
5. d (pp. 544, 545)
6. b (p. 545)
7. c (p. 545)
8. a (p. 548)
9. Assess the victim; terminate exposure to the poison; identify the poison; call poison control center for immediate advice (p. 548; Emergency Treatment box)
10. b (p. 548)
11. a (p. 550; Family-Centered Care box)
12. b (p. 549)
13. c (p. 548)
14. Lead; mercury; iron (p. 550)
15. c (p. 551; Nursing Alert box)
16. c (pp. 551, 552; Box 14-3)
17. T (p. 552), T (p. 552), T (p. 551), F (p. 551), T (p. 553), F (p. 552), T (p. 553), T (p. 554), T (p. 551), T (p. 551), F (p. 551), F (p. 552), T (p. 552)
18. b (p. 555)
19. a (pp. 553, 554; Table 14-2)
20. d (p. 554; Table 14-2)
21. a (p. 555)
22. d (p. 557), g (p. 557), i (p. 556), c (p. 557), b (p. 557), h (p. 555), a (p. 556), e (p. 557), f (p. 557)
23. a (p. 558)
24. b (p. 558)
25. a (p. 558)
26. e (p. 558), d (p. 559), a (p. 558), b (p. 558), c (p. 558)
27. F, T, T, F, F, F, T (p. 559)
28. c (p. 559)
29. d (pp. 560, 561; Nursing Alert box)
30. d (p. 559)
31. d (p. 560)
32. a (p. 561)
33. c (p. 563)
34. d (pp. 563, 564)
35. d (pp. 560-562; Box 14-6)
36. a (p. 561)
37. d (pp. 563, 565; Nursing Care Plan box)
38. a (pp. 560, 563, 566; Applying Evidence to Practice box)

CHAPTER 15

1. c (p. 569)
2. Begins with shedding of the first deciduous tooth; ends at puberty with the acquisition of final permanent teeth (with the exception of the wisdom teeth) (p. 569)

3. a (p. 569)
4. T (p. 570), F (p. 570), T (p. 570), F (p. 570), T (p. 570), F (p. 570), T (p. 569), F (p. 570), T (p. 570), T (p. 571),
5. b (p. 570)
6. b (p. 571)
7. d (p. 571)
8. d (p. 571)
9. a (pp. 572, 573)
10. c (p. 571)
11. d (pp. 570, 571)
12. a (pp. 571-573)
13. c (p. 572)
14. b (p. 573)
15. c (p. 572)
16. f (p. 573), g (p. 573), e (p. 573), c (p. 573), d (p. 573), b (p. 573), a (p. 573), h (p. 576), j (p. 573), i (p. 573)
17. c (p. 575)
18. b (p. 575)
19. b (p. 577)
20. d (p. 576)
21. d (p. 578)
22. c (p. 578; Community and Home Health Considerations box)
23. Their own self-assessment and what they interpret as the opinion of family members and outside social contacts (p. 579)
24. a (pp. 577, 578)
25. a (p. 580)
26. c (p. 579)
27. Children learn to subordinate personal goals to group goals. Children learn that division of labor is an effective strategy for the attainment of a goal. Children learn about the nature of competition and importance of winning. Children will work hard to develop skills needed to become members of a team, thus improving their social, intellectual, and skill growth (p. 582).
28. d (p. 582)
29. F (p. 583), T (p. 583), T (p. 583), T (p. 583), F (p. 583), T (p. 585), F (p. 585), T (p. 585), T (p. 585), F (p. 586)
30. c (p. 586)
31. To help the child interrupt or inhibit forbidden actions; to help child identify an acceptable form of behavior so that he or she can identify what is right in future situations; to provide understandable reasons as to why one action is appropriate and another action is not; to stimulate child's ability to empathize with the victim (p. 586)
32. a (p. 587)
33. b (p. 588)
34. b (p. 589)
35. Children in elementary school who are left to care for themselves without adult supervision before or after school (p. 589)
36. Hygiene, nutrition, exercise, recreation, sleep, safety (p. 591)
37. c (pp. 591, 592)
38. a (p. 593)

295

Answer Key

39. a (p. 593)
40. c (p. 594)
41. T (p. 593), F (p. 593), F (p. 593), F (p. 593), T (p. 593), T (p. 596), T (p. 597), T (p. 597), T (p. 594), T (p. 595), F (p. 595), F (p. 602), T (p. 602), F (p. 602), T (p. 603), T (p. 605), T (p. 605), T (p. 602)
42. Limit media time, monitor game selection and content, and increase access to games and information that are educational (p. 596)
43. Health appraisal, health promotion, emergency care and safety, communicable disease control, counseling and guidance, adjustment to individual student needs (p. 598; Box 15-7)
44. c (p. 600)
45. c (pp. 582, 591, 592, 594, 595; Family-Centered box, 602, 603)
46. a (pp. 569, 579, 584, 601; Table 15-2)
47. a (pp. 591, 592)
48. b (p. 579)
49. b (pp. 591, 592)
50. The bike should be sized to fit the child. The child should be able to stand with the balls of both feet on the ground when seated on the bike, to place both feet flat on the ground when straddling the center bar, and to grasp the brake lever easily and comfortably. The helmet should be hard shelled and lined with Styrofoam; it should be adjusted to the child's head and fit securely without limiting the child's vision or hearing; it should be brightly colored for better visibility and carry the U.S. Consumer Product Safety Commission seal (p. 603).

CHAPTER 16

1. d (p. 609)
2. Contact with injurious agents to the skin as a toxic chemical, physical trauma, allergens or infectious organism; hereditary factors; systemic disease where the lesions are a cutaneous manifestation (p. 609)
3. c, b, e, a, d (p. 610)
4. j (p. 610), f (p. 610), h (p. 610), a (p. 610), b (p. 610), d (p. 610), c (p. 610), e (p. 610), i (p. 610), g (p. 610), k (p. 611)
5. d (p. 615; Nursing Alert)
6. c (p. 611)
7. b (p. 612)
8. c (p. 611)
9. a (p. 612)
10. c (p. 612)
11. b (pp. 612, 616)
12. d (pp. 613-615; Nursing Alert box)
13. a (p. 615)
14. b (pp. 613, 614)
15. c (p. 615)
16. Increased erythema, especially beyond the wound margin; edema; purulent exudate; odor; pain; increased temperature (p. 615; Nursing Alert box)
17. d (p. 616)
18. b (p. 618)

19. d (p. 620)
20. c (p. 620)
21. a (p. 621)
22. c (p. 621)
23. d (p. 621), c (p. 621), h (p. 618), f (p. 620), e (p. 620), b (p. 622), a (p. 622), g (p. 622)
24. b (p. 622)
25. d (p. 623)
26. 7 days; almost immediately; penicillin and sulfonamides (p. 623)
27. c (p. 624)
28. b (pp. 624, 626; Table 16-4)
29. b (pp. 625-627; Box 16-1; Table 16-4)
30. c (p. 625)
31. c (p. 624)
32. a (p. 626; Table 16-4)
33. b (pp. 627, 628; Table 16-5)
34. a (p. 629; Table 16-5)
35. d (p. 627)
36. b (p. 629)
37. a (pp. 629, 630; Table 16-5)
38. b (p. 630)
39. b (p. 630)
40. c (p. 631; Nursing Alert box)
41. d (p. 631)
42. b (pp. 631, 632, 633)
43. c (p. 633)
44. d (p. 633)
45. d (p. 634; Emergency Treatment box)
46. b (p. 637)
47. d (p. 638)
48. a (p. 640)
49. a, b, c (p. 641)
50. c (p. 642)
51. d (p. 642)
52. d (p. 644)
53. c (p. 644)
54. b (p. 645)
55. a (p. 646)
56. b (p. 647)
57. genetic characteristics, gestational and birth complications and winter birth (pp. 647, 648)
58. b (pp. 615, 616, 620)
59. c (p. 620)
60. a (pp. 616, 617, 619, 620)
61. d (pp. 616-620)
62. b (pp. 617, 619, 620)

CHAPTER 17

1. a (pp. 651, 652; Table 17-1)
2. d (p. 652)
3. a (p. 653)
4. h (p. 654), f (p. 651), d (p. 653), a (p. 654), i (p. 656), e (p. 655), j (p. 657), k (p. 657)b (p. 654), c (p. 654), g (p. 653)
5. c (p. 654)
6. b (pp. 655, 657; Figure 17-6)
7. a (pp. 653, 656)

8. b (p. 654; Figure 17-4)
9. d (p. 657; Figure 17-6)
10. b (p. 657)
11. c (p. 658)
12. d (pp. 659, 666, 668)
13. b (p. 659)
14. b (p. 659)
15. b (p. 660)
16. c (p. 660)
17. c (p. 660)
18. a (p. 661)
19. d (p. 661)
20. d (p. 663)
21. Realization of romantic or erotic attractions; erotic daydreaming; romantic partners or dates without sexual activity; sexual activity with others; self-identification of the orientation that best fits one's current circumstances and understanding; publicly self-identifying sexual orientation; intimate committed sexual relationship (p. 664)
22. b (p. 664)
23. a (p. 665)
24. d (p. 665)
25. Authoritative parenting is characterized by parental expectations of mature behavior on the part of the adolescent and setting and enforcing reasonable limits for behavior; this type of parenting is related to greater psychosocial maturity and school performance and less substance abuse among adolescents (p. 665).
26. a (p. 667)
27. a (pp. 665, 666)
28. b (p. 667)
29. d (p. 667)
30. Motor vehicle injuries, other injuries, homicide, suicide (p. 669)
31. a (p. 669)
32. c (p. 669)
33. d (p. 670)
34. c (p. 671)
35. d (p. 669)
36. a (pp. 669, 670)
37. b (pp. 672, 673)
38. Giving adolescents written materials during "teachable moments"; directing the adolescent to health resources in the community and on the Internet; teaching adolescents how the health care system works and how to keep their own personal health information (p. 672)
39. c (p. 674)
40. b (p. 674)
41. c (p. 674)
42. c (p. 675)
43. b (p. 675)
44. d (pp. 675, 676)
45. c (p. 677)
46. b (pp. 676, 677)
47. The adolescent has a specific plan (p. 678).
48. a (p. 678)
49. hypertension, smoking, obesity, elevated serum cholesterol and triglyceride levels (p. 679)

50. a (p. 679)
51. c (p. 680)
52. c (p. 680)
53. b (pp. 682, 683)
54. c (pp. 662, 676)
55. c (pp. 676, 677, 679)
56. d (pp. 652, 661; Table 17-1)
57. c (pp. 679)
58. c (pp. 677, 682)

CHAPTER 18

1. c (p. 687)
2. d (p. 688)
3. a (p. 690)
4. a (pp. 688-690)
5. c (p. 690)
6. b (p. 690)
7. c (p. 691)
8. a (p. 691)
9. d (p. 693; Box 18-2)
10. d (p. 693), a (p. 692), d (p. 693), e (p. 690), b (p. 692), g (p. 691), c (p. 692), b (p. 692), f (p. 691), c (p. 692), a (p. 692)
11. d (p. 695), e (p. 695), a (p. 694), c (p. 694), b (p. 694)
12. decrease the intensity or duration of her training; modify her diet to include the appropriate nutrition for her age (a daily calcium intake of 1200 to 1500 mg plus 400 to 800 International Units of vitamin D and 60 to 90 mg of potassium and a 20% increase in caloric intake have been recommended); explain the consequences of low bone density, osteoporosis, and stress fractures; discuss ways to prevent stress in her life and possible lifestyle changes (p. 695)
13. c (pp. 696, 697)
14. k (p. 701), b (p. 700), c (p. 698), d (p. 701), h (p. 703), i (p. 710), j (p. 699), a (p. 710), e (p. 703), f (p. 704), g (p. 702)
15. antibiotic therapy, broad-spectrum antibiotics such as ampicillin, tetracycline, cephalosporins and metronidazole; diabetes especially uncontrolled in pregnancy; obesity; diets high in refined sugars or artificial sweeteners; use of corticosteroids and exogenous hormones, and immunosuppressed states; also tight clothing and underwear or pantyhose made of nonabsorbent materials create an environment in which a vaginal fungus can grow (p. 703)
16. d (p. 707)
17. HPV and hepatitis B (p. 708)
18. d (pp. 705, 708; Table 18-4)
19. c (p. 711)
20. a (pp. 701, 718; Box 18-3)
21. b (p. 712)
22. d (pp. 713, 714)
23. b (pp. 714-716)
24. T (p. 717), T (p. 717), F (p. 717), F (p. 717), T (p. 717), T (p. 717), F (p. 718), F (p. 718), T (p. 718), T (p. 718), T (p. 717), F (p. 717)
25. d (p. 718)

26. c (pp. 719, 720)
27. b (p. 720)
28. Preventing subsequent pregnancies and enhancing life outcomes for the adolescents and infant (p. 721)
29. a (p. 721)
30. d (p. 722)
31. Allowing adolescents to role-play refusal skills (for sexual activity) in a safe environment (pp. 724, 725)
32. d (p. 726; Box 18-7)
33. a (p. 727)
34. c (p. 729), d (p. 729), e (p. 729), f (p. 739), a (p. 728), b (p. 728)
35. d (pp. 728, 729, 730)
36. d (pp. 730, 731)
37. c (pp. 728, 731, 732)
38. a (p. 732)
39. d (pp. 732, 733)
40. b (p. 728)
41. c (pp. 733, 734, 735)
42. c (pp. 736, 737)
43. b (pp. 736, 737)
44. Reduce the quantity eaten by purchasing, preparing, and serving smaller portions; alter the quality consumed by substituting low-calorie, low-fat foods for high-calorie foods, especially for snacks; eating regular meals and snacks, particularly breakfast; severing the association between eating and other stimuli such as eating while watching television (p. 736)
45. a (pp. 733, 737)
46. a (pp. 736, 737)
47. a. A strong fear of becoming fat, a distorted body image, and progressive weight loss (p. 737)
    b. Repeated episodes of binge eating followed by inappropriate compensatory behaviors, such as self-induced vomiting; misuse of laxatives, diuretics or other medications; fasting; or excessive exercise (p. 737)
48. d (p. 739)
49. d (pp. 739, 740)
50. a (p. 740)
51. c (p. 741)
52. Reinstitution of normal nutrition or reversal of the malnutrition; resolution of disturbed patterns of family interaction; individual psychotherapy to correct deficits and distortions in psychologic functioning (p. 741)
53. c (p. 741)
54. a (p. 742)
55. d (p. 742)
56. T (p. 746), T (pp. 745, 746), F (p. 746), T (p. 746), T (p. 746), T (p. 746), T (747), T (p. 747), T (p. 748)
57. a (pp. 746, 747; Community and Home Health Considerations box)
58. c (pp. 747, 748)
59. a. Crack (or rock) (p. 748)
    b. Constricted pupils, respiratory depression, cyanosis, and needle marks seen on extremities of chronic users (p. 749)

c. Flunitrazepam (Rohypnol) (p. 749)
d. Methamphetamine (p. 749)
e. Rapid loss of consciousness, respiratory arrest, fatal cardiac arrhythmias (p. 749)
60. a (p. 750)
61. c (p. 751), d (p. 751), b (p. 751), a (pp. 751, 752), e (p. 752)
62. b (p. 751)
63. d (p. 752)
64. d (pp. 753, 754)
65. d (pp. 751-753; Box 18-17)
66. c (p. 753)
67. a (p. 753)
68. c (p. 753)

CHAPTER 19

1. f (p. 763), b (p. 762), h (p. 764), a (p. 762), d (p. 762), i (p. 763), c (p. 763), j (p. 763), g (p. 762), e (p.762)
2. a (p. 761)
3. d (p. 762)
4. b (p. 762)
5. d (p. 763)
6. a (p. 764)
7. d (p. 765)
8. e, c, a, b, d (pp. 766-767)
9. b (pp. 763, 772)
10. b (p. 772)
11. b (p. 776)
12. c (p. 773)
13. a (p. 773)
14. d (p. 774)
15. c (p. 775)
16. b (p. 775)
17. Possible responses: Share complete information. Share information in manageable doses. Be sensitive to parents' reactions. Listen carefully. Provide technical information in understandable terms. Offer to share information. Provide information about resources (p. 776).
18. a (p. 777)
19. Home, school (p. 777)
20. a (p. 779)
21. c (p. 780)
22. d (p. 780)
23. b (p. 780)
24. False reassurance; assuring parents that the child will grow out of the problem when the parents are struggling to accept reality (p. 781)
25. Approach behaviors: a, c, e, f, g
    Avoidance behaviors: b, d (pp. 782-783)
26. b (p. 783)
27. d (p. 783)
28. c (p. 784)
29. d (p. 784)
30. a (p. 784)
31. Possible answers: Facilitate support from professionals; encourage expression of emotions; describe the behavior; give evidence of understanding; give evidence of

298

Answer Key

caring; help parents focus on feelings; facilitate parent-to-parent support (pp. 774-776)

32. b (p. 776)
33. d (p. 785)
34. c (pp. 784-785)
35. Possible answers: Makes many sacrifices; helps the child even when the child is capable; provides inconsistent discipline; is dictatorial; hovers and overdoes praise; protects the child from every discomfort; restricts play; denies the child opportunities for growth; sets goals too high or too low; monopolizes the child's time (p. 785)
36. a (p. 787)
37. d (p. 785)
38. d (p. 778)
39. a (p. 786)
40. a (p. 786)
41. b (p. 787)
42. a (p. 788)
43. a (p. 788)
44. a (p. 776)
45. c (Nursing Process)
46. c (pp. 767-768, 775)
47. b (pp. 765, 762, 767-768)
48. d (pp. 766-768)

CHAPTER 20

1. h (p. 802), d (p. 802), e (p. 792), c (p. 802), b (p. 800), a (p. 818), f (p. 811), g (p. 817)
2. c (p. 791)
3. Possible answers: Listen for an "invitation" to talk about the situation; use open-ended, nonjudgmental questions to explore the family's wishes; answer questions honestly; address fantasies or misunderstandings; remain neutral (p. 795; Box 20-2).
4. a (p. 792)
5. c (p. 793)
6. Pain control—withheld for fear of addiction and opioid side effects; Chemotherapy or Treatment—may be withheld to minimize side effects and pain of treatment itself; Resuscitation—family often refuses to give up or stops CPR, believing child has suffered enough; Withholding nutrition for fear that child will starve to death, or administration which may cause nausea and vomiting and discomfort; autopsy—parents may fear body desecration or disfiguring but it may help establish a cause of death (p. 793, Table 20-1)
7. c (p. 795)
8. d (p. 796)
9. a (pp. 795-796)
10. c (p. 799)
11. a (p. 798)
12. b (p. 798)
13. d (p. 799)
14. c (p. 800)
15. Children who are dying are allowed the opportunity to remain with those they love and with whom they feel secure. Many children who were thought to be in imminent danger of death have gone home and lived longer than expected. Siblings can feel more involved in the care and often have a more positive perception of the death. Parental adaptation is often more favorable, as is shown by their perceptions of how the experience at home affected their marriage, social reorientation, religious beliefs, and views on the meaning of life and death. Parents who have used home hospice feel significantly less guilt after the child's death than those whose child died in the hospital (p. 801).
16. d (p. 802)
17. b (pp. 802-803)
18. d (pp. 804-805)
19. d (p. 805)
20. Loss of senses; confusion; muscle weakness; loss of bowel and bladder control; difficulty swallowing; change in respiratory pattern; weak, slow pulse (pp. 806-807)
21. d (p. 807)
22. Recall events that were important with their family; draw pictures or leave messages for important friends and family; reassure parents and others that they are not afraid and are ready to die; experience visions of "angels"; mention that someone is waiting for them (pp. 806-807).
23. c (p. 813)
24. a (p. 806)
25. a (pp. 810-811)
26. All the statements are false (p. 812).
27. d (pp. 812-813)
28. a (pp. 813)
29. c (p. 814)
30. c (p. 814)
31. d (p. 813)
32. d (p. 813)
33. d (p. 816)
34. Possible answers: Denial, anger, depression, guilt, ambivalence (pp. 817-818)
35. b (p. 818)
36. a (pp. 804, 807-808)
37. c (p. 808)
38. d (pp. 808, 810)
39. a (pp. 807-809)

CHAPTER 21

1. Infections and intoxications (e.g., alcohol, rubella)
   Trauma or physical agent (e.g., traumatic brain injury)
   Metabolic or nutritional abnormality (e.g., phenylketonuria)
   Gross postnatal disease (neurofibromatosis)
   Unknown prenatal condition (e.g., microcephaly)
   Chromosomal abnormality (e.g., Fragile X syndrome)
   Gestational disorder (e.g., extreme preterm birth)
   Psychiatric disorder with onset during childhood (e.g., autism)
   Environmental influences (e.g., hereditary and environmental factors) (p. 825)

2. Either the Bayley Scales of Infant Development or the Mullen Scales of Early Learning (p. 825)
3. Maintain current immunizations; obtain genetic counseling with known risk factors present; avoid rubella infection in perinatal period; obtain adequate prenatal care; ensure adequate folic acid intake prior to and during all pregnancies; counsel mothers about danger of alcohol and nicotine in pregnancy (p. 825)
4. a (p. 824)
5. Nonresponsiveness to contact; poor eye contact during feeding; diminished spontaneous activity; decreased alertness to voice or movement; irritability; slow feeding (p. 826)
6. c (p. 827)
7. Fading means to take the child physically through each sequence of the desired activity and gradually fade out physical assistance so that the child becomes more independent (p. 827).
8. Shaping means to wait for the child to give a response that approximates the desired behavior, and then reinforce the child by gestures of social approval, such as touching or talking to him or her (p. 827).
9. d (p. 828)
10. c (p. 828)
11. Task analysis means to break the process of a skill into its components. It is used when teaching a cognitively impaired child to help the child master one step of a skill at a time, building on the parts that the child has mastered already (p. 827).
12. d (p. 831)
13. The child should be able to sit quietly for 3 to 5 minutes; to watch what he or she is doing while working on a task; to follow physical gestures or cues; to follow verbal commands; to relate clothing with the appropriate body part; and to be willing to participate (p. 832).
14. b (pp. 832-833)
15. c (p. 834)
16. b (p. 833)
17. Separated sagittal suture; oblique palpebral fissures (upward, outward slant); small nose; depressed nasal bridge (saddle nose); high, arched narrow palate; excess and lax neck skin; wide space between big and second toes; plantar crease between big and second toes; hyperflexibility; muscle weakness (p. 834).
18. c (p. 837)
19. Congenital heart defects, Hirschprung disease, renal agenesis, tracheoesophageal fistula, duodenal atresia, hip subluxation, atlantoaxial instability (p. 835)
20. a (p. 837)
21. b (p. 838)
22. Autism-like behavior such as gaze aversion; hyperactivity; potentially aggressive behavior; short attention span; intolerance to changes in routine; mouthing behaviors; mild to severe cognitive impairment (p. 838)
23. c (p. 839)
24. d (p. 839)
25. d (p. 840)
26. d (p. 840)

27. b (p. 841)
28. a (p. 841)
29. d (p. 843)
30. d (p. 843)
31. a (p. 844)
32. b (p. 847)
33. d (p. 847)
34. f, d, b, a, e, c (pp. 845-846)
35. Talk to the child about everything that is occurring. Emphasize aspects of procedures that are felt and/or heard. Approach the child with identifying information. Explain unfamiliar sounds. Encourage rooming-in for parents. Encourage parents to participate in the care. Bring familiar objects from home. Orient the child to the immediate surroundings. If the child has sight on admission, use this opportunity to point out significant aspects of the room and to have the child practice ambulating with the eyes closed. (pp. 849-850)
36. b (p. 850)
37. a (p. 851)
38. b (p. 851)
39. b (p. 853)
40. c (p. 853)
41. a (p. 853)
42. d (p. 853)
43. c (p. 857)
44. b (p. 858)
45. c (p. 858)
46. c (p. 859)
47. d (pp. 835-837, 858)
48. d (pp. 835-837)
49. b (pp. 835-837)
50. c (pp. 835-837)

CHAPTER 22

1. i (p. 874), b (p. 864), g (p. 868), f (p. 875), e (p. 864), d (p. 864), c (p. 864), a (p. 865)
2. b (p. 865)
3. c (p. 866)
4. a (p. 865)
5. d (p. 864)
6. Opportunities to master stress and feel competent in their coping abilities; new socialization experiences; broadened interpersonal relationships (p. 867)
7. b (p. 868)
8. Provides diversion; brings about relaxation; helps child feel secure; helps lessen stress; provides a means for tension release; encourages interaction; helps develop positive attitudes; acts as an expressive outlet; provides a means for accomplishing therapeutic goals; places child in active role; gives more control and choices to the child (p. 875)
9. Possible answers: Include family in care planning; observe for negative effects of continuous visiting by parents (encourage the parents to leave for brief periods; arrange for sleeping quarters on the unit but outside the child's room; plan a schedule of alternating

300

Answer Key

visits with the other parent or with another family member); provide information; provide a therapeutic presence; complement and augment the parents' caregiving responsibilities (p. 865; 868)
10. c (p. 871)
11. b (p. 873)
12. b (p. 872)
13. c (p. 873)
14. c (p. 873)
15. c (p. 873)
16. a (p. 876)
17. Allows for creative expression; allows nurse to assess adjustment and coping; serves as a springboard for discussion; provides distraction, diversion (p. 876)
18. d (p. 869)
19. d (p. 869)
20. Encourage parents to stay with their child. Provide information about child's condition in understandable language. Establish a routine that maintains some similarity to daily events in child's life whenever possible. Schedule undisturbed times. Reduce stimulation (p. 878).
21. c (p. 874)
22. d (p. 870)
23. c (p. 871)
24. d (p. 877)
25. d (p. 877)
26. c (p. 879)
27. a (p. 880)
28. c (p. 880)
29. a (pp. 869-872)
30. d (p. 873)
31. d (p. 873)
32. a (pp. 873-874)

CHAPTER 23

1. m (p. 895), h (p. 898), j (pp. 898-899), k (p. 899), a (p. 895), e (p. 896), b (p. 896), d (p. 896), c (p. 896), i (p. 899), l (p. 899), f (p. 896), g (p. 898)
2. d (p. 883)
3. a (p. 884)
4. c (p. 884)
5. d (p. 884)
6. b (p. 885)
7. c (p. 885)
8. a (p. 886)
9. b (p. 888)
10. d (p. 889)
11. Expect success. Have extra supplies handy. Involve the child. Provide distraction. Allow expression of feelings. Provide positive reinforcement. Use play in preparation and postprocedure (pp. 888-889).
12. Examples of appropriate responses:
    a. Ambulation: Give a toddler a push-pull toy.
    b. Range-of-motion exercises: Touch or kick balloons.
    c. Injections: Make creative objects out of syringes.
    d. Deep breathing: Practice band instruments.

e. Extending the environment: Move the patient's bed to the playroom.
f. Soaks: Put marbles or coins at the bottom of bath container.
g. Fluid intake: Make freezer pops using the child's favorite juice (p. 891).
13. b (p. 890)
14. c (p. 890)
15. a (p. 892)
16. d (p. 892 and Chapter 5, p. 176)
17. c (p. 892)
18. d (p. 893)
19. b (p. 892)
20. c (p. 894)
21. c (pp. 894-895)
22. c (p. 895)
23. c (p. 895)
24. b (p. 896)
25. c (p. 896)
26. c (p. 897)
27. a (p. 897)
28. a (p. 898)
29. a (p. 899)
30. d (p. 899)
31. a (p. 899)
32. How to treat the fever (antipyretic; no tepid bath, alcohol sponging or ice water bath)
    How to take the child's temperature
    How to read the thermometer used in the home accurately
    When to call the primary practitioner (p. 900)
33. Falls risk assessment; on admission and throughout hospitalization (p. 901)
34. If a toy or item is small enough to be placed in a toilet paper tube (usually less than 1¾ inches in diameter) it is a choking hazard for children younger than 3 years of age (p. 901)
35. d (p. 902)
36. d (pp. 902-903)
37. b (p. 905)
38. d (p. 906)
39. c (p. 907)
40. c (p. 904)
41. b (p. 904)
42. d (p. 907)
43. b (p. 909)
44. a (p. 912)
45. c (p. 913)
46. d (p. 914)
47. a (p. 914)
48. b (p. 915)
49. a (p. 915)
50. d (pp. 918-919)
51. a (p. 921)
52. d (p. 933)
53. a (p. 931)
54. b (p. 931)
55. c (p. 934)
56. Implanted port (p. 924)

57. Skin-level gastrostomy (p. 938)
58. a (p. 940)
59. b (pp. 890-891)
60. b (pp. 890-891)
61. a (p. 892)
62. d (pp. 892-894)

CHAPTER 24

1. c (p. 945), b (p. 945), a (p. 945), t (p. 979), u (p. 980; Drug Alert box), f (p. 947; Box 24-1), g (p. 947; Box 24-1), d (p. 947; Box 24-1), e (p. 951), k (pp. 945, 948), l (p. 946), m (p. 956), p (p. 954), i (p. 945), n (p. 956), j (p. 945), o (p. 956), h (p. 945), s (p. 961), r (p. 962), q (p. 958)
2. d (p. 946)
3. a (p. 947)
4. d (pp. 947, 948)
5. b (p. 948)
6. c (p. 948)
7. Isotonic (p. 952)
8. Hypotonic, less (p. 952)
9. Hypertonic, less, intake, more (p. 952)
10. b (p. 952)
11. c (p. 953; Table 24-3)
12. c (p. 953)
13. d (p. 954)
14. c (p. 955)
15. c (p. 955)
16. b (p. 955)
17. Anasarca (p. 956)
18. b (p. 956)
19. c (p. 957; Figure 24-4)
20. a (p. 957)
21. d (pp. 957, 958)
22. b (p. 951; Table 24-2)
23. a. Hypovolemic (pp. 958, 959; Box 24-3)
    b. Cardiogenic (pp. 958, 959; Box 24-3)
    c. Distributive (vasogenic) (pp. 958, 959; Box 24-3)
    d. Anaphylactic (pp. 958, 959; Box 24-3)
    e. Septic (pp. 958, 959; Box 24-3)
    f. Neurogenic (p. 958)
24. b (p. 960)
25. Oxygenation and ventilation, fluid administration, improvement of the pumping action of the heart (vasopressor support) (pp. 961, 962; Emergency Treatment box)
26. c (p. 962)
27. a (p. 962)
28. a (p. 964; Table 24-7)
29. c, a, b (p. 963)
30. c (p. 965)
31. a (pp. 955, 956; Box 24-6)
32. d (p. 967)
33. d (p. 967; Box 24-7)
34. Wash hands before inserting the tampon; do not use a soiled or dropped tampon; insert carefully to avoid vaginal abrasion; alternate use with sanitary napkins (e.g., use tampons during the day and sanitary napkins during the night); young girls are advised not to use superabsorbent tampons; do not leave tampon in the body longer than 4 to 6 hours; remove the tampon immediately with development of sudden fever, rash, vomiting, diarrhea, muscle pain, dizziness, or feeling of near-fainting (p. 968; Nursing Alert box).
35. Extreme heat sources, exposure to cold, electricity; chemicals, radiation (p. 968)
36. d (p. 968)
37. a (p. 969)
38. b (pp. 969, 971; Figure 24-6)
39. d (p. 970)
40. a (p. 969)
41. b (p. 970)
42. c (pp. 969, 970, 971)
43. c (p. 973; Figure 24-10)
44. b (p. 972)
45. d (p. 973)
46. b (p. 974)
47. d (p. 974
48. b (pp. 974, 975)
49. a (p. 975)
50. a (p. 975)
51. b (p. 976)
52. c (p. 977)
53. c (p. 978)
54. b (p. 978)
55. b (p. 979)
56. a (p. 979)
57. b (p. 981)
58. a (p. 982; Box 24-11)
59. d (pp. 982, 983)
60. b (p. 983)
61. a (pp. 985, 987; Nursing Care Plan)
62. d (pp. 985, 988: Nursing Care Plan)
63. c (p. 989)
64. d (p. 992)
65. c (p. 952)
66. d (p. 957)
67. d (p. 953; Box 24-3)
68. c (p. 954)
69. c (p. 961)

CHAPTER 25

1. F (p. 996), T (p. 996), T (p. 996), F (p. 996), F (p. 996), T (p. 997), T (p. 998), T (p. 998), T (p. 998), T (p. 998), T (p. 998), T (p. 1005), T (p. 1005), F (p. 1006; Research Focus box), F (p. 1003; Box 25-2)
2. Anatomic integrity of the lower urinary tract, detrusor control, and competence of the urethral sphincter mechanism (p. 1000)
3. A, N, A, A, N, N, A (p. 1002; Table 25-1)
4. c (p. 999), f (p. 1004; Box 25-2), h (p. 1004; Box 25-2), j (pp. 1003, 1009, 1010; Table 25-2), k (pp. 1152, 1156, 1163), b (p. 999), d (p. 1000), i (p. 1004; Box 25-2), e (p. 1000), g (p. 1004; Box 25-2), a (p. 1004;

Box 25-2), m (p. 1025), l (p. 1029), o (p. 1024), n (p. 1026)

5. a (p. 1004; Table 25-2)
6. d (p. 1004; Table 25-2)
7. a (pp. 1009, 1010)
8. d (p. 1005)
9. d (p. 1006; Box 25-3)
10. b (p. 1007; Nursing Tip box)
11. a. Eliminate the current infection.
    b. Prevent complications.
    c. Reduce the likelihood of renal damage (p. 1007).
12. a (p. 1006)
13. d (p. 1007)
14. d (p. 1007)
15. a (p. 1007; Table 25-4)
16. b (p. 1010)
17. c (p. 1011)
18. a. that the administration of antibiotics prophylaxis will result in sterile urine and that reflux of sterile urine does not cause renal damage (p. 1011)
    b. Amoxicillin is used in infants less than 2 months of age because it is safer in this age group but not used in older infants because of the increased likelihood of resistant organisms. (p. 1011)
19. b (p. 1013)
20. b (p. 1013)
21. Hypertensive encephalopathy, acute cardiac decompensation, acute renal failure (p. 1014)
22. b (p. 1015)
23. a (p. 1016)
24. b (p. 1016)
25. a (pp. 1017, 1018)
26. a (p. 1017)
27. c (p. 1019)
28. Children with nephrotic syndrome should receive pneumococcal conjugate vaccine (PCV13) and pneumococcal polysaccharide vaccine (PPSV-23). Live vaccine should not be given while the child is on steroid therapy. (pp. 1018, 1019)
29. c (p. 1019)
30. a (p. 1019)
31. c (p. 1020)
32. b (p. 1021)
33. a (p. 1021)
34. b (p. 1021)
35. c (p. 1023)
36. a (p. 1023)
37. a (p. 1024)
38. c (p. 1025)
39. b (p. 1025)
40. a (pp. 1025, 1026, 1027; Table 25-7)
41. c (p. 1028)
42. Monitoring and assessing fluid and electrolyte balance (p. 1029)
43. b (p. 1030)
44. b (p. 1032)
45. c (p. 1032)
46. d (p. 1032)
47. c (p. 1033; Family-Centered Care box)

48. a. Hemodialysis; peritoneal dialysis; hemofiltration (p. 1034)
    b. life-threatening electrolyte abnormalities; severe volume overload; bilateral neoplastic disease or bilateral nephrectomies (p. 1034)
    c. Peritonitis (p. 1037)
    d. Continuous venovenous hemodialysis (CVVHD) (p. 1038)
49. b (p. 1035)
50. a (p. 1039)
51. a (p. 1040), j (p. 1041), e (p. 1040), b (p. 1041), c (p. 1042), d (p. 1044), f (p. 1046), i (p. 1047), g (p. 1040), h (p. 1046)
52. b (p. 1041)
53. b (p. 1044)
54. c (pp. 1044, 1045)
55. c (p. 1047)
56. b (p. 1017)
57. d (pp. 1008, 1020; Quality Patient Outcomes)
58. c (pp. 1017-1021)
59. d (p. 1020)
60. Teach the family to recognize signs of relapse and to bring the child for treatment at the earliest indications of relapse; provide instruction about testing urine for albumin, administration of medications, side effects of medications, and prevention of infection; emphasize the importance of restricting salt (e.g., no additional salt during relapse and steroid therapy), followed by a regular diet for the child in remission (p. 1020).
61. Teach the family and Darlene about the disease, its implications, and the therapeutic plan; the possible psychologic effects of the disease and the treatment; the technical aspects of the procedure, including possible complications and changes to observe for (pp. 1037, 1038).
62. Provide dietary instructions for foods that reduce excretory demands on kidneys and provide sufficient calories and protein for growth. Encourage intake of carbohydrates to provide calories for growth and foods high in calcium to prevent bone demineralization. Recommend foods that are rich in folic acid and iron because anemia is a complication of chronic renal failure. Limit phosphorus, salt, and potassium as needed and prescribed. Teach parents and Darlene how to read food labels carefully for content and to modify meals. Arrange for renal dietitian to meet with Darlene and her family to help them understand dietary needs and to assist Darlene in independent formulation of dietary allowances when she is away from home (pp. 1031, 1032, 1033, 1034).
63. Serum creatinine is the best predictor of renal function because the BUN can be elevated from dehydration, hemorrhage, high protein intake, and corticosteroid therapy. The serum creatinine is an indicator of the end product of protein metabolism in muscle and is thus a more stable and better indicator of renal function (p. 1004; Table 25-3).

303

CHAPTER 26

1. b (pp. 1051, 1052; Box 26-1)
2. F, T, T, T, T, F (p. 1052)
3. a. Digestion, absorption, metabolism (p. 1052)
   b. Enzymes, hormones, hydrochloric acid, mucus, water, and electrolytes (p. 1052)
   c. Small intestine (p. 1053)
4. Measurement of intake and output, measurement of height, measurement of weight, abdominal examination, laboratory studies of urine and stool (p. 1054)
5. c (p. 1058; Box 26-4)
6. b (p. 1058)
7. Intractable diarrhea of infancy (p. 1058)
8. c (p. 1058; Box 26-4)
9. a (p. 1061; Box 26-5)
10. T (p. 1061), T (p. 1067), T (p. 1067), F (p. 1061), F (p. 1061), T (p. 1061), T (p. 1064)
11. d (p. 1062)
12. b (p. 1062)
13. a. *Clostridium difficile* (p. 1062)
    b. Bacterial gastroenteritis or inflammatory bowel disease (p. 1062)
    c. Glucose intolerance (p. 1062)
    d. Fat malabsorption (p. 1062)
    e. Parasitic infection or protein intolerance (p. 1062)
14. a (p. 1062)
15. Assessment of fluid and electrolyte imbalance; rehydration; maintenance fluid therapy; reintroduction of adequate diet (p. 1062)
16. a (pp. 1062, 1063, 1064; Box 26-7; Nursing Alert box)
17. d (p. 1064)
18. c (p. 1064)
19. c (pp. 1066, 1067; Nursing Care Plan)
20. d (p. 1067)
21. d (p. 1068)
22. a (p. 1057, 1090; Table 26-1)
23. b (p. 1057; Table 26-1)
24. j (p. 1056; Table 26-1), f (p. 1052; Box 26-2), g (p. 1052; Box 26-2), h (p. 1052; Box 26-2), m (p. 1091), a (p. 1069), l (p. 1052; Box 26-2), n (p. 1107), d (p. 1052; Box 26-2), e (p. 1052; Box 26-2), b (p. 1052; Box 26-2), i (p. 1052; Box 26-2), k (p. 1055; Table 26-1), c (p. 1052; Box 26-2),
25. b (pp. 1069, 1070)
26. d (p. 1070)
27. b (p. 1072)
28. b (p. 1073)
29. d (pp. 1070, 1072-1074)
30. b (pp. 1072-1074)
31. d (p. 1074)
32. c (p. 1075)
33. d (p. 1074; Box 26-11)
34. d (p. 1075)
35. b (p. 1076)
36. b (p. 1078)
37. b (p. 1077)
38. a (p. 1078)
39. Periumbilical pain, followed by nausea, right-sided lower quadrant pain, and then later vomiting with fever (p. 1079)
40. d (p. 1079; Nursing Alert)
41. a. McBurney point (p. 1079)
    b. Midway between the right anterosuperior iliac crest and the umbilicus (p. 1079)
    c. Rebound tenderness (p. 1079)
42. c (p. 1081)
43. a (pp. 1084, 1086)
44. In CD the chronic inflammatory process may involve any part of the GI tract, from the mouth to the anus, but most commonly affects the terminal ileum. It can affect segments of the intestine with intact mucosa in between. CD involves all layers of the wall. The inflammation may result in ulcerations, fibrosis, adhesions, stiffening of the bowel wall, and obstruction. In UC the inflammation is limited to the colon and rectum, with the distal colon and rectum often the most severely affected. UC involves the mucosa and submucosa; it also involves continuous segments with varying degrees of ulceration, bleeding, and edema. Long-standing UC can cause shortening of the colon and strictures (pp. 1084, 1085).
45. c (p. 1086)
46. b (p. 1086)
47. b (p. 1087)
48. a (p. 1090)
49. c (p. 1088)
50. c (p. 1088)
51. (1) Bismuth, clarithromycin, and metronidazole; (2) lansoprazole, amoxicillin, and clarithromycin; (3) metronidazole, clarithromycin, and omeprazole (p. 1090)
52. b (p. 1090)
53. b (p. 1091)
54. d (p. 1093)
55. a (p. 1093)
56. a (pp. 1093, 1094; Box 26-17)
57. a (p. 1094; Nursing Alert box)
58. c (p. 1094)
59. Malrotation, volvulus (p. 1094)
60. a (p. 1095)
61. c (p. 1095)
62. d (p. 1097)
63. a (p. 1099)
64. a (p. 1100), a (pp. 1100, 1101; Table 26-7), e (p. 1102), c (p. 1102), d (p. 1102), c (pp. 1101, 1102), b (pp. 1100, 1101), b (pp. 1100, 1101; Table 26-7), e (p. 1102)
65. a (p. 1102)
66. a (pp. 1102, 1103)
67. c (p. 1103)
68. b (p. 1104)
69. c (p. 1106)
70. c (p. 1107)
71. a (p. 1108)
72. c (pp. 1107, 1108)
73. d (pp. 1112, 1113, 1114)
74. b (p. 1114), e (p. 1116), a (p. 1114), a (p. 1114), c (p. 1115), d (p. 1116), g (p. 1110), f p. 1116)

75. Questions about the patient's pain: When did the pain start? Has it been constant or intermittent? What were you doing when the pain started? Where did the pain start, and does the pain radiate or move to other areas? How would you describe the pain intensity and quality? What makes the pain better? What makes it worse? How have you tried to treat the pain? Has there been change in normal activities because of the pain?

Questions about related symptoms or review of associated symptoms: Is there nausea or vomiting? If there is, did it start before or after the pain? Is there diarrhea or constipation? How would you describe your last stool? When did it occur? Are there urinary tract signs and symptoms such as frequency, difficulty with flow, burning? Is there fever? If so, how much fever? How long has the fever been present? Have you taken medications for the fever? If so, when was the last dose taken? Is there hunger or lack of hunger?

Questions about the reproductive system: For females—When was your last menstrual period? For males and females—Are you sexually active? Do you have any genital discharge? (pp. 1080, 1081; also Chapter 5)

76. b (p. 1079)
77. d (pp. 1080, 1081)
78. A white blood cell count with a differential elevated greater than 10,000/mm^3, with an elevated number of bands indicating a shift to the left; C-reactive protein elevation that rises within 12 hours of the onset of infection (p. 1080)
79. a (p. 1082; Nursing Care Plan)
80. a (pp. 1080-1082; Nursing Care Plan)

CHAPTER 27

1. b (p. 1124)
2. a (p. 1122)
3. c (p. 1123)
4. b (p. 1122).
5. c (p. 1122), e (p. 1122), g (p. 1126), m (p. 1133), s (p. 1133), r (p. 1133), d (p. 1122), f (p. 1122), a (p. 1126), b (p. 1122), h (p. 1125), j (p. 1125), l (p. 1133), n (p. 1132), k (p. 1134), q (p. 1156), i (p. 1139), o (p. 1133), t (p. 1140), p (p. 1142)
6. b (p. 1123)
7. Fewer number of alveoli, smaller size of the alveoli, more shallow air sacks, decreased surface area for gas exchange (p. 1125)
8. b (p. 1126)
9. a (p. 1126)
10. b (p. 1126)
11. d (p. 1127)
12. a (p. 1133)
13. c (p. 1134)
14. b, c, a, c, b, a (p. 1135, Table 27-4)
15. a (p. 1130)
16. carbon dioxide (p. 1129)

17. Compensation (p. 1129)
18. (p. 1130)
   pH—7.35-7.45
   PCO_2—32-45 mm Hg (girls)
         35-48 mm Hg (boys)
   HCO_3—22-26 mEq/mL
   BE (base excess)—+2 to −4
19. b (p. 1130)
20. c (p. 1132)
21. base bicarbonate, metabolic acidosis (p. 1131)
22. carbon dioxide, respiratory alkalosis (p. 1131)
23. HCl (hydrochloric acid), metabolic alkalosis (p. 1132)
24. a (p. 1133)
25. d (p. 1137)
26. b (p. 1139)
27. c (pp. 1138-1139)
28. b (p1141)
29. a (pp. 1142-1143)
30. a (p. 1143)
31. d (p. 1143)
32. c (p. 1145)
33. b (p. 1148)
34. b (pp. 1145-1146)
35. d (p. 1146)
36. a (pp. 1146-1147)
37. D (displacement): tube has come out of the trachea; O (obstruction): tube may be obstructed by mucus, secretions; P (pneumothorax): child may have air in the pleural space preventing adequate lung expansion; E (equipment): equipment failure; check oxygen tubing, correct concentration being delivered (p. 1149)
38. Work of breathing, breath sounds, LOC, capillary refill, skin color, vital signs including pulse oximetry and blood pressure (p. 1149)
39. Remove air or fluid from the pleural or pericardial space.
   Prevent the backflow (or rebreathing) of air or fluid into the pleural or pericardial space (p. 1150).
40. The fluid collection chamber collects drainage from the patient's pleural or pericardial space. The water seal chamber is directly connected to the fluid collection chamber and acts as a one-way valve, protecting patients from air returning to the pleural or pericardial space. The suction chamber may be a dry suction or calibrated water chamber. It is connected to external vacuum suction set to the amount of suction ordered; the suction establishes a pressure gradient to the fluid collection chamber to prevent rebreathing air or aspiration of fluid into the lung (p. 1150).
41. d (p. 1151)
42. a (p. 1153)
43. b (p. 1154)
44. Possible answers: Avoid toys, blankets, clothing, and pets that shed fine hair or lint. Avoid aerosols, powder, dust, and smoke. Eliminate toys with small removable parts. Clothing should have loose-fitting collars that do not cover the tracheostomy tube opening. When the child is outside, the artificial collar or a thin cloth is used to prevent cold air, dust, dirt, or sand from

305

entering the tube. Bathe the child in a tub filled with shallow water; no water or soap should enter the tube (p. 1145).

45. a (pp. 1155-1156)
46. d (p. 1157)
47. a (p. 1157)
48. A nonrebreathing or partial rebreathing mask would be the best option (p. 1142).
49. Noninvasive pulse oximetry on a fingertip would be the best way to monitor his oxygenation status (pp. 1138-1139).
50. Assess his work of breathing, use of accessory muscles, listen to breath sounds bilaterally, observe respiratory rate, observe for any clinical manifestations indicative of respiratory failure (hypopnea, apnea) (pp. 1132-1133).
51. Respiratory acidosis
52. Use the DOPE mnemonic to troubleshoot the problem: Displacement of the ET tube; Obstruction of the ET tube (suction); Pneumothorax (auscultate breath sounds and observe chest movements); Equipment failure—check oxygen source, use bag and mask to ventilate, check status of ventilator (p. 1149).

CHAPTER 28

1. d (p. 1171), i (p. 1173), e (p. 1171), m (p. 1174), g (p. 1173), h (p. 1173), p (p. 1176), l (p. 1174), f (p. 1173), a (p. 1177), n (p. 1176), c (p. 1171), j (p. 1173), b (p. 1177), o (p. 1176), k (p. 1173)
2. b (p. 1164)
3. c (p. 1164)
4. c (p. 1166)
5. c (p. 1165)
6. b (p. 1170)
7. Increased respiratory rate makes it difficult to take in fluids or nurse; fever increases total body fluid turnover; nasal secretions block nasal passages and make it difficult to breathe and therefore to drink or nurse (p. 1169).
8. a (p. 1170)
9. b (p. 1171)
10. c (pp. 1171-1172)
11. b (p. 1172)
12. d (p. 1171)
13. d (p. 1173)
14. d (p. 1174)
15. c (p. 1174)
16. c (p. 1174)
17. a (p. 1175)
18. c (p. 1175)
19. c (p. 1176)
20. c (p. 1176)
21. b (p. 1176)
22. a (p. 1177)
23. 24 to 48 (p. 1178)
24. b (p. 1178)
25. a (p. 1178)
26. a (p. 1179)
27. d (p. 1180)

28. a (p. 1180)
29. b (p. 1181)
30. a (p. 1181)
31. d (p. 1181)
32. b (p. 1182)
33. c (p. 1182)
34. c (p. 1187)
35. d (p. 1185)
36. c (p. 1185)
37. a (p. 1185)
38. b (p. 1185)
39. a (p. 1186)
40. c (p. 1185)
41. a (p. 1190)
42. b (p. 1190)
43. c (p. 1196)
44. b (p. 1196)
45. b (p. 1198)
46. c (p. 1200)
47. e (p. 1211)
48. d (p. 1206)
49. a (p. 1208)
50. Prevent and control asthma symptoms, reverse airflow obstruction, and reduce the frequency and severity of acute exacerbations (p. 1222).
51. d (p. 1227)
52. Maintain normal activity levels, maintain normal pulmonary function, prevent chronic symptoms and recurrent exacerbations, provide optimal drug therapy, with minimal or no adverse effects, and assist the child in living as normal a life as possible (p. 1221).
53. b (p. 1236)
54. e (pp. 1237-1241)
55. Ineffective airway clearance
Interrupted family processes
Fluid deficit
Risk for injury
(pp. 1169-1170)
56. Administer oxygen via nasal cannula or small mask (pp. 1188-1191).
57. Suction her nose to clear secretions (maintain patent airway).
Monitor oxygenation status.
Administer an antipyretic to decrease her fever—acetaminophen would be appropriate at her age.
Prevent spread of infection with droplet, standard, and contact precautions.
Administer ordered nebulized bronchodilator medications (as ordered).
Allow mother to hold Jessica and to stay with her daughter.
Keep mother informed of Jessica's progress and explain treatments (pp. 1190-1191).
58. Administer IV fluids for hydration (pp. 1190-1191).
59. Instill normal saline nose drops before feedings and placing to sleep; suction the infant's nose before feedings and sleep; administer small amounts of fluids frequently; encourage Jessica's mother to breastfeed her. (pp. 1190-1191)

60. She would benefit from antibiotics to treat the otitis media, but antibiotics are not effective for RSV as it is a viral infection. (p. 1190)

CHAPTER 29

1. g (p. 1266), f (p. 1266), e (p. 1266), b (p. 1266), d (p. 1266), a (p. 1265), c (p. 1266)
2. a (p. 1252)
3. a (p. 1252)
4. b (p. 1252)
5. c (p. 1252)
6. a (p. 1252)
7. b (p. 1255)
8. d (p. 1255)
9. a (p. 1256)
10. b (p. 1256)
11. c (p. 1257)
12. c (p. 1258)
13. b (p. 1259)
14. Pulses, especially below the catheterization site, for equality and symmetry (pulse distal to the site may be weaker for the first few hours after catheterization but should gradually increase in strength)
    Temperature and color of the affected extremity, since coolness or blanching may indicate arterial obstruction
    Vital signs, which may be taken as frequently as every 15 minutes, with special emphasis on the heart rate, which is counted for 1 full minute for evidence of dysrhythmias or bradycardia
    Blood pressure, especially for hypotension, which may indicate hemorrhage from cardiac perforation or bleeding at the site of initial catheterization
    Dressing for evidence of bleeding or hematoma formation in the femoral or antecubital area
    Fluid intake, both intravenous and oral, to ensure adequate hydration (blood loss in the catheterization laboratory, the child's preprocedure NPO status, and diuretic actions of contrast material used during the procedure put the child at risk for hypovolemia and dehydration) (p. 1260)
15. d (p. 1260)
16. c (p. 1262)
17. c (p. 1264)
18. d (p. 1264)
19. c (p. 1265)
20. a (p. 1265)
21. c (p. 1266)
22. d (p. 1271)
23. c (p. 1271)
24. d (p. 1272)
25. Administer 100% oxygen by face mask
    Place in knee-chest position
    Administer morphine SQ or IV if IV route is available
    Comfort and soothe infant (p. 1273)
26. b (p. 1273)
27. b (p. 1273)

28. a (p. 1273)
29. c (p. 1278), d (p. 1278), c (p. 1277), d (p. 1279), b (p. 1283), c (p. 1277), d (p. 1277), a (p. 1280), d (p. 1279), a (p. 1281), d (p. 1279), b (p. 1283), c (p. 1276), b (p. 1281), b (p. 1282)
30. c (p. 1277)
31. d (p. 1284)
32. b (p. 1280)
33. b (pp. 1276-1283)
34. c (p. 1282)
35. a (pp. 1285-1286)
36. c (p. 1286)
37. d (pp. 1264-1265)
38. Secondary to a structural defect that results in increased blood volume and pressure within the heart (p. 1262)
39. a (dosage calculation)
40. Signs and symptoms of heart failure, activity restrictions and/or guidance, nutritional guidelines, medications, immunizations (p. 1287)
41. c (p. 1288)
42. a (p. 1288)
43. a (p. 1289)
44. d (p. 1289)
45. d (p. 1289)
46. d (p. 1289)
47. a (p. 1290)
48. b (p. 1290)
49. d (p. 1290)
50. c (p. 1317)
51. d (p. 1290)
52. d (p. 1291)
53. c (p. 1291)
54. b (p. 1294)
55. a (p. 1294)
56. a (p. 1296)
57. d (p. 1297)
58. d (p. 1296)
59. d (p. 1297)
60. b (p. 1298)
61. a (p. 1300)
62. c (p. 1302)
63. b (p. 1302)
64. 95th (p. 1305)
65. d (p. 1306)
66. c (p. 1306)
67. d (p. 1308)
68. a (p. 1315)
69. a (p. 1316)
70. b (p. 1313)
71. c (p. 1287)
72. a (nursing diagnosis)
73. d (p. 1288)

CHAPTER 30

1. b (p. 1322), k (p. 1328), e (p. 1324), n (p. 1328), g (p. 1325), l (p. 1328), i (p. 1328), c (p. 1322), j (p. 1328), a (p. 1322), m (p. 1328), h (p. 1328), d (p. 1322),

f (p. 1324), o (p. 1325), q (p. 1325), p (p. 1352), s (p. 1326; Table 30-1), r (p. 1325), t (p. 1326; Table 30-1), u (p. 1324), v (p. 1326; Table 30-1), x (p. 1325), w (p. 1325)

2. F (p. 1322), F (p. 1326; Table 30-1), F (p. 1326; Table 30-1), T (p. 1324), T (p. 1324), T (p. 1324), T (p. 1324), F (p. 1324), T (pp. 1325, 1326; Table 30-1), F (p. 1325), T (p. 1324), F (p. 1325), T (p. 1324), T (p. 1326; Table 30-1), T (p. 1324)

3. c (pp. 1329, 1330)

4. Inadequate production of RBCs or RBC components, increased destruction of RBCs, excessive loss of RBCs (p. 1329)

5. Decrease in the oxygen-carrying capacity of blood and consequently a reduction in the amount of oxygen available to the cells (p. 1329)

6. Can result from any tissue destruction such as bacterial or viral infections, hemorrhage, neoplastic disease, toxicity, operative procedures, burns, or tissue ischemia (p. 1325)

7. a (p. 1330)

8. b (p. 1329)

9. b (pp. 1330, 1331)

10. c (p. 1333)

11. b (pp. 1332, 1333; Table 30-2)

12. a (p. 1335)

13. a (p. 1336)

14. b (p. 1335)

15. d (p. 1336)

16. a (pp. 1337, 1338; Drug Alert and Nursing Alert)

17. "This is a normally expected change and usually means that an adequate dosage of iron has been reached" (p. 1338).

18. b (p. 1338)

19. b (p. 1339)

20. d (p. 1339)

21. c (pp. 1339, 1340)

22. Dehydration, acidosis, hypoxia, temperature elevation (p. 1339)

23. c (p. 1340; Box 30-4)

24. b (pp. 1339, 1340)

25. c (p. 1342)

26. d (p. 1343)

27. d (p. 1343)

28. b (p. 1346)

29. d (p. 1347; Drug Alert)

30. a (p. 1346)

31. c (p. 1349)

32. d (p. 1353)

33. a (p. 1354)

34. Primary, or congenital; secondary, or acquired (p. 1354)

35. a. Bone marrow aspiration, which demonstrates the conversion of red bone marrow to yellow, fatty bone marrow (p. 1355)
    b. Anemia; leukopenia; low platelet counts (p. 1355)
    c. Immunosuppressive therapy; bone marrow transplant (p. 1355)

36. d (p. 1355; Drug Alert)

37. d (p. 1358; Table 30-5), g (p. 1356), e (p. 1356; Table 30-5), a (p. 1356; Table 30-5), b (p. 1356; Table 30-5), c (p. 1356; Table 30-5), f (p. 1356)

38. a (p. 1357)

39. a (p. 1358)

40. b (p. 1359; Drug Alert)

41. d (pp. 1359, 1360; Table 30-7)

42. a (pp. 1361, 1362)

43. c (p. 1362)

44. a (p. 1362)

45. d (p. 1363; Drug Alert)

46. a (p. 1364)

47. b (pp. 1363, 1364; Box 30-7)

48. a (p. 1365)

49. Nonthrombocytopenic purpura, arthritis, nephritis, abdominal pain (p. 1366)

50. a. IgM; b. IgG (p. 1367)

51. d (pp. 1368, 1369)

52. Lymphadenopathy, hepatosplenomegaly, oral candidiasis, chronic or recurrent diarrhea, failure to thrive, developmental delay, parotitis (p. 1369; Box 30-8)

53. Slowing growth of the virus, preventing and treating opportunistic infections and providing nutritional support and symptomatic treatment (p. 1370)

54. a (pp. 1369, 1370)

55. c (p. 1371)

56. ELISA and Western blot will be positive because of presence of maternal antibodies derived transplacentally. Maternal antibodies may persist in the infant up to 18 months of age (p. 1370).

57. d (p. 1372)

58. b (p. 1371)

59. a (p. 1372)

60. a (p. 1374)

61. c (p. 1340)

62. Plan preventive schedule of medication around the clock, not only when needed to prevent pain; prevent resistance to administration by reassuring child and family that analgesics, including opioids, are medically indicated, that high doses may be needed, and that children rarely become addicted; patient-controlled analgesia (PCA) could be used to reinforce the patient's role and responsibility in managing the pain and provides flexibility; combine pain management program with psychologic support to help the child deal with the depression, anxiety, and fear that accompany the disease. (pp. 1347, 1348)

63. d (pp. 1343, 1347)

64. a (p. 1433)

CHAPTER 31

1. e (p. 1380), g (p. 1382), a (p. 1380), b (p. 1380), c (p. 1398), f (p. 1385), d (p. 1391)

2. g (p. 1391), f (p. 1391), e (p. 1391), d (p. 1391), c (p. 1390), b (p. 1390), a (p. 1390)

3. c (p. 1391), e (p. 1395), f (p. 1395), a (p. 1391), d (p. 1394), b (p. 1391)

4. c (p. 1380)
5. a (p. 1381)
6. b (p. 1400)
7. c (p. 1383)
8. DNA or RNA (p. 1383)
9. a (p. 1384)
10. c (p. 1384)
11. Gastrointestinal tract—Nausea and vomiting; give antiemetic around the clock.
    Skin—Alopecia; introduce idea of wig; stress necessity of scalp hygiene.
    Head—Xerostomia (dry mouth); stress oral hygiene and liquid diet.
    Urinary bladder—Cystitis; encourage liberal fluid intake and frequent voiding (pp. 1384-1385).
12. a (pp. 1385-1386)
13. b (p. 1386)
14. Unusual mass or swelling; unexplained paleness and loss of energy; sudden tendency to bruise; persistent, localized pain or limping; prolonged, unexplained fever or illness; frequent headaches, often with vomiting; sudden eye or vision changes; excessive, rapid weight loss (p. 1381)
15. Colony-stimulating factor (p. 1391)
16. b (p. 1391)
17. 350/mm^3 (p. 1391)
18. c (p. 1393)
19. a (p. 1394)
20. Liberal oral and/or parenteral fluid intake; frequent voiding immediately after feeling the urge, including immediately before bed and after arising; administration of drug early in the day to allow for sufficient fluid and frequent voiding; administration of mesna, a drug that inhibits the urotoxicity of cyclophosphamide and ifosfamide (p. 1395)
21. c (p. 1393)
22. d (p. 1395)
23. a (p. 1395)
24. d (p. 1396)
25. d (p. 1397)
26. c (p. 1397)
27. d (p. 1399)
28. Anemia from decreased erythrocytes
    Infection from decreased neutrophils
    Bleeding from decreased platelet production (p. 1400)
29. d (p. 1400)
30. b (p. 1401)
31. c (p. 1400)
32. c (p. 1400)
33. c (p. 1401)
34. c (p. 1401)
35. d (p. 1403)
36. a (p. 1403)
37. b (p. 1403)
38. d (p. 1404)
39. c (p. 1404)
40. b (pp. 1404-1405)
41. b (p. 1406)

42. e, c, d, b, a (all p. 1406)
43. d (p. 1408)
44. d (p. 1407)
45. Possible answers: Braid the hair if it is long; then cut it and save the braid. Show child how he or she looks at each stage of the process. Give the child a cap or scarf to wear. Ensure privacy during the procedure. Emphasize that the hair will begin to grow back after surgery. Introduce the idea of wearing a wig (pp. 1408-1409).
46. d (p. 1410)
47. c (p. 1409)
48. a (p. 1412)
49. d (p. 1413)
50. b (p. 1413)
51. b (p. 1413)
52. b (p. 1414)
53. c (p. 1416)
54. a (p. 1415)
55. Spread cancer cells to adjacent organ or distant sites (p. 1416)
56. d (p. 1417)
57. a (p. 1418)
58. b (p. 1418)
59. b (p. 1419)
60. c (p. 1391)
61. d (p. 1393)
62. Suggest that Cory's mother meet with the school teacher and devise a plan for Cory to be able to do some school work at home if she is too tired to attend school. Some make-up work could be planned for the summer months so Cory could stay in the same class with her peers. (p. 1402)

CHAPTER 32

1. r (p. 1427), j (p. 1427), c (p. 1425), l (p. 1427), e (p. 1426), n (p. 1427), g (p. 1427), s (p. 1427), h (p. 1427), b (p. 1425), i (p. 1427), f (p. 1426), k (p. 1427), m (p. 1427), t (p. 1427), o (p. 1427), d (p. 1426), p (p. 1427), a (p. 1426), q (p. 1427)
2. b (p. 1430; Box 32-2), d (p. 1430), a (p. 1429), f (p. 1430), l (p. 1432), e (p. 1430), h (p. 1430), c (p. 1429), n (p. 1432), i (p. 1430), r (p. 1434), j (p. 1431), t (p. 1434; Figure 32-4), m (p. 1432), o (p. 1433), k (p. 1432), p (p. 1433), g (pp. 1430, 1431; Box 32-4), q (p. 1433), s (p. 1434; Figure 32-4)
3. k (p. 1445), c (pp. 1443, 1444), a (p. 1443), q (p. 1447), o (p. 1445), m (p. 1445), i (p. 1444), e (p. 1443), b (p. 1443), r (p. 1447), n (p. 1445), f (p. 1447), d (pp. 1443, 1444), g (p. 1447), s (p. 1447), h (p. 1444), l (p. 1445), j (p. 1444), p (p. 1446)
4. i (p. 1457), b (p. 1454), j (p. 1462), d (p. 1454), c (p. 1462), e (p. 1459), g (p. 1454), a (p. 1454), h (p. 1457), f (p. 1460)
5. b, f, l, g, k, c, i, e, m, d, h, j, a (p. 1436; Table 32-1)
6. a (p. 1425)
7. b (p. 1464), i (p. 1468), a (p. 1464), k (p. 1465), m (pp. 1465, 1466; Box 32-10), f (pp. 1465, 1466;

Box 32-10), h (p. 1464), v (p. 1473), c (p. 1465), d (p. 1465), e (p. 1465), j (pp. 1465, 1466; Box 32-10), l (p. 1467), n (p. 1467), o (p. 1467), g (p. 1468), u (p. 1473), p (p. 1466; 1473; Box 32-10), r (p. 1469), s (p. 1469), q (p. 1467), t (p. 1473)

8. d (p. 1428)
9. c (pp. 1428, 1429; Box 32-1)
10. b (pp. 1430, 1431; Box 32-4)
11. Function of the cerebral cortex is permanently lost; eyes follow objects only by reflex or when attracted to the direction of loud sounds; all four limbs are spastic but can withdraw from painful stimuli; hands show reflexive grasping and groping; the face can grimace; some food may be swallowed; the child may groan or cry but utters no words (p. 1431; Box 32-4).
12. a (p. 1432; Nursing Care Guidelines box)
13. d (p. 1439)
14. c (p. 1434)
15. c (p. 1434)
16. b (p. 1430; Box 32-3)
17. a (pp. 1435, 1436; Table 32-1)
18. c (p. 1437; Table 32-1)
19. b (p. 1437)
20. d (pp. 1437, 1438)
21. b (p. 1438)
22. c (pp. 1438, 1439)
23. a (p. 1440)
24. d (p. 1442)
25. a (p. 1443)
26. c (pp. 1446, 1445; Figure 32-8)
27. c (p. 1444)
28. a (p. 1446)
29. c (p. 1446; Table 32-3)
30. d (p. 1449)
31. a (p. 1448; Emergency Treatment box)
32. b (p. 1448; Box 32-5)
33. d (p. 1450)
34. d (p. 1451)
35. The need for adequate supervision (pp. 1452, 1454)
36. a (pp. 1452, 1453)
37. d (p. 1453)
38. c (p. 1454)
39. a (p. 1456)
40. b (p. 1457; Nursing Alert; Figure 32-10)
41. b (pp. 1457, 1459)
42. d (pp. 1459, 1460)
43. a (p. 1461)
44. b (p. 1461)
45. a (p. 1462)
46. b (p. 1462)
47. c (p. 1463)
48. a (p. 1463)
49. b (p. 1463)
50. a (p. 1464; Box 32-9)
51. a (p. 1465; Table 32-5)
52. b (p. 1465)
53. b (pp. 1466, 1467, 1469; Box 32-10)
54. a (p. 1469)

55. b (p. 1469)
56. c (p. 1470)
57. a (p. 1472; Nursing Alert box)
58. b (p. 1472)
59. a (p. 1473)
60. d (p. 1474)
61. c (p. 1478; Emergency Treatment; Nursing Care Plan)
62. d (p. 1478; Nursing Care Plan; Emergency Treatment)
63. b (p. 1479)
64. c (p. 1481)
65. a (p. 1481)
66. d (p. 1483)
67. c (p. 1483)
68. a (p. 1483)
69. a (p. 1484)
70. c (p. 1485)
71. a (p. 1487)
72. c (p. 1489)
73. d (p. 1437)
74. b (pp. 1441, 1442, 1450, 1451)
75. c (p. 1441)
76. b (pp. 1441, 1442, 1450, 1451)

CHAPTER 33

1. d (p. 1495)
2. c (p. 1496)
3. d (p. 1497)
4. c (p. 1499)
5. a (p. 1499)
6. c (p. 1499)
7. c (p. 1499)
8. Acromegaly results from hypersecretion of growth hormone that occurs after epiphyseal closure. Hyperfunction of the pituitary that occurs before the epiphyseal closure is not considered acromegaly (p. 1501).
9. c (p. 1502)
10. b (p. 1503)
11. enuresis and excessive thirst (p. 1503)
12.

Diabetes Insipidus	Diabetes Mellitus Type 1
enuresis	polyuria
polyuria	polydipsia
polydipsia	polyphagia
infant irritability	elevated serum glucose
dehydration	glycosuria
	dehydration only in DKA (usually)

13. d (pp. 1502-1503)
14. c (p. 1504)
15. a (p. 1506)
16. d (p. 1507)
17. c (p. 1508)
18. c (p. 1509)
19. b (p. 1509)
20. a (p. 1511)
21. b (p. 1512)

22. d (p. 1514)
23. b (p. 1516)
24. a (p. 1518)
25. c (p. 1518)
26. d (p. 1519)
27. d (p. 1520-1521)
28. a (p. 1521)
29. c (p. 1524)
30. To maintain near-normal blood glucose values while avoiding frequent episodes of hypoglycemia (p. 1524)
31. b (p. 1526)
32. c (p. 1528)
33. Give 10 to 15 g of simple carbohydrate, such as a tablespoon of table sugar, fruit juice, 8 oz of milk, Insta-Glucose (cherry-flavored glucose), carbonated sugar-containing drinks (not sugarless), sherbet, gelatin, cake icing, sugar-containing candy (LifeSavers, Charms), or glucose tablets (p. 1529)
34. c (p. 1529)
35. c (p. 1530)
36. a (p. 1530)
37. d (p. 1532)
38. c (p. 1530)
39. c (p. 1533)
40. d (p. 1533)
41. a (p. 1534)
42. c (p. 1535)
43. b (p. 1536)
44. d (p. 1537)
45. b (p. 1538)
46. b (pp. 1520-1521)
47. c (pp. 1531-1533)
48. c (p. 1534)
49. d (pp. 1534-1535)

CHAPTER 34

1. a. Falls; being struck by or against an object; motor vehicle accidents; fires and burns; drowning; pedestrian-vehicle accidents; bicycle injuries; firearm injuries; sports injuries, especially for school-age children and adolescents; poisonings, especially for young children (pp. 1544-1545)
   b. Become active in legislative efforts, assist with public awareness campaigns, provide individual prevention counseling for children and family, implement home visits to identify potential sources of danger in the home, administer screening questions about safety issues on admission and discharge from the hospital or health clinic visits (pp. 1544-1545).
2. b (p. 1544)
3. b (p. 1545)
4. The cervical spine is immobilized by holding the head in a neutral position and not allowing movement of the head or body in any direction (p. 1545).
5. a (p. 1547)
6. Orthostatic hypotension, increased workload of the heart, thrombus formation (pp. 1548-1549)

7. Numbness, tingling, changes in sensation, loss of motion (p. 1551)
8. a (p. 1552)
9. a (p. 1563), f (p. 1564), b (p. 1563), j (p. 1564), e (p. 1564), h (p. 1564), i (p. 1564), g (p. 1564), d (p. 1564), l (p. 1565), k (p. 1565), c (p. 1565)
10. a (p. 1554)
11. c (p. 1565)
12. Financial strains decrease or eliminate family resources; focus of attention is placed on the affected child and other family members' needs may not be met; family members may have difficulty accepting child's altered body image; family members may be unable to express feelings and may have difficulty coping with crises; parents often experience guilt and have the perception of failing to protect the child (p. 1552).
13. b (p. 1551)
14. Instruct patients to change position frequently; sit in a bedside chair or ambulate; dorsiflex feet and rotate ankles; wear antiembolism stockings or intermittent compression devices; passive ROM of upper and lower extremities; anticoagulant therapy (p. 1553)
15. Poor nutrition; Friction; Moist skin (p. 1552)
16. d (p. 1570)
17. b (p. 1572)
18. pain, paralysis, paresthesia, pallor, pulselessness (p. 1573)
19. b (p. 1573)
20. To regain alignment and length of the bony fragments by reduction; to retain alignment and length by immobilization; to restore function to the injured parts; to prevent further injury (p. 1572)
21. d (pp. 1558-1559)
22. Calm and reassure the child and parents.
    Inquire about the method of injury.
    Apply a temporary splint if not already in place.
    Evaluate the extent of the injury. (p. 1572).
23. Keep the extremity elevated.
    Assess the neurovascular integrity by checking peripheral pulses, assessing the color and temperature of the extremity, having the child wiggle fingers, evaluate for edema.
    Contact the practitioner if there are abnormal findings such as cool extremity, absence of pulse, color changes.
    If the extremity becomes edematous have parents call the practitioner who placed the cast.
    Avoid inserting anything in the cast if it itches. Instead, take a mild antihistamine.
    Keep the cast dry. (p. 1559)
24. b, d, e, f, j, i, a, c, k, g, h (all on p. 1569)
25. c (p. 1557)
26. c (pp. 1572-1573)
27. Severe pain (not always present)
    Absence of pulses in the extremity
    Pallor or cyanosis of the extremity
    Edema
    Loss of sensation

Paralysis of extremity involved
(p. 1573)
28. b (p. 1562)
29. b (p. 1573)
30. b (p. 1574)
31. b (pp. 1574-1575)
32. c (p. 1577), i (p. 1577), g (p. 1579), a (p. 1577),
e (p. 1578), h (p. 1579), f (p. 1577), b (p. 1577),
d (p. 1578)
33. d (p. 1577)
34. a (p. 1578)
35. Ligaments, physis, or growth plate (p. 1578)
36. c (p. 1580)
37. b (p. 1581)
38. b (p. 1580)
39. a (pp. 1582-1583)
40. a (p. 1584)
41. Amenorrhea, osteoporosis, low caloric intake (or low
energy availability) (p. 1582)
42. a (p. 1585)
43. d (p. 1595)
44. a (p. 1596)
45. d (pp. 1592-1593)
46. c (p. 1593)
47. a (p. 1598)
48. b (p. 1599)
49. d (pp. 1599-1600)
50. b (p. 1601)
51. d (p. 1601)
52. d (p. 1587)
53. Realignment and straightening with internal fixation
and instrumentation, along with bony fusion of the
realigned spine (p. 1588)
54. b (p. 1587)
55. a (p. 1588)
56. a (pp. 1602-1603)
57. a. Diet: Eat a well-balanced diet without exceeding
caloric expenditure and maintain appropriate
weight on corticosteroids. A low-salt diet may be
required if the patient becomes nephritic or hypertensive. A low-fat diet is indicated in children with
dyslipidemia. Maximizing peak bone mass in adolescent SLE is essential with a diet rich in calcium
and vitamin D (p. 1610).
b. Sun exposure: Avoid excessive exposure; use sunscreen (with a sun protection factor of at least 30),
hat, and protective clothing; schedule outdoor
activities in morning and evening (p. 1610).
c. Birth control medications: Pregnancy is a potential
trigger for disease flare; because estrogen can trigger disease flare, low-dose estrogen or progester-
one-only contraceptives are preferred (p. 1610).
58. To minimize disease activity with appropriate medications; to help child and family cope with the complications of the disease and treatment (p. 1609)
59. Corticosteroids (p. 1609)
60. Fostering adaptation and self-advocacy skills (p. 1610)
61. d (p. 1602)
62. c (p. 1604)

63. a (p. 1605, 1607)
64. c (p. 1607)

CHAPTER 35

1. a (p. 1617)
2. b (p. 1617)
3. e, g, a, d, b, c, f (p. 1619 for all)
4. a (p. 1619)
5. d (p. 1619)
6. d (p. 1620) c
7. a (p. 1621)
8. b (p. 1621)
9. Establish locomotion, communication, and self-help.
Gain optimum appearance and integration of motor
functions.
Correct associated defects as early and effectively as
possible.
Provide educational opportunities adapted to the individual child's needs and capabilities.
Promote socialization experiences with other affected
and unaffected children. (p. 1622)
10. T (p. 1622), T (p. 1622), F (p. 1623), T (p. 1623),
T (p. 1623), T (p. 1624), T (p. 1624), F (p. 1624), F
(p. 1624), T (p. 1625), T (p. 1625)
11. Drowsiness, fatigue, and muscle weakness (p. 1623)
12. They often have increased energy expenditure
They often cannot feed themselves
They often have associated problems that interfere
with normal nutrition such as gastroesophageal reflux,
feeding and swallowing difficulties, chronic constipation, and subsequent anorexia (p. 1627)
13. c (p. 1641)
14. a (p. 1641)
15. c (p. 1641)
16. c (pp. 1641-1642)
17. a. Scoliosis; hip subluxation and dislocation (p. 1641)
b. To assist the child and family in dealing with the
illness while progressing toward a life of normalization within the child's capabilities (p. 1642)
18. c (p. 1643)
19. b (p. 1644)
20. a (p. 1644)
21. d (p. 1644)
22. Progressive stiffness and tenderness of the muscles in
the neck and jaw, with difficulty opening the mouth
and spasms of facial muscles (p. 1646)
23. b (p. 1645)
24. d (p. 1647)
25. d (p. 1647)
26. b (p. 1647)
27. Administration of human botulism immune globulin
intravenously (BIG-IV) (p. 1648)
28. d (p. 1648)
29. a (p. 1649)
30. c (p. 1649)
31. b (p. 1634)
32. b (p. 1634)
33. b (p. 1632)

34. a. Preserve renal function (p. 1635).
    b. Preserve renal function and achieve maximum urinary continence (p. 1635).
35. d (p. 1636)
36. a (pp. 1637-1638)
37. c (p. 1635)
38. c (p. 1653)
39. b (p. 1655)
40. The paraplegic individual who has function down to and including the quadriceps muscle or who has muscle function below the L3 level will have little difficulty learning to walk with or without braces and crutches. (p. 1656)
41. FES may enable the child to sit, stand, and walk with the aid of crutches, or a walker; can be used to elicit grasp and release from the hand; helps cardiovascular conditioning; decreases pressure ulcers and increases blood flow; helps to reduce complications due to bladder and bowel incontinence; assists males in achieving penile erection. (pp. 1656-1657)
42. d (p. 1659)
43. b (p. 1662)

44. b (p. 1663)
45. d (pp. 1666-1667)
46. Contractures, scoliosis, disuse atrophy, infections, obesity, and respiratory and cardiopulmonary problems (pp. 1665-1666)
47. c (p. 1667)
48. d (p. 1665)
49. d (p. 1667)
50. b (p. 1667)
51. d (p. 1668)
52. Kevin will acquire mobility within personal capabilities, acquire communication skills or use appropriate assistive devices, engage in self-help activities, receive appropriate education, develop a positive self-image, and receive appropriate nutrition and feeding assistance. The family members will receive appropriate education and support in their efforts to meet Kevin's needs. Kevin will receive appropriate care if hospitalized or in the community (p. 1668)
53. c (p. 1668)